Genetic Immunization

Genetic Immunization

Constantin A. Bona
Mount Sinai School of Medicine
New York, New York

and

Adrian I. Bot
Alliance Pharmaceutical Corp.
San Diego, California

Kluwer Academic / Plenum Publishers
New York, Boston, Dordrecht, London, Moscow

Library of Congress Cataloging-in-Publication Data

Bona, Constantin A.
   Genetic immunization/by Constantin A. Bona and Adrian Bot.
     p. ; cm.
   Includes bibliographical references and index.
   ISBN 0-306-46226-5
    1. DNA vaccines. I. Bot, Adrian. II. Title.
   [DNLM: 1. Vaccines, DNA. 2. Immunization. QW 805 B697g 2000]
   QR189.5D53 B36 2000
   615′.372—dc21

                           99-051913

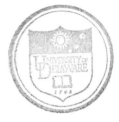
ISBN 0-306-46226-5

©2000 Kluwer Academic/Plenum Publishers, New York
233 Spring Street, New York, N.Y. 10013

http://www.wkap.nl/

10 9 8 7 6 5 4 3 2 1

A C.I.P. record for this book is available from the Library of Congress

Preface

Wolf's discovery demonstrating that a reporter gene is expressed in myocytes subsequent to injection of naked DNA, was exploited by immunologists and vaccinologists to develop a new generation of vaccines.

This observation galvanized the research and in a short lapse of time, an oceanic volume of knowledge has been accumulated.

The research carried out in a variety of animal models showed the efficacy of genetic immunization against viruses, bacteria, and some parasites by the ability to induce a strong priming effect resulting from long-lasting persistence of plasmid as episomes. Furthermore, it was demonstrated that newborn or infant immune unresponsiveness to classical vaccines can be corrected by genetic immunization. The applications of genetic immunization for prophylaxis of infections was extended to immunotherapy, namely, cancerous, auto-immune, and allergic diseases. Immunologists have provided pertinent information on the cellular basis of the immune responses elicited by genetic immunization, and molecular biologists have established the molecular basis of intrinsic adjuvant properties of plasmids.

As always, the experimental systems provide to scientists pertinent, valuable, and important information. However, the success of a discovery depends on whether this information can be translated into practical terms. In the case of genetic immunization, it would be important to establish whether the naked DNA can be used for the development of a new generation of vaccines or efficient immunotherapeutics for the treatment of persistent infections and allergic diseases or cancers. The final verdict for the usefulness of genetic immunization for the health of the human kingdom will be provided by the information resulting from clinical trials in humans.

In this monograph, we present extensive information on this area, in the hope of helping a large readership to find the information in the haystack of multiplicities derived from experimental findings.

If we succeed in this venture, we hope that the information will help "to continue to cultivate the garden" as Voltaire said, namely, to continue the development of research in the area of genetic immunization.

Contents

Genetic Immunization

Chapter 1

Approaches for Development of New Vaccines

1.1. INTRODUCTION

Vaccination is one of most spectacular achievements of medicine. The conquest of small-pox resulted from the preparation of vaccine by Jenner, two hundred years ago. The World Health Organization (WHO) estimates that vaccination against polio, diphtheria, measles, and hepatitis prevents the death of three million people yearly.

The studies of Pasteur on antirabies vaccine and of Ramon on toxoids led to formulation of a "golden rule" for the development of vaccines: The microbe or toxin used as vaccine should be devoid of pathogenicity but should have its immunogenicity preserved.

After Jenner's and Pasteur's seminal discoveries, there has been no hiatus in the effort to develop new vaccines. However, there are microbes such as HIV, HSV, or Hepatitis C virus, and respiratory and enteroviruses or parasites such as plasmodium, against which no efficient vaccine is available and the associated death rate is still very high.

Vaccine development was a wellspring of research that contributed to an understanding of how the immune system reacts to foreign antigens in general.

The lymphocytes mediate the immune response against antigens as well as vaccines, and are divided into two populations: *B*-cells responsible for humoral response, and *T*-cells that mediate cellular responses. *B*-cells can recognize a particular epitope on the surface of the native antigen molecule via their antigen-specific Ig receptor. In some cases, the antigen can directly activate the *B*-cell. This is the case of *T*-independent antigens such as polysaccharides, which, by virtue of repetitive epitope, can cross-link Ig receptors and provide a positive signal for the activation. In the case of *T*-dependent antigens, the *B*-cells need a second activation signal delivered by *T*-cells. The second lymphocyte population is represented by *T*-cells that are divided into two subsets: CD4 and CD8 *T*-cells. These subsets exhibit two major roles in immune responses elicited by vaccination:

a. A regulatory role that alerts *B*-cells to make antibodies or arm the macrophages to efficiently kill the microbes.
b. An effector role that attacks and destroys infected cells.

1

In contrast with *B*-cells, *T*-cells can recognize only fragments of protein antigens in association with major histocompatibility complex (MHC) molecules. CD4 *T*-cells recognize peptides in association with Class II molecules. The peptides recognized by CD4 *T*-cells are generated in endosomes from digestion of molecules engulfed by professional antigen presenting cells (APCs). CD8 *T*-cells recognize the peptides in association with Class I molecules. These peptides derive from the processing of cytoplasmic (endogenous) proteins fragmented by proteasomes and then transported to the endoplasmic reticulum (ER) by transporter peptide (TAP) molecules. In the ER, the peptides are released from TAP molecules and bind to Class I molecules. Class II-peptide complexes formed in endosomes, as well as class I-peptide complexes formed in the ER, are transferred to cell surfaces where they are recognized by T-cell receptor (TCR) of *T*-cells. Fig. 1.1 illustrates the mechanism of endogenous and exogenous pathways of generation of peptides.

It should be mentioned that CD4 *T*-cells are divided into three distinct subsets called Th1, Th2, and Th3. This subdivision is based on the pattern of lymphokine production. Th1 secretes IL-2 and INFγ. Th2 secretes IL-4 and IL-10, and Th3 secretes mainly tumor growth factor (TGFβ). These lymphokines display various physiological effects not only on the cells of the immune system but also on other somatic cells. The protective response elicited by vaccines comes from generation of *B*- and *T*-memory cells. Whenever the vaccine activates the lymphocytes, some of them differentiate into memory cells, which can respond promptly and more efficiently to infectious agent.

1.2. FIRST GENERATION OF VACCINES

Development of first-generation vaccines was based on the principle that a vaccine should be devoid of pathogenicity without altering its immunogenicity. During the last nine decades, efforts were focused upon generation of vaccines able to induce production of antibodies. The rationale of this approach followed the progress in immunological knowledge demonstrating that opsonine-antibodies facilitate the phagocytosis, that antibodies can prevent localization of bacteria into tissues or binding of viruses to viral cell receptors, that they can lyse the microbes in the presence of the complement, can immobilize bacteria at site of entry, and can neutralize the toxins produced by bacteria.

The toxoides (i.e., toxins inactivated by formalin) elicit strong neutralizing antibody responses leading to preparation of efficient vaccines against tetanus, diphtheria, and botulin toxins.

The live-attenuated vaccines were produced by growing pathogenic viruses under special conditions leading to loss of pathogenicity. The development of such vaccines was possible after Enders introduced the tissue culture to grow and attenuate the viruses. Ensuing years saw the efficiency of this approach leading to preparation of vaccines against polio, measles, rubella, mumps, chicken pox viruses, yellow fever, and tuberculosis. Live-attenuated vaccines can elicit a strong humoral response, activate CD4 *T*-cells and CD8 cytotoxic *T*-cells consequent to replication within the cells. The proteins are then processed and peptides are presented to *T*-cells.

The inactivated vaccines are produced by killing the infectious agent with chemicals or heat. The majority of inactivated vaccines induce a poor antibody response that can be

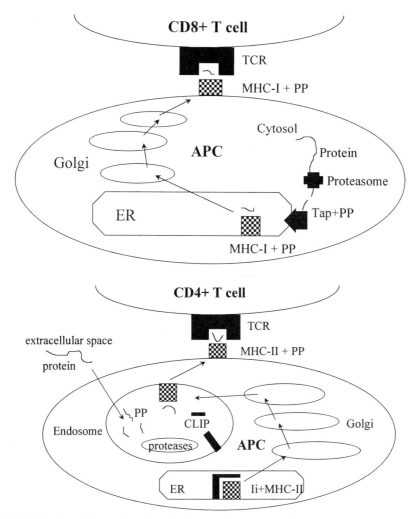

Figure 1.1. Mechanisms of processing of proteins in the endogenous and exogenous pathways and the presentation of peptides to CD4 and CD8 *T*-cells.

strengthened by several boosts. While they can activate CD4, they fail to activate CD8 *T*-cells, since the peptides recognized by cytotoxic T lymphocytes (CTLs) are produced subsequent to the processing of proteins synthesized within the cytoplasm. Such vaccines proved to be effective against influenza and polio viruses, as well as *B. pertussis*, *R. prowatzeki*, *S. typhi*, and *Y. pestis*.

Table 1.1 compares the properties of live-attenuated and inactivated vaccines. Progress in the development of immunochemistry allowed for an accurate characterization of epitopes able to induce a protective response. These studies opened a new avenue consisting in purification of macromolecules from microbes that were then used as subunit vaccines.

Table 1.1. Properties of Live-Attenuated, Inactivated, and Subunit Vaccines

	Live-attenuated	Inactivated	Subunit
Booster requirement	Single	Multiple	Multiple
Reverse mutation	Possible	No	No
Stability	Less	Stable	Very stable
Induction of humoral response	High	Less	Less
CD4	High	Poor	Null
CD8	High	Null	Null

While the subunit vaccines can induce production of protective antibodies, they fail to activate both CD4 and CD8 *T*-cells. The subunit vaccines elicit predominantly the synthesis of IgM antibodies. Generally, IgM antibodies display poor protective properties. To bypass this limitation, a new generation of polysaccharide–subunit vaccines were produced by conjugation of sugar moiety with a protein carrier. The protein–polysaccharide conjugates more efficiently stimulate CD4 *T*-cells and are able to induce memory cells. Subunit vaccines proved to be efficient against some bacteria, such as *H. influenza*, *N. meningitides*, *S. pneumoniae*, and *B. anthracis*. Table 1.2 illustrates currently used vaccines.

1.3. SECOND GENERATION OF VACCINES

While the efficacy of the first generation of vaccines was well proven, these vaccines are not completely devoid of side effects. In addition, because of the complexity of microbial membranes, composed of myriad macromolecules endowed with antigenic properties, the protective response can be diluted by production of antibodies or *T*-cell mediated response against nonprotective epitopes. It is well documented that only a few epitopes are capable of eliciting protective responses (Wiley et al., 1977). The major goal in the preparation of a second generation of vaccines was to produce safer and more efficient vaccines.

Table 1.2. Vaccines against Various Infectious Agents Currently Used

Live-attenuated	Inactivated vaccines	Subunit
Measles	*B. pertussis*	*H. influenzae*
Mumps	*S. typhi*	*N. meningitides*
Rubella	*R. prowatzekii*	*S. pneumoniae*
Yellow fever	*B. anthracis*	Hepatitis B virus
Polio virus	Polio virus	
Chicken pox	*Y. pestis*	
Adenoviruses (types 4 and 7)	Rabies virus	
S. typhi	Hepatitis A	
V. cholera	Influenza virus	
M. tuberculosis	Microbial toxins	
F. tularense		

Several factors contributed to the development of a new generation of vaccines. First, the advance of peptide chemistry made possible large-scale preparation of synthetic peptides. Second, the advance of molecular biology provided a revolutionary technology for creation "a la carte" molecules expressing microbial genes, minigenes, or peptides. Third, the advance of immunobiology, and particularly the understanding of molecular and cellular events of antigen recognition, provided a background for targeting the vaccines on induction of protective responses.

1.3.1. Recombinant Protein Vaccines

The utilization of recombinant proteins as vaccines represents an extension of subunit concept that the protective epitopes are expressed on a limited number of microbial molecules. The principle of this approach is to isolate the gene(s) encoding a protein and to clone it in bacteria, yeast, or mammalian cells. Recombinant proteins are prepared either from transfected cells or from culture medium. While some recombinant proteins elicit a strong immune response when administered in saline, others require adjuvants. The first protein recombinant vaccine used in humans was against Hepatitis B. The vaccine was developed by cloning the gene encoding the surface antigen in yeast cells and subsequently purifying it from disruption of cells by high pressure. The vaccine induces a strong protective immune response and is currently used not only for prophylactic purposes but also for therapeutics in chronic carriers to prevent major sequels such as cirrhosis or hepatocarcinomas.

1.3.2. Recombinant Vector Vaccines

The preparation of this type of vaccine is based on the possibility of introduction and expression of genes, encoding a major gene of a pathogen into an attenuated virus or bacterium. Vaccinia virus was initially used as vector because DNA recombination occurs extensively during replication of poxviruses and therefore facilitates the insertion of foreign DNA into the vaccinia genome. Recombinant vaccinia vectors are prepared by infection of permissive cells with vaccinia virus and transfection with a plasmid expressing a foreign gene. Since the recombination process is likely, and about 0.1% of virions incorporate the foreign gene, the recombinant virons are easily selected by common procedures. The genes of more than 20 RNA viruses, of more than 10 DNA viruses, bacterial, parasitic genes, or those coding tumor-associated antigens, were successfully expressed in vaccinia vector (Moss, 1992). A number of other organisms have been used as vaccine vectors: adenovirus (Graham et al., 1992), attenuated polio virus (Evans et al., 1989), attenuated AroA Salmonella strain (Dougan et al., 1987), and Bacille Calmette Guerin (BCG) (Stover et al., 1991). Recently, a nonpathogenic strain of *B. anthracis* (Stern strain) which contains pXO1 plasmid coding for toxin and lacking the pXO2 plasmid required for the expression of capsular polysaccharide, was used to deliver into cytoplasm the listeriolysin that bears the major epitopes recognized by CD8 *T*-cells (Sirard et al., 1997).

Recombinant vector vaccines can elicit a strong cellular response and sometimes a good humoral response. The major drawback of this approach is a strong immune response against the vector itself, which precludes an efficient boost response.

1.3.3. Peptide-Based Vaccines

The development of peptide synthesis technology raised hopes for preparation of safer and more efficient vaccines because the peptides are devoid of side effects and peptides corresponding to protective epitopes were supposed to induce a strong protective immunity. Peptide-based immunization initiated by Atassi (1975), and continued by others, failed. The failure was related to two factors: (a) fast clearing and poor immunogenicity of peptides. Addition of adjuvants or coupling the peptide to strong carriers has not seen an improvement of immune response comparable to that elicited by classical vaccines, with the exception of vaccination against foot and mouth disease (Brown, 1994); (b) linear-peptide vaccines' inability to elicit a response against conformational *B*-cell epitopes, which apparently represent the majority of protective epitopes.

In contrast, the advance in *T*-cell immunobiology knowledge resurrected the interest for peptide-based vaccines, because *T*-cells are activated subsequent to interaction of TCR with MHC-peptide complex (Townsend et al., 1986; Chesnut et al., 1982; reviewed in Braciale and Braciale, 1992). This advance opened a new avenue for the development of *T*-cell vaccines.

Currently used vaccines can be divided into three categories:

1. *B*-cell vaccines eliciting neutralizing antibodies. This is the case of toxoids and vaccines against poliovirus (Salk vaccine), hepatitis A and B viruses, or some bacteria (*S. pneumoniae, H. influenze, N. meningitides*, etc.).
2. *T*-cell vaccines able to induce cellular immune responses. Retrospectively, Jenner's vaccinia vaccine and the Calmette–Guerin BCG vaccine are genuine *T*-cell vaccines, since the protective immunity against smallpox or *M. tuberculosis* is mediated by *T*-cells.
3. Vaccines able to elicit both humoral and cellular immunity.

1.3.4. *T*-Cell Vaccines

Various approaches were undertaken to present *T*-cell epitopes in various platforms aimed at circumventing both the short life and poor immunogenicity of peptides. These approaches are as follows:

1. Recombinant proteins bearing *T*-cell epitopes. The generation of such molecules was carried out by insertion of oligonucleotide sequences encoding *T*-cell epitopes into bacterial organelles such as fimbriae (Jennings et al., 1989), flagella (Bruce et al., 1994), or LamB outer membrane protein, or into genes encoding proteins secreted by *E. coli*, such as MalE protein (O'Callaghan et al., 1990). The protective immune responses induced by recombinant molecules can be diluted by competitive responses against a multitude of *T*-cell epitopes borne on host molecules.

2. Chimeric viruses bearing *T*-cell epitopes inserted in various genes. The rationale of development of these viruses was to create a multivaccine able to vaccinate people simultaneously against various microbes. Initially, *B*-cell epitopes were inserted in the genes of DNA viruses (Clarke et al., 1987) as well in plus (Hahn et al., 1992) or minus (Enami and Palese, 1991) strand RNA viruses. More recently, *T*-cell epitopes derived from the *Plasmodium circumsporozite* protein, the V3 loop of HIV-1, or nucleoprotein of influenza viruses were expressed in the hemagglutinin of influenza viruses. Such transfectant viruses were able to induce a strong cellular response against not only inserted peptide but also the virus itself (Li et al., 1993), demonstrating that the dream of designing multivaccines can become a real possibility.

3. Receptor peptide approach based on delivery of peptides chemically coupled to natural ligands to APCs that process the complexes and present the peptide to *T*-cells. This approach was used to create anti-Class II or anti-Ig-peptide conjugates able to bind to the MHC or Ig receptor of APCs (Casten and Pierce, 1988), as well as peptides linked to α 2 macroglobulin (Mitsuda et al., 1995) or transferrin (McCoy et al., 1993) internalized via the corresponding receptors.

4. Self molecules expressing *T*-cell epitopes. Genes encoding Igs or MHC molecules were used to express viral epitopes. The first successful attempt was performed by Zaghouani et al., who replaced the complementary determining region 3 (CDR3) of a (Vh) gene with an influenza nucleoprotein recognized by CD8 *T*-cells in association with Class I molecules (Zaghouani et al., 1992), and later an epitope of influenza hemagglutinin recognized in association with Class II molecules (Zaghouani et al., 1993b). These molecules were able to induce a peptide-specific cellular response in various *in vitro* or *in vivo* experimental systems (Zaghouani et al., 1993). Chimeric Class I (Abastado et al., 1993) or Class II (Kozono et al., 1994; Casares et al., 1997) peptide molecules were obtained by genetic engineering in which the peptides were covalently linked and set into grooves as natural peptides derived from the processing of endogenous or internalized proteins. Experiments carried out in various laboratories are evaluating potential vaccinating capacity of such chimeric self-peptide molecules.

T-cell vaccines can be useful against obligatory intracellular microbes such as *Mycobacterium*, *Salmonella*, *Listeria*, *Francisella* or *Brucella*, all rickettsia species, and the vast majority of viruses. They also may be suitable for vaccination against fungi and protozoa in cases in which cellular responses are the major arm of host defense reactions.

1.3.5. DNA Vaccines

The principle of genetic immunization is based on observation that parenteral administration of naked DNA may lead to *in vivo* transfection. Stasney et al. (1950) and Ito et al. (1961) demonstrated appearance of tumors in mice injected with a crude preparation of DNA extracted from tumors. These observations were forgotten until Wolff et al. (1990) demonstrated that a plasmid DNA expressing a reporter gene was transcribed and translated subsequent to intramuscular injection.

During the early 1960s Atanasiu (1962) showed that subcutaneous injection of polioma virus DNA in newborn hamsters resulted not only in appearance of tumors but also in the production of antiviral antibodies. This remarkable observation was buried for several decades, until Johnston (Tang et al., 1992) showed that the injection with a plasmid-expressing bovine growth hormone leads to production of specific antibodies. This basic information was appealing for vaccinologists, who further exploited the immunization with naked DNA as a potentially new approach for development of a new generation of vaccines (Ulmer et al., 1993). Ensuing years have seen an explosion of research in this area, leading to clinical human trials of genetic vaccines.

The galvanized interest stirred by genetic immunization led to rapid progress in knowledge of this area. Molecular studies contributed to definition of the best parameters of vectors to be used: insertion in vectors of strong promoter required to drive the synthesis of proteins, spacing between regulatory and inserted genes, and stability of RNA transcripts and the minimum number of copies necessary for the synthesis of immunogenic amounts of antigen. The utilization of polymerase chain reaction (PCR) showed long-lasting persistence of plasmid as episomes in the cells transfected *in vivo*.

Immunological studies allowed for determining the characteristics of immune response with respect to (1) magnitude of antibody synthesis and the isotype pattern, (2) the ability to stimulate antigen-specific CD4 *T*-cells, (3) the ability to prime the CD8 *T*-cell, and (4) the efficiency of various routes of immunization. Thus, genetic immunization exploited the progress in both molecular biology and immunobiology.

Several advantages made genetic immunization very appealing for vaccinologists:

1. DNA is as stable as subunit vaccines and more stable than live attenuated vaccine.

2. Low-cost manufacturing procedures for cheap vaccines are particularly suitable for global vaccination programs, taking into account that third-world developing countries cannot afford the high cost of some vaccines.

3. The amount of plasmid necessary to induce an immune response is generally small, on the order of micrograms.

4. That vectors can be rapidly constructed is an important property for preparation of vaccines against microbes exhibiting natural genetic variation. In addition, there is a possibility of inserting in the same vectors multiple microbial genes expressing protective epitopes, or lymphokines or chemokines known to play a critical role in the immune response. Virtually, any DNA sequence can be inserted into a plasmid that has multiple cloning sites. Grifantini et al. (1998) showed that multiplasmid vaccination avoids the antigen competition inherent in immunization with several antigens. Comparison of magnitude of antibody response for a single antigen following immunization with either one or four plasmids showed that antibody response was enhanced after immunization with a mixture of four plasmids.

5. Regarding the possibility of expression of *T*- or *B*-cell epitopes, Brumeanu et al. (1996) constructed for the first time a doubly antigenized molecule by replacing the CDR2 of a Vh gene with an epitope of influenza virus hemagglutinin recognized by *B*-cells, and the CDR3 with an epitope recognized by *T*-cells. Casares et al. (1997a) inserted the chimeric Vh gene in a plasmid that was then used to immunize mice. Immunized mice produced antibodies specific for hemagglutinin, and their lymphocytes proliferated upon *in vitro* incubation with peptide. In addition, the mice immunized with plasmid-expressing chimeric gene exhibited an increased rate of survival after challenge with a lethal dose of virus.

6. Long-lasting persistence of plasmid results in sustained synthesis of antigen at low levels. This property indicates that genetic immunization precludes the induction of high dose tolerance and drives the immune response to memory cells, and, therefore, may obviate the requirement for boosts.

7. Lack of proteins in plasmids may preclude the induction of side effects such as allergic reactions.

8. Naked DNA has the ability to elicit both humoral and cellular responses subsequent to processing of endogenous proteins by APCs that present the peptide to CD4 and CD8 *T*-cells.

9. Genetic immunization is able to overcome the unresponsiveness of immature lymphocytes.

10. Genetic immunization does not require adjuvants, because the plasmids are themselves endowed with immunostimulatory sequences (Raz et al., 1996; Klinman et al., 1996).

These promising findings make genetic immunization a new, attractive approach, offering the prospect of a new way to vaccinate at a global level. However, there are two important, potential side effects of DNA immunization. First, there is the possibility to induce anti-DNA antibodies. Such antibodies are spontaneously produced by both humans afflicted by systemic lupus erythematosus (SLE) and mice that develop an SLE-like syndrome. There is no hard evidence that mammals produce anti-ss or -ds DNA autoantibodies following injection of bacterial DNA. However, the DNA can function as hapten, since the immunization of mice with methylated-BSA complexes in Friend's complete adjuvant (FCA) effectively induced anti-DNA antibody responses (Gilkeson et al., 1991, 1998). We examined sera from 1-day-old, 2-week-old, and 1-month- or 2-month-old BALB/c mice immunized with pHA plasmid. No anti-ss or -ds DNA antibodies were found in the sera of these mice. These results clearly show that neonates, infants, and adults do not produce anti-DNA antibodies subsequent to genetic immunization.

The second potentially serious drawback of genetic immunization is the integration of plasmid into host genome, which may have devastating consequences by inducing mutations in essential structural genes, or in protooncogens favoring the development of tumors. Numerous studies showed long-lasting persistence of plasmids within the cytoplasm of transfected cells. Dowty et al. (1995) have studied the intracellular traffic of plasmid microinjected in the myotubule cytoplasm. The plasmid was found in karyoplasm of postmitotic nuclei with intact membrane. However, most of injected plasmid remained in the cytoplasm. The cytoplasm sequestration prevented nuclear accumulation of plasmid, most likely due to binding to cytoskeleton elements that function as a cytoplasmic sieve. Even if a small fraction of plasmid DNA migrates into the nucleus, there is no hard evidence for the integration of injected plasmids. A single study reported by Xiong et al. (1997b) claimed the integration into *B*-cell genome but not in the genome of other somatic and germinal cells of a plasmid expressing a chimeric Vh gene of an autoantibody in which a segment of *P. falciparum* circumsporozoite protein (CSP) gene was added to CDR3. However, the results of this study are at best confusing, and show that the half-life of integration was identical to the half-life of persistence of plasmid as episomes. The integration should be permanent during the life span, if some mysterious event leading to the loss of integrated gene does not take place. The integration concept was based on failure of authors to amplify by PCR the entire plasmid sequence of about 15 kb. Generally, it is difficult to amplify by PCR a 15 kb DNA. In these experiments, an Xba-1-digested DNA was relegated and then used as a template for PCR. This experiment did not take into consideration that Xba-1-digested fragments of chimeric Vh gene, either from episomal or integrated plasmid, represent less than 10^{-6} of genomic Xba-1 fragments generated (15 kb of plasmid in 5×10^6 kb of genomic DNA). Because the number of transfected cells *in vivo* has been reported to be below 1%, the rate of chimeric gene:genomic DNA would be 10^{-8}, which makes PCR amplification difficult.

Taking into account the low rate of heterologous recombination, the failure to demonstrate the integration of plasmids into host genome by other investigators, and the confusing data reported by Xiong et al. (1997b), at the present time, we conclude that parenteral administration of plasmid DNA does not lead to integration in the mammalian genome.

Chapter 2

Genetic Vaccination

Routes and Formulations

2.1. GENETIC VACCINES: VECTORS

Proper expression vectors are crucial for immunogenicity of nucleic-acid-based vaccines. Ideally, they should have the following properties: (1) sufficient expression of the foreign gene; (2) prolonged expression; (3) selective expression in APC; (4) low immunogenicity by themselves; (5) no side effects; (6) allow regulation of expression in terms of on–off. Evidently, various vectors differ in these regards and sustained effort is being dedicated to improvement of mammalian expression vectors (Table 2.1). These efforts are fueled by the necessity to design superior delivery systems for gene therapy as well. However, it is important to stress that requirements for effective vectors in genetic vaccination may not be as stringent as in the case of gene therapy, simply because the levels of expression required for immunity are lower than those that lead to therapeutic effects. Thus, this discrepancy apparently defines a window of opportunity for genetic vaccination in terms of vectors: Nucleic-acid-based vectors, in spite of their lower expression level, may be of greater usefulness for genetic vaccination than most of the viral vectors associated with more side effects. We first discuss the functional structure of classical nucleic-acid-based vectors, followed by a brief comparison with other types of vectors and efforts to improve nucleic-acid-based vectors.

The smallest vector unit comprises the antigen sequence and regulatory elements that differ in the case of DNA- versus RNA-based vectors. In the case of DNA vectors, the most common structure is the bacterial plasmid that comprises a promoter and a polyadenylation signal, regulatory elements that are functional in mammalian cells. Whereas the rest of the plasmid that usually bears various restriction enzyme sites and selection elements has limited effect on the level of expression, the nature of both the promoter and polyadenylation signal is crucial. Pioneering studies compared the expression levels of reporter genes inserted into plasmid vectors, conferred by different viral promoters–enhancers—cytomegalovirus (CMV), Rous sarcoma virus (RSV), Simian virus 40 (SV40), adenovirus and nonviral actin, myocite creatin kinase (MCK), α-globin, dihidrofolate reductase, troponin-C, immu-

Table 2.1. Vectors for Genetic Vaccines

Type of vector	DNA-based (plasmids)
	RNA-based (mRNA)
Promoters	Promiscuous (viral)
	Tissue specific
Open reading frame inserts	Reporters
	Microbial antigens
	Tumor-associated antigens
	Self-antigens
	Immune regulatory molecules

noglobulin, and metallothionein (Manthorpe et al., 1993; Davis et al., 1993b; Prigozy et al., 1993; Cheng et al., 1993; Gerloni et al., 1997). As a result of these studies, most of the subsequently used plasmid vectors had the initial early-CMV (IE-CMV) promoter and termination sequences like the bovine growth hormone polyadenylation signal. Use of reporter genes allowed great improvement of mammalian expression vectors over two orders of magnitude. For example, usage of IE-CMV promoter and intron A, as well as removal of the SV40 origin of replication and optimization of termination sequence, allowed significant improvement of the transfection ability (Norman et al., 1997). They were shown to provide the highest and most reproducible expression levels upon *in vivo* administration of plasmids that carry them.

An alternative for plasmid-based expression vectors is represented by messenger RNA (mRNA) expression vectors. Usually, the mRNA should be capped and polyadenylated. Ideally, it should comprise stabilizing untranslatable 5' and 3' sequences. There are two potential advantages for RNA vectors: (1) the lack of likelihood for insertion into genome, and (2) the possibility to immunize against transforming proteins without side effects, due to the limited persistence of RNA. However, the instability of RNA may be an important limiting factor for the magnitude of immunity. Furthermore, preparation of such vectors is more tedious compared to plasmids. Thus, only a few studies approached the issue of mRNA vectors, demonstrating *in vitro* and *in vivo* transfection as well as immune responses subsequent to lipid- or particle-mediated delivery (Lu et al., 1994; Conry et al., 1995c; Qiu et al., 1996). More recently, attempts were carried out to enhance the stability of such RNA vectors by condensation with protamine prior to formulation in liposomes (Hoerr et al., 2000).

Alternatives for nucleic acid vectors are recombinant viruses that have the advantage of increased cellular uptake and expression but two disadvantages: side effects due to cellular infection, and immune response to simultaneously expressed viral antigens. It is not clear yet if safer viral vectors will prove a better solution compared with nucleic acid vectors for the purpose of vaccination. Efforts are ongoing to improve retroviral vectors (Warner et al., 1995), adenovirus and adeno-associated virus vectors (Berns and Giraud, 1995; Ambriovic et al., 1997), Semliki Forest virus vectors (Zhou et al., 1994), Sindbis virus vectors (Johanning et al., 1995) and alphavirus vectors (Frolov et al., 1996). An emerging approach to improve the immunogenicity of DNA vaccines consists in the "replicon" technology. Based on regulatory elements from alphavirus (i.e., Sindbis or Semliki Forest viruses), such plasmid elements, upon transfection, launch multiple rounds of self-replication without leading to the generation of infectious particles. Delivery of replicons via viral-like particles (coated by virus surface proteins) offers the additional advantage of facilitated entrance into host cells, a potentially limiting aspect in the case of "naked" DNA. Immune responses are triggered at doses 100 to 1000-fold lower compared to naked plasmid; however, surprisingly, this is not necessarily due to enhanced antigen expression but perhaps to more effective access of antigen to professional antigen presenting cells (Leitner et al., 2000). A somewhat similar, exciting technology has been recently tested in the herpes simplex virus model. Bacterial artificial chromosomes ("BAC") bearing 152 kbp of the HSV-1 genome, devoid of packaging signals, can induce substantial cytotoxic T lymphocyte (CTL) and antibody immunity in animal models (Suter et al., 1999). The DNA can still replicate and generate virus-like particles that are devoid of infectious ability. The obvious advantage of this strategy is the possibility of accommodating multiple and sometimes poorly understood immunogenic elements from more complex microbes, in order to generate broader immunity.

A new and interesting area receiving a lot of attention approached bacterial-mediated delivery of plasmids as a method to increase the efficiency of DNA vaccination. The proof of concept is based on the ability of certain bacteria to reach the cytosol, thus increasing the efficiency of plasmid delivery in the cell. The first studied vehicle was an attenuated *Shigella* strain (Sizemore et al., 1995) that was able to deliver plasmids to mucosal epithelial cells as well as to induce immunity against epitopes expressed by plasmid, subsequent to intranasal inoculation of the bacteria (Sizemore et al., 1997). Another effective bacterial shuttle was shown to be an attenuated strain of *S. typhimurium*, namely, AroA (Darji et al., 1997). Even single immunization via the oral route with this attenuated bacterium, transformed with plasmids expressing *Listeria monocytogenes* antigens, resulted in excellent humoral and cellular responses as well as protection against infectious challenge. A recent study described an even more versatile bacterial-based, plasmid-delivery vehicle: an attenuated *Listeria monocytogenes* strain that bears a phage-derived suicide factor, namely, lysin (Dietrich et al., 1998). *In vitro* experiments showed effective shuttling of plasmids inside macrophages as well as self-destruction of the microbe in the cytosol. The enhanced delivery rate was associated with plasmid integration in macrophage genome, with a frequency of 10^{-7}. Such a low integration rate, even when cell transfection is facilitated, may explain the difficulty in detecting similar events in the case of inoculation of naked DNA. Refinement of this strategy is possible: For example, engineering of inducible lysis systems (i.e., lambda lysis genes S and R in case of potential bacterial vectors such as *Vibrio cholerae* and *Salmonella entarica*) facilitates the release of plasmid upon cellular entrance of bacterial vectors (Jain and Mekalanos, 2000).

Simultaneously, with efforts to characterize the immunity triggered by genetic vaccination, ongoing studies addressed and continue to approach the issue of creating superior plasmid-based vectors bearing characteristics that make them more effective in certain circumstances. For example, one direction is designing plasmids that coordinately express two proteins from a single promoter, thus allowing for concomitant expression of multiple antigens in the same cells (Clarke et al., 1997). Such strategies take advantage of "internal ribosomal entry sites" (IRES sequences). Another direction is designing plasmids that can replicate as extrachromosomal units, thus avoiding their dilution in proliferating cells. Epstein–Barr virus–based episomal vectors were shown to lead to more persistent expression of cytokine genes in proliferating human lymphoma cells (Mucke et al., 1997). Steps toward designing regulable expression vectors have been pursued. One candidate is the tetracycline-regulated expression system that comprises the bacterial tetracycline responsive element (tet). Decrease of expression was triggered by tetracycline administration. Administration of such expression vectors allowed *in vivo* modulation of expression levels over two orders of magnitude (Dhawan et al., 1995). Another strategy aimed at limiting the *in vivo* expression of the foreign gene had the advantage of not requiring continuous administration of repressors. It employed an expression vector bearing the bacteriophage T7 promoter, concomitantly administered with the T7 RNA polymerase (Selby et al., 1997). The shorter *in vivo* half-life of the polymerase resulted in limited expression from T7 promoter that nevertheless allowed for the generation of immune responses. However, a disadvantage of this second system consists in the difficulty to regulate precisely the inhibition of expression.

2.2. ADMINISTRATION OF GENETIC VACCINES

Various routes and strategies of administration have been explored for genetic vaccines (Table 2.2). Earlier studies focused on methods to improve the efficiency of *in vitro* transfection, particularly by formulating the nucleic acids with compounds that promote their uptake by cells (Malone et al., 1989; Felgner and Ringold, 1989). Accumulating observations, particularly during the previous decades, suggested that inoculation of DNA into various organs leads to transfection and synthesis of foreign proteins. Thus, it was shown that inoculation of cloned DNA corresponding to Hepatitis B virus (HBV) genome into chimpanzees (Will et al., 1982), ground squirrel hepatitis virus into Beechey squirrels (Seeger et al., 1984) and polyoma into mice (Dubensky et al., 1984), resulted in synthesis of viral proteins and infection. However, theoretically, a single *in vivo* transfected cell could have accounted for the resulting infection. Although these types of observations documented the phenomenon of *in vivo* transfection, only subsequent studies approached the issue of efficacy.

Nonreplicating RNA and DNA expression vectors were first tested for *in vivo* transfection of mouse muscle during the late 1980s. Inoculation of such vectors without special delivery systems (naked DNA) was followed by expression of reporter genes in the muscle

Table 2.2. Routes and Means of Delivery for Genetic Vaccines

Routes		Means of delivery
In vivo	Intradermal	Injection via needle
	Subcutaneous	Particle-mediated administration
	Intramuscular	Jet injection
	Intravenous	Puncture-mediated transfer
	Intratumoral	Topical exposure
	Mucosal	
	Internal organs	
Ex vivo	*In vitro* transfection and adoptive transfer of cells	Lipid-mediated transfection
		Particle-mediated transfection

at levels comparable with those subsequent to *in vitro* transfection (Wolff et al., 1990). Furthermore, the expression lasted at least 2 months subsequent to injection. A more recent report extended the time interval of expression in muscle to 19 months (Wolff et al., 1992b). Furthermore, it was shown that inoculation in the muscle of a plasmid bearing a 12-kilobase insert, corresponding to human dystrophin, resulted in expression of the gene in approximately 1% of the myofibers at the inoculation site (Acsadi et al., 1991a). Another study, while extending the principle of *in vivo* transfection by naked DNA administration to myocardial cells, showed that other tissues may display less prolonged expression of the foreign gene (Acsadi et al., 1991b). These studies compared the ability of different tissues to express foreign genes after naked DNA administration. They concluded that the myocytes only, due to unique features such as T tubules, may have inherent ability to uptake nucleic acids in the absence of special delivery systems. *In vitro* studies with primary rat muscle cells apparently supported this hypothesis (Wolff et al., 1992b). Importantly, elegant controls carried out in the same study showed that administration via needle does not lead to direct delivery of DNA through sarcolemma, but an uptake mechanism is likely to be involved. Age and sex exert slight effects on the ability of rodent myocytes to express foreign genes subsequent to naked DNA inoculation (Wells and Goldspink, 1992).

Formulation of DNA with cationic lipids resulted in uptake and expression by other types of cells, such as neurons (Ono et al., 1990) and embryonic cells (Demeneix et al., 1991). Only more recently, *in vitro* and *in vivo* studies showed that other cells, such as bone-marrow-derived antigen presenting cells and keratinocytes, are able to uptake naked plasmids and to synthesize foreign proteins (Rouse et al., 1994; Raz et al., 1994; Casares et al., 1997b). This achievement has been promoted by the shift in interest from gene therapy to genetic immunization, subsequent to understanding that while levels of expression conferred by naked DNA inoculation might not be sufficient to replace defective proteins, they are certainly enough to generate immunity against important pathogens (Ulmer et al., 1993; Wang et al., 1993b; Montgomery et al., 1993).

Many subsequent studies confirmed that uptake and expression of foreign proteins subsequent to naked DNA inoculation are not an exclusive property of rodent myocytes. Thus, an initial study reported that both Type I and II myofibers expressed reporter genes delivered as naked DNA into muscle of nonhuman primates (Jiao et al., 1992). However, a reduced level of expression compared to rodents was attributed to increased thickness of perimysium. Since then, numerous reports, discussed in subsequent chapters, extended this observation to other species, including humans.

In parallel with studies describing expression of foreign genes subsequent to injection of naked DNA via needle, another strategy of gene delivery has been initiated with the observation that tungsten microprojectiles coated with nucleic acids and accelerated into living cells may be used to enhance the transfection efficiency of cultured cells (Armaleo et al., 1990). As an essential element, this strategy, biolistic (from biological–ballistic) delivery of DNA, comprises high velocity (500 m/s) acceleration of submicronic particles, leading to intracellular penetration. The acceleration of metal particles to such speed can be achieved using strong electrostatic fields, provided by devices called gene-guns, or by expansion of compressed gases. The rate of gene transfection using this procedure was increased to the order of $1/10^3$ to $1/10^5$. Subsequent studies extended the initial observations, carried out with tungsten particles in cultured cells of *Saccharomyces cerevisiae*, to gold particles in rodents or cultured mammalian cells (Johnston, 1990; Yang et al., 1990).

Importantly, the study of reporter gene expression after biolistic DNA administration into the skin showed that the microprojectiles can penetrate and transfect several layers of epidermal cells up to the subcutaneous tissue, without evidence of injury and with a transfection rate of 10% to 20% of cells at the site of delivery (Williams et al., 1991). Two factors may explain the numerous subsequent reports showing increased immunity relative to the dose of plasmid in the case of administration via biolistic means, as compared to inoculation into muscles via needle: (1) The rate of *in vivo* transfection at the site of administration that is 1–2 log higher, and (2) the direct delivery of foreign genes to Langerhans cells that are potent professional APC. Importantly, such a method and variations such as, for example, *in vivo* transfection promoted by jet injection of plasmid DNA solution (Furth et al., 1992), administration of DNA-coated projectiles via pneumatic gun (Vahlsing et al., 1994), or puncture-mediated gene transfer to skin (Ciernik et al., 1996b), may circumvent the limited ability of cells to uptake naked DNA. The implications are quantitative and qualitative: First, the number of *in vivo* transfected cells is simply higher, and second, the categories of transfected cells are broader, leading to potentially new consequences. Furthermore, from the perspective of possible side effects of genetic immunization, the requirement for smaller doses of plasmid is likely to be associated with decreased risks of chromosomal integration.

Another strategy originating in promoted uptake of nucleic acids into cells that normally have decreased ability to incorporate naked genetic material is based on formulation with special compounds, an issue that will be discussed in the following paragraph.

Administration via both needle and gene-gun has been tested for gene delivery to various tissues. Administration of nucleic acids via needle comprises either naked or formulated material. Besides muscle, other sites have been explored as well: intradermal (Raz et al., 1994), subcutaneous (Fynan et al., 1993b), intravenous (Zhu et al., 1993), intra-arterial (Nabel et al., 1992b), into viscera such as the spleen, liver (Dubensky et al., 1984; Hickman et al., 1994), brain (Ono et al., 1990), heart (Acsadi et al., 1991b), or intratumoral (Nabel et al., 1993). However, particularly when the immune response was followed as read out, administration via needle was more successful and reproducible in the case of intramuscular, intradermal and, less frequently, intravenous administration (Fynan et al., 1993b; Raz et al., 1994). The other routes, namely, subcutaneous and intraperitoneal, were either nonimmunogenic or poorly investigated from this point of view. As a particular route involving topical administration of nucleic-acid-based vectors, mucosal delivery received special attention due to its important implications for immunization. Administration of DNA-expressing microbial antigens, even without adjuvant formulation, resulted in induction of local and/or systemic immunity (Fynan et al., 1993b). Numerous, more recent studies examined various formulations of nucleic acids that were aimed at increasing the immunity subsequent to mucosal immunization. This issue, together with the one regarding attempts to selectively target nucleic acids by encapsulation in coated microvesicles, will be discussed in the next paragraph concerning formulations.

Direct intracellular delivery via gene-gun has been pursued, particularly for skin administration, because of practical suitability as well as excellent results in terms of immunity. Interestingly, transfection of epidermal cells rather than dermal cells, achieved by increasing the propelling speed, resulted in increased immune responses (Eisenbraun et al., 1993). Together with the observation that intradermal inoculation via needle was not as effective compared to gene-gun immunization (Fynan et al., 1993b), this observation argues that cells distributed throughout the epithelial layer, if directly transfected, have potent immune-priming abilities. However, their capacity to pick up naked DNA might be a limiting factor. Few reports described gene-gun-mediated immunization at different sites, such as mucosa of the genital tract (Livingston et al., 1995). Other studies approached biolistic delivery of genes into cultured cells (Johnston and Tang, 1993), with the general aim of *ex vivo* engineering. Rat neurons and glial cells in primary cultures were effectively transfected via particle bombardment with genes expressing either luciferase or rat tyrosine hydroxylase (TH), a candidate for treatment of Parkinson's disease (Jiao et al., 1993). Importantly, freshly excised and bombarded fetal brain tissue expressed the foreign gene up to 2 months after implantation into rat brain stem (Jiao et al., 1993). The obvious limitation of this strategy is the transient nature of gene expression. This might not be an important problem when immune therapy is aimed. *Ex vivo* transfection by gene-gun of human peripheral blood mononuclear cells, as well as murine T lymphocytes or macrophages, resulted in rapid expression of the foreign reporter gene (Burkholder et al., 1993). Together, these pioneering studies validated a new method for direct *in vivo* or *ex vivo* transfection of cells, independent of the stage of cell cycle.

2.3. FORMULATIONS

In spite of the fact that naked DNA is taken up by and leads to expression of foreign genes, particularly in muscle cells but in other cells as well, the relatively low transfection efficiency promoted studies regarding formulations that enhance *in vivo* and *ex vivo* transfection (Table 2.3). Many of these studies have been focused on administration of DNA formulated in cationic lipids to nonmuscle cells, particularly epithelial cells of mucosal origin. Other formulations, including molecular adjuvants such as cytokine-expressing plasmids, will be discussed as well. It is important to note that microbial DNA itself, and in particular, unmethylated CpG motifs, exerts strong Th1-promoting adjuvant activity. This issue is detailed in a subsequent chapter.

Before discussing more elaborate formulations, we approach early studies that looked at simple parameters such as type of solution, volume of injection, tonicity, speed of injection, needle type, or the physiological condition of muscles. Interestingly, normal

Table 2.3. Adjuvants and Formulations for Genetic Vaccination

Categories	Examples
Formulations that enhance the transfection rate	Cationic or noncationic liposomes
	DNA pellets
	Formulation in hypo- or hypertonic solutions
	Pre- or coadministration of agents inducing tissue regeneration[a]
	Encapsulation in microvesicles[a]
	Bacterial mediated delivery[a]
Formulations that enhance or modulate the responsiveness of lymphocytes	Cytokine- and chemokine-expressing plasmids
	Plasmids expressing costimulatory molecules

[a]May act by both increasing transfection rate and modulating immune responsiveness.

saline as injection fluid seems to be optimal for gene expression in the case of intramuscular inoculation (Wolff et al., 1991), although other groups employed hyper- (Davis et al., 1993b) or hypotonic formulations. For example, water was a more effective vehicle for reporter genes when the target organ was lung (Sawa et al., 1996). Induction of muscle regeneration was reported to have enhancing effects on gene expression following the inoculation of nucleic acid vectors. Local anesthetics such as bupivacaine (Wells, 1993), or cobra venom cardiotoxin (Danko et al., 1994), when inoculated a few days prior to administration of expression vectors, resulted in expression levels that were up to one magnitude higher as compared with nonregenerating muscles. Such regenerating–inducing agents did not easily find their way to clinical trials of genetic vaccines because of practical as well as safety considerations.

We can formally divide the types of formulations into two general categories: formulations that enhance the uptake of DNA by cells (i.e., cationic liposomes) or formulations that promote the recruitment and activation of APC and lymphocytes (i.e., cytokine-expressing plasmids).

Liposome formulations were shown to promote translocation of vesicle content through the cell membrane due to the fusion of lipid shell with the plasma membrane. Liposomes can be designed as uni- or multilamellar structures, having an internal aqueous environment. Most of the formulations regarding DNA comprise cationic lipids that are thought to attach to nucleic acids on the internal surface of vesicles, through the quaternary ammonium group. Long alkyl chains comprising approximately 20–30 carbon residues are preferred, since they are more hydrophobic. Apart from cationic liposomes that fuse readily with cell membrane, noncationic liposomes, although not as fusogenic, may offer effective vehicles for macrophage/APC delivery. However, *in vitro* studies showed that cationic liposomes are endocytosed via coated pits and vesicles, resulting in delivery of lipid/DNA complexes into endosomes, followed by translocation into cytoplasm and nucleus (Friend et al., 1996).

Liposome-mediated delivery of genes was extensively developed during the 1980s and offered a more effective strategy for *in vitro* transfection (Malone et al., 1989; Felgner and Ringold, 1989) compared to more classical approaches such as DNA precipitation with calcium phosphate, dextran, or electroporation. This strategy initially focused on gene therapy simply because an increased effectiveness of transfection was required to achieve therapeutic effects. Pioneering studies showed that inoculation of nucleic acids complexed with cationic lipids into mouse brain (Ono et al., 1990), intratumorally, intravenously, or intra-arterially (Stewart et al., 1992; Nabel et al., 1992a), was followed by *in vivo* expression of foreign genes. A subsequent study showed generalized expression for at least 9 weeks of a reporter gene after intravenous inoculation of DNA complexed with cationic liposomes (Zhu et al., 1993). An early clinical trial using DNA-mediated immunotherapy showed *in vivo* expression of a gene expressing HLA-B7 introduced into melanoma tumors as DNA complexed with cationic lipids (Nabel et al., 1993). Difficult biodegradation of liposomes was associated with increased *in vivo* toxicity and consequently limited ability of liposomes to deliver DNA. This promoted further optimization of liposome structure: It was found that novel cationic lipids in combination with neutral lipids structured in large (300–700 nm) multilamellar vesicles displayed improved activity/safety profiles (San et al., 1993; Felgner et al., 1994). More recent findings allowed further optimization of liposome structures based on the assumption that two parameters are critical for the activity: ability to fuse with plasma membranes and to protect the DNA content from enzymatic degradation prior to cellular uptake (Gregoriadis et al., 1996; Lewis et al., 1996). Use of cholesterol as neutral lipid in the structure of liposomes resulted in enhanced expression following systemic delivery (Liu et al., 1997).

Parenteral inoculation of liposome-formulated nucleic-acid-based vectors demonstrated transfection of embryonic cells (Watanabe et al., 1994), T-cells, bone-marrow-derived cells (Philip et al., 1993), lung cells, and hepatocytes (Thierry et al., 1997). An interesting recent study compared the magnitude of cellular and humoral immunity subsequent to intramuscular inoculation with HBsAg-expressing DNA entrapped in liposomes, complexed with liposomes or in saline (Gregoriadis et al., 1997). Intramuscular delivery via liposomes containing DNA was followed by significantly increased immunity compared with the other formulations. This indicates that liposomes facilitate the priming of lymphocytes only if they contain DNA, indirectly suggesting that they act by increasing the uptake of, as well as shielding, nucleic acids. Furthermore, even in the muscle, a limiting factor may be the uptake and expression of DNA.

Numerous studies approached mucosal administration of nucleic acids formulated with lipids as a method to enhance the expression of foreign genes subsequent to topical administration. In a first stage, different formulations were tested for the efficiency of *in vivo* transfection. Such read out may be considered predictive for the immune-enhancing properties, although several studies suggested the lack of direct relationship between the level of expression and the magnitude of immunity. Both administration of reporter genes formulated with cationic lipids, either via intranasal instillation (Wheeler et al., 1996) or aerosol administration (Eastman et al., 1997a, 1997b), resulted in limited but detectable lung expression, namely, that approximately 1% of the alveoli displayed transfected cells and the total level of expression corresponded to picograms of reporter protein/lung. Importantly, liposome formulation resulted in a level of expression ten times higher as compared with saline formulation (Wheeler et al., 1996).

More recent studies approached the characterization of immune responses elicited by mucosal vaccination with liposome-formulated DNA. An interesting study defined local expression and immunity elicited by nasal application of luciferase-expressing DNA formulated with cationic lipids (Klavinskis et al., 1997). Importantly, nasal administration of DNA resulted in systemic induction of CTL and B-cell responses, as well as local immunity in the genital tract. Formulation with cationic lipids allowed a 100-fold increase in the expression of a reporter gene subsequent to intranasal administration (Norman et al., 1997). Other studies looked at the immunity elicited by a prototype vaccine against HIV-1, comprising plasmids that express gp160 and rev. It has been shown that intranasal administration of liposome-formulated DNA was followed by induction of CTL and mucosal IgA antibodies (Okada et al., 1997). Furthermore, coadministration of plasmids that express Interleukin-12 (IL-12) or granulocyte-monocyte colony stimulating factor (GM-CSF) resulted in enhanced CTL immunity. The immunity provided by such DNA vaccine formulated with cationic lipids was significantly higher compared to the one afforded by saline-formulated DNA. This observation was generalized to parenteral routes, including intramuscular injection (Ishii et al., 1997a). Thus, the formulation itself seems to promote a more efficient exposure of lymphocytes to the antigen, probably by increasing its expression. A more elaborate formulation, comprising mannan-coated liposomes loaded with plasmids expressing HIV-1 antigens, was aimed at optimizing the targeting of vesicles to mannan-receptor$^+$ APC (Toda et al., 1997). Both CTL activity and delayed type hypersensitivity (DTH) response were enhanced in an IFN-γ dependent manner by formulation of plasmids in mannan-coated liposomes. Such studies probably mark the beginning for a new avenue that consists of the design of vesicle-based carriers for genetic vaccines that selectively target specific APC subpopulations.

Another explored route for mucosal immunization is oral administration. Encapsulation of plasmids in poly(DL-lactide-co-glycolide) and oral administration resulted in significant IgA responses (Jones et al., 1997). More importantly, oral immunization with DNA-expressing VP6 antigen of rotavirus, encapsulated in similar particles, resulted in induction of mucosal IgA and partial protection against virus challenge (Chen et al., 1998a). Consistent results were obtained in BALB/c mice by oral vaccination with poly-lactide-glycosyl (PLG)-encapsulated DNA expressing gp160 (Kaneko et al., 2000). It is not clear yet if such capsules protect the DNA from degradation and/or facilitate the uptake by intestinal epithelial or M-cells.

In general, the interest for mucosal routes of DNA vaccination was amplified by two factors: (1) the essential role of the local or mucosal-associated lymphoid system, and (2) the assumption that the protection levels obtained by DNA vaccination could be improved using alternate routes of delivery, particularly in the case of microbes entering the body via mucosal areas. Nasal delivery of DNA expressing the L1 protein of the human papillomavirus-16 was able to prime local responses in remote areas, such as the vagina (Dupuy et al., 1999). More specialized administration of DNA vaccines to the oral mucosa by jet injection (Lundholm et al., 1999) or to the salivary glands (Kawabata et al., 1999) was able to trigger not only local antibody responses but also systemic cellular and humoral responses. Thus, potential advantages emerge for the mucosal route of vaccination: generation of immunity at the port of entry, including remote mucosal areas and induction of systemic immunity as well.

Improved lipid-based adjuvants for DNA vaccines were introduced based on the observation that lipopolyamines spontaneously condense DNA on a cationic lipid layer (Barthel et al., 1993). Subsequent studies demonstrated *in vivo* transfection of embryos with lipospermine-compacted DNA (Demeneix et al., 1994). *In vivo* efficiency of transfection was increased by DNA condensation with polyamines and polyethylene glycol phospholipids prior to incorporation in liposome structures (Hong et al., 1997). Further refinement of lipid–polyamine formulation by chemical modification has been reported (Erbacher et al., 1997).

An interesting adjuvant seems to be monophosphoryl lipid A (MPL), reported to enhance the cellular and humoral responses subsequent to mucosal or intramuscular inoculation or DNA-based expression vectors encoding the env and rev genes of HIV-1 (Sasaki et al., 1997, 1998b). However, the enhancement of immunity did not correlate with the level of expression at the site of immunization, suggesting that MPL acts through different mechanisms, possibly direct activation of APC or lymphocytes.

Genetic engineering strategies have been employed to design delivery vectors endowed with enhanced transfection abilities. For example, a nonlipid formulation of DNA complexed with recombinant peptide comprising a histone fragment and the SV40 T Ag nuclear localization signal resulted in transfection efficiency that was similar to conventional liposome formulations (Fritz et al., 1996). More recently, a group designed cationic alpha-helical peptides endowed with the ability to complex and transport DNA into cells (Niidome et al., 1997).

Other studies described manipulation of antigen targeting by attaching or removing signal sequences to foreign antigens expressed by plasmids. This usually resulted in strong modulation of immunity, resulting from the segregation of processing pathways with the type of immune response. For example, engineering of a plasmid that expressed ubiquitin-ated viral protein resulted in enhanced CTL induction but abrogation of humoral response subsequent to genetic immunization of mice (Rodriguez et al., 1997). Interestingly, removal or addition of ER export signals to the expressed protein does not have major effects on the T helper or isotype profile (Inchauspe et al., 1997). However, antibody titers are usually higher in the case of secreted variants, obtained by the manipulation of leader signals, probably because the exposure of B-cell receptors to antigen is optimized (Weiss et al., 1999; Svanholm et al., 1999), although there may be exceptions to this rule in case of antigens that do not fold correctly in the ER (Rice et al., 1999). This rule seems to hold, as expected, in primates, namely, that DNA vaccination of macaques with a truncated version of E2 antigen from HCV, exported to the cell surface, triggered enhanced humoral responses (Forns et al., 1999). Another recent study carefully examined differences in the humoral and cellular responses generated by DNA vaccination of antigenic variants either retained in the cell or exported at the cell surface: Interestingly, extracellular export led to the induction of Th2 immunity and IgG1 antibodies, whereas cellular retainment led to Th1 response associated with IgG2a antibodies (Lewis et al., 1999).

Targeting of released antigen to specific cells via receptor–ligand interaction is another area under current investigation. Targeting of antigen to FcR$^+$ APC, by attaching Ig-binding motifs of microbial origin to a protein expressed by a plasmid-based vector, resulted in strong modulation of immunity (Lobell et al., 1998). Attachment of CTLA-4, a natural ligand for B7 molecules on APC, to a bacterial antigen (*Corynebacterium pseudo-tuberculosis* phospholipase D) resulted in enhanced humoral responses upon DNA vaccination of sheep (Chaplin et al., 1999). In a papillomavirus system, it was recently shown that the attachment of E7 antigen to the *M.tb.* heat shock protein 70 leads to significant protection against E7-expressing tumors via generation of stronger CTL responses, probably by cross-priming (Chen et al., 2000).

In the category of molecular adjuvants, we discuss cytokines and costimulatory factors (Table 2.3). By providing such factors, the immunity triggered by antigen-expressing plasmids should be enhanced or modulated. Clearly, the most important driving force for such studies was the necessity to increase the immunity afforded by genetic vaccines. An early study demonstrated that intramuscular injection of plasmids expressing cytokines, such as TGF-β1, IL-2, or IL-4, was followed by systemic effects in terms of modulation of cellular versus humoral response to antigens inoculated into remote sites (Raz et al., 1993). These results were attributed to persisting levels of cytokines in the blood due to ectopic expression. The strategy was optimized by subsequent studies that addressed the issue of cytokine-mediated modulation of immunity through protocols comprising coadministration of plasmids expressing antigens and cytokines. Coadministration of plasmids expressing GM-CSF usually resulted in increased humoral responses (Xiang and Ertl, 1995; Kim et al., 1997b). Coadministration of IL-2 or TNF-α resulted in enhanced cellular and humoral responses (Chow et al., 1997; Kim et al., 1998). A more selective effect is exhibited by coadministration of IL-12: increased Th1, CTL as well as IgG2a antibody induction (Iwasaki et al., 1997b; Kim et al., 1997b; Chow et al., 1998; Lee et al., 1998). Interestingly, one study reported decreased humoral responses after IL-12 coadministration (Kim et al., 1997b). IL-4-expressing plasmid suppressed Th1 and CTL responses, while shifting the isotype profile toward IgG1 (Chow et al., 1998). Other Th2-promoting cytokines such as IL-5 and IL-10 were shown to enhance the humoral responses to antigens coadministered via plasmid expression vectors (Kim et al., 1998). Besides IL-12 and IL-2, other cytokines such as TNF-α and IL-15 were shown to enhance CTL responses (Kim et al., 1998). The ability of plasmids expressing IFN-γ to enhance cellular responses is disputed (Xiang and Ertl, 1995; Xiang et al., 1997). Interestingly, another study showed that the enhanced T-cell response followed by IL-12 coinoculation was dependent on endogenous IFN-γ production (Tsuji et al., 1997b). Delivery of cytokines has been achieved by three different means: inoculation of distinct plasmids expressing antigens and cytokines, of bicistronic plasmids coexpressing antigens and cytokines, or plasmids expressing antigen–cytokine fusion proteins. The last two methods optimize the coexpression of antigens and cytokines in the same cellular environment. More recent reports, while confirming the general principle of immune modulation by codelivery of cytokines together with antigen via DNA vaccination into primates (Kim et al., 1999a), extended this type of observations to the world of chemokines. For example, a recent report shows that coadministration of MIP-1α with the gp160 antigen in a mouse model resulted in enhanced CTL and humoral immunity, probably due to the increased employment at the site of injection of professional APC (Lu et al., 1999).

Genetic immunization with cytokine–fusion constructs resulted in significant modulation of immunity: IL-12 and IL-1β constructs led to increased CTL response, whereas the IL-4 construct primed antibody responses (Maecker et al., 1997). These observations elegantly demonstrate the possibility of designing chimeric molecules that comprise active cytokines.

In the same line, coadministration of membrane-bound stimulatory molecules that participate in the process of T-cell priming was shown to enhance or modulate the immune responses afforded by genetic vaccines. Coadministration of B7-2, and to a lesser extent of B7-1 molecules, was followed by enhanced induction of specific CTL (Iwasaki et al., 1997a). Both bicistronic plasmids as well as mixtures of plasmids expressing antigens and B7-2 resulted in enhanced CTL induction (Iwasaki et al., 1997b; Kim et al., 1997c; Tsuji et al., 1997c). This might suggest that coexpression of antigen and B7-2 by the same cell is not a requirement. The humoral response was not affected, but Th response was slightly increased by codelivery of B7-1 (Kim et al., 1997c). Interestingly, the enhancement of CTL response noted in the case of B7-2 codelivery depended on endogenous IFN-γ and, as expected, CD28 engagement (Tsuji et al., 1997c). Two nonmutually exclusive mechanisms may account for these observations: First, nonprofessional APC may acquire the ability to express B7-2 molecules thus becoming potent priming cells, and second, resident or migratory professional APC may upregulate their B7-2 expression following direct transfection. Another study showed enhanced humoral and cellular responses following coadministration of plasmids expressing CD40L and LacZ (Mendoza et al., 1997). Presumably, engagement of CD40 on migrant APC by ectopic CD40L leads to more rapid and effective activation of APC. Naturally, a variant of these strategies is represented by *ex vivo* transfection of professional APC with foreign genes that express antigens, followed by inoculation into the organism (Manickan et al., 1997a). More recently, it was shown that even codelivery of intercellular adhesion molecules (ICAM-1), together with the antigen, by DNA vaccination, may improve the Th and CTL immunity via a costimulatory pathway independent of CD86/CD28 but likely comprising the upregulation of β-chemokines (Kim et al., 1999).

Altogether, while demonstrating the proof of concept regarding coinoculation of cytokines and costimulatory molecules, the studies just mentioned used strong microbial or other foreign antigens. This strategy would be of particular importance in the case of weak antigens, such as tumor-associated antigens, or in the case of limited responsiveness of lymphocytes, for example, in neonates. Pre- and coadministration via genetic immunization of GM-CSF or B7-1 with carcinoembryonic antigen (CEA) resulted in enhanced cellular and humoral responses (Conry et al., 1996a). Similar results were obtained in a melanoma model employing MAGE-1 and MAGE-3 antigens (Bueler and Mulligan, 1996). Thus, a new generation of molecular adjuvants may find its use in vaccination against tumors or microbes. However, more advanced vectors that allow control of gene expression would be critical in eliminating the possibility of side effects due to uncontrolled or longtime expression of cytokines.

An important body of evidence suggests that DNA vaccines are more potent in inducing cellular rather than humoral responses. Furthermore, the T-cell responses elicited by genetic immunization consist of CTL and Th1 cells. Some groups exploited this characteristic of genetic vaccines, combined with more conventional vaccines, in order to design potent immunization regimens. Most of the resulting schedules involve priming with genetic vaccines followed by boost with recombinant viruses or subunit protein vaccines. There may be at least two reasons that such regimens are more successful: First, priming with DNA vaccines leads to induction of Th1 immunity that will further amplify during boost, and second, whereas genetic vaccines trigger stronger T-cell responses, conventional vaccines are more potent inducers of humoral immunity. Thus, the overall immunity conferred by such combination regimens is superior compared to any of the individual vaccination strategies. The proof of concept has been demonstrated in the case of (1) vaccination against HIV-1, with DNA vaccine followed by multipeptide vaccination (Okuda et al., 1997); (2) vaccination against *Taenia ovis*, with a prototype DNA vaccine followed by recombinant protein administration (Rothel et al., 1997), and (3) experimental vaccination against *Plasmodium berghei*, consisting of DNA immunization followed by boost with recombinant virus (Schneider et al., 1998). It is very likely that such combination regimens that consist of priming by DNA vaccines, followed by boosts employing more conventional approaches, are a better alternative for the future.

Chapter 3

Intrinsic Adjuvant Properties
of Plasmid DNA

3.1. INTRODUCTION

While parental administration of highly purified proteins, peptides, or hapten-carrier conjugates fails to elicit an immune response, coinjection with adjuvants induces both humoral and cellular responses.

The adjuvants are a heterogeneous class of substances with different gross chemical structure, originating from various sources and with various modes of action. Therefore, the adjuvants are defined only by functional criteria, namely, their ability to enhance the immune responses. There are only a few Thymus-independent, TI-2, antigens exhibiting both immunogenic and adjuvant properties (i.e., lipopolysaccharides, flagellin). The adjuvant activity of DNA and oligodeoxynucleotides (ODN) was described in the early 1960s. Braun and Nakano (1961) showed for the first time that the injection of calf thymus DNase-digested DNA with sheep red blood cells (SRBC) into AKR mice elicited a two to three times higher plaque-forming cell (PFC) response compared to that induced by injection of antigen alone. Later, Nakano and Braun (1967) demonstrated that poly(A-U) nucleotides also can increase the early rate of production of PFC in mice immunized with SRBC. Poly(A-U) nucleotides were able to enhance primary as well as secondary immune responses.

Several investigators showed that ODN can stimulate the *T*-cells. Hamaoka and Katz (1973) showed that the ODNs are able to expand carrier-specific *T*-cells and Allison (1973) showed that they are able to enhance mixed lymphocyte reactions.

The interest for adjuvant properties of DNA or ODN vanished during the past decades, leading to the paradigm that the DNA is immunologically inert and rapidly degraded in body fluids by nucleases.

Interest was recently resurrected by two observations. First, in the demonstration that bacterial DNA is endowed with polyclonal stimulatory properties, Messina et al. (1991) and Sun et al. (1997) showed that the bacterial DNA induces T-independent proliferation and polyclonal synthesis of immunoglobulin by murine B lymphocytes. This effect was observed with ss-, ds-DNA, and even with a 100 bp DNA fragment. Since the effect of DNA resembled that of endotoxins, it was proposed that both substances stimulate the innate immunity by triggering inflammatory reactions.

The second observation was the discovery of immunostimulatory sequences (ISS) by Tokunaga et al. (1984). The ISS were discovered initially in mycobacteria. Mycobacteria, and particularly the Bacille Calmette Guerin (BCG), were extensively used as non-specific agents in antitumor therapy. The antitumor activity of Mycobacteria was related to various substances such as mycolates, peptidoglycans cord factor, etc. (Adam, 1985). Tokunaga isolated from *M. tuberculosis* a fraction called MY-1, which when injected in tumor-bearing mice caused the regression of tumor. Gross chemical analysis showed that the fraction contains 70% DNA and its activity was abolished by DNase. The DNA contained in this fraction was rich in CpG motifs. This was not surprising, since it was shown that in contrast with eukaryote DNA, the prokaryotic DNA is rich in unmethylated CpG motifs. Yamamoto et al. (1992) used 30-mer single-stranded ODNs to determine the structure of DNA required for stimulatory activity. They demonstrated that the presence of unique palindromic sequences such as GACGTC, AGCGT, and AACGTT were essential for the immunostimulatory activity of ODN.

The presence of ISS in plasmids became important for study of the immune responses induced by genetic immunization because of the striking discrepancy between the small amount of proteins secreted by transfected cells (pg-ng) and the excellent responses induced by plasmid DNA.

3.2. IMMUNOSTIMULATORY SEQUENCES OF PLASMID DNA

Bacterial ISS are made of short, 6-base DNA fragments with CpG motifs. The ISS occur more frequently in bacterial (1:16) than in mammalian (1:50) DNA. The C and G bases occur less frequently in tandem in mammalian DNA, a phenomenon known as CpG suppression (Bird, 1987). The ISS are composed of two 5′ purines-CpG–two 3′ pyrimidine bases. In contrast to mammalian DNA, in which 70–90% of cytosines are methylated at C5 position, less than 5% are methylated in bacterial DNA. The role of ISS in adjuvanticity of plasmids was demonstrated in three pioneering experiments.

Sato et al. (1996) have studied the immune response against β-galactosidase elicited by two plasmids expressing Lac Z gene. One plasmid contained kanR gene and the other ampR gene. While ampR gene expresses CpG motifs, the kanR gene did not. Only the animals immunized with plasmid expressing kanR gene were able to induce an immune response. Inability of the plasmid carrying ampR gene to induce antibody synthesis was restored subsequent to coinjection of both plasmids. These results strongly suggested that ISS are able to enhance the immune responses. Klinman et al. (1997) demonstrated that the adjuvanticity of plasmid requires unmethylated ISS in a series of experiments aimed at studying the synthesis of lymphokines subsequent to injection of a plasmid. The treatment of plasmid with a reagent that methylates the CpG dinucleotides reduced the ability of plasmid to activate cytokine-secreting cells.

Finally, the experiments of Roman et al. (1997) and Klinman et al. (1997), using CpG-rich ODN and control ODN, formally proved that palindromic single-strand unmethylated CpG sequences are responsible for the enhancement of innate and specific immunity. These pioneering studies showed that immunogenicity of plasmids depends on two units: the transcriptional unit made up of the promoter and the foreign gene inserted into plasmid, and a second unit comprising the ISS.

While CpG motifs play a major role in the adjuvant activity of plasmids, the structure of 5' and 3' flanking regions of palindrome may also contribute to adjuvanticity. Kimura et al. (1994) noted that the immunostimulatory property of AACGTT palindrome was enhanced by presence of dG in 5' and 3' flanking region. Runs of dG are potentially able to form unconventional pairs favoring the formation of of unusual structures such quadriplex DNA.

3.3. EFFECT OF ISS ON CELLS INVOLVED IN INNATE IMMUNITY

Professional antigen-presenting cells and natural killer (NK) cells are the effectors of innate immunity that are able to recognize dangerous or aberrant signals.

Plasmid DNA triggers maturation of murine dendritic cells (DCs; Sparwasser et al., 1998). These authors demonstrated that bacterial DNA, or CpG ODN, caused maturation of immature DCs and activation of mature DCs to produce cytokines such as IL-12, IL-6, and TNFα. Induction of maturation of DCs and cytokine production shows that the bacterial DNA or CpG ODN are able to render effective the DCs for the initiation of T-cell-mediated cellular immune responses. Stacey et al. (1996) showed that intact rather than DNase-treated plasmid induced TNFα in bone-marrow-derived macrophages or the macrophage RAW264 line. In addition, plasmid induces the expression of IL-1β and PAI-2 genes, a phenomenon characteristic for activated macrophages.

Chace et al. (1997) found that bacterial DNA induces the production of IFNγ by NK cell and that this process was dependent on two factors: first, the presence of unmethylated CpG motifs, and second, the secretion of IL-12 by macrophages. Macrophages treated with DNA produce IL-12 accompanied by an increase of IL-12 p40 mRNA level. These experiments show that unmethylated CpG-rich bacterial DNA stimulated the production of IL-12 by macrophages, which in turn stimulate IFNγ synthesis by NK cells. NK cells spontaneously lyse certain transformed or virally infected cells but do not kill normal cells. Thus, the NK cells participate in the innate defense mechanisms against some viruses such as hepatitis virus or neoplastic cells.

Cowdery et al. (1996) showed that bacterial, but not calf thymus, DNA induce a rapid increase of splenic cell population producing IFNγ and that over 90% of cells producing this cytokine were identified by surface marker as NK cells. The role of ISS was demonstrated in an experiment in which the bacterial DNA was replaced with a 20-base CpG ODN. These results strengthen those reported by Yamamoto et al. (1992), who showed that a 30-mer single-strand ODN corresponding to a sequence of a mycobacterial antigen induced IFNγ and augmented NK cell activity. The requirement of CpG motif for activation of NK cells was demonstrated by using structurally different ODN. All ODN with GACGTC palindromic sequences were active. Furthermore, when 6 nucleotides of ODN devoid of stimulatory activity were replaced with other palindromic sequences (GACGTC, AGCGCT or AACGTT), the ODN acquired the ability to activate the NK cells. Another palindromic sequence, ACCGGT, was devoid of effect. These results strongly suggested that the presence of unique palindromic sequences are essential for the augmentation of NK activity.

Ballas et al. (1996) found that unmethylated CpG motifs, rather that the palindromic sequences, are more important in NK activation. This study also showed that the augmentation of NK activity is not due to a direct effect of ODN on NK cells, but rather to activation of production of NK-stimulating cytokines such as IFNα and β, TNFα, or IL-12 by macrophages.

3.4. EFFECT OF ISS ON B-CELLS

B-cells display two major functions in the body. First, they are able to take up exogenous antigens, process them, and present the peptides to T-cells. Second, the B-cells are the effectors of humoral immunity by virtue of their capacity to synthesize immunoglobulins.

Davis et al. (1998) showed for the first time the upregulation of the expression of MHC Class II, B7.2, and Ly-6C on sorted B-cells incubated in vitro with CpG ODN, or from animals injected with ODN. Class II and B.7 are key molecules involved in both the activation of T-cells and the cooperation processes between T- and B-cells in immune responses elicited by T-dependent antigens. Class II molecules are required for antigen presentation, and B7 molecules, subsequent to interaction with CD28 expressed on the surface of T-cells, deliver costimulatory signals required for the activation of T-cells. The expression of these molecules is not dependent on T-cells, as shown by the ability of sorted B-cells to be activated by CpG ODN. Apparently, CpG ODN display the same properties as other B-cell polyclonal activators. This was further demonstrated by Krieg et al. (1995) who compared the capacity of bacterial DNA and ODN containing unmethylated CpG motifs to activate the B-cells. The activation of B-cells is T-independent, as observed in highly purified B-cells by sorting. B-cell activation was measured by ^{3}H-uridine incorporation. Increased incorporation was evident by 4 hours and peaked at 24 hours. Cell-cycle analysis demonstrated that more that 95% of B-cells enter the cycle.

The CpG ODN exert the immunomodulatory properties not only on small resting mature cells but also on immature B-cells. This was shown in studies carried out on WEHI-231 cells, which exhibit a phenotype characteristic for immature B lymphocytes (Yi et al., 1996b; MacFarlane et al., 1997). In these experiments, the authors studied the effect of CpG ODN on survival of WEHI cells incubated with anti-Ig antibodies, which crosslink the surface Ig receptor leading to apoptosis. The CpG ODN prevents apoptosis even if added up to 8 hours after incubation with anti-Ig antibodies. The antiapoptotic effect was not affected by inhibitors of protein kinase C, indicating that the ODN did not exert the effect via protein kinases. In contrast, these cells exhibited an augmented expression of c-myc and bcl-x$_L$ genes. It was reported that the expression of c-myc may prevent apoptosis in various cells (Fischer et al., 1994). The prevention of anti-IgM-induced apoptosis of immature B-cells suggests that ODN may play a role in preventing deletion processes of autoreactive B-cells. This capacity is related to polyclonal activation of B-cells. There are other examples demonstrating that polyclonal B-cell mitogens can break down either natural tolerance or anergy. Murakami et al. (1994) showed that oral administrating of lipopolysaccharide (LPS) induced hemolytic anemia in transgenic mice, which otherwise do not produce anti-red blood cells (RBC) autoantibodies. We also showed that another polyclonal activator, nocardia water soluble mitogen (NWSM), was able to breakdown the anergy of B-cells from maternally allotype-suppressed rabbits (Bona and Cazenave, 1977).

ODN can serve as adjuvant for the induction of humoral responses against protein antigens. Thus, the adjuvant properties of CpG-rich ODN was demonstrated *in vivo* in animals injected with various antigens plus ODN. Significantly increased concentration or titers of specific antibody was noted in the case of immunization with influenza virus vaccine (Romal et al., 1997). Lipford et al. (1997a) observed a similar effect on anti-ovalbumin antibody response. These experiments showed that ODN potentiated antibody response and induced class switching toward IgG2a and IgG2b. Davis et al. (1998) also reported an increased titer of antihepatitis B surface antigens in mice immunized with a recombinant surface antigen and ODN.

It therefore clearly appears that the CpG-rich bacterial DNA as well as ODN are endowed with adjuvant properties similar to those exhibited by other microbial polyclonal activators such as LPS or NWSM. It would be of great interest to find out whether the adjuvant activity of ODN observed in small rodents can be demonstrated in nonhuman primates and man.

3.5. EFFECT OF ISS ON *T*-CELLS

Bacterial DNA exhibits an adjuvant effect also on *T*-cells. Leclerc et al. (1997) have studied the immune response elicited by soluble β-galactosidase or Hepatitis B surface antigen (HBs) recombinant protein and noted that the antibody response was higher when the immunization was carried out with a mixture of plasmid DNA and soluble antigens compared with the response elicited by immunization with antigens in saline. However, this study failed to address seminal questions, namely, the molecular structure of plasmid sequences responsible for the activation of *T*-cells.

The role of ISS on activation of CD4 *T*-cells was demonstrated by *in vivo* or *in vitro* studies that evaluated the phenotype of *T*-cells activated by ISS and by determining the isotypes of antibodies produced following genetic immunization. Figure 3.1 illustrates the mechanisms of the priming of Th1 cells by plasmid DNA. The general conclusion of several studies is that the Th1 cells that drive isotype switching to IgG2a and IgG2b are stimulated by ISS (Chu et al., 1997; Roman et al., 1997; Lipford et al., 1997a; Davis et al., 1998). In all these experiments, activation was observed with CpG ODN but not with control ODN lacking CpG motifs.

Apparently, the CpG ODN can also stimulate the CD8 cytotoxic *T*-cells. Generally, the cytotoxic *T*-cells cannot be activated by exogenous antigen or by peptides. Sato et al. (1996) showed that a plasmid containing CpG motifs and Lac Z gene was able to induce a specific cytotoxic response. Similarly, Lipford et al. (1997a) showed that the immunization of mice with the immunodominant K^b-restricted ovalbumin (OVA) peptide and CpG ODN induced a specific primary CTL response.

3.6. EFFECT OF ISS ON CYTOKINE PRODUCTION

Numerous findings demonstrated that immune systems respond to ISS by activating in a coordinated manner the production of cytokines important for both humoral and cellular immune responses.

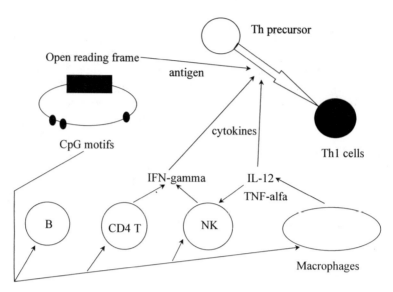

Figure 3.1. Priming of Th1 cells by plasmid-based expression vectors.

3.6.1. CpG ODN-Induced Synthesis of Cytokines by CD4 *T*-Cells

CD4 *T*-cells produce a large variety of cytokines, such as IL-2, IFNγ, IL-3, IL-4, IL-5, IL-9, IL-10, and IL-17.

While the ISS activate the synthesis of IFNγ, which is produced by Th1 cells, they do not induce the production of IL-3, IL-4, IL-5, which are synthesized by other Th cells. This strongly suggests that ISS function as a Th1 promoting adjuvant.

Roman et al. (1997) reported a striking increase of IFNγ synthesis by *in vitro* cultured CD4 *T*-cells from mice injected with a plasmid-bearing ISS. Klinman et al. (1997) demonstrated that CpG ODN triggers the synthesis of IFNγ by CD4 populations enriched by MACS. In this excellent study, a series of 151 synthetic ODNs were tested. Optimal stimulation was induced when central CpG was flanked at 5' by two purines (GpA or ApA) and at 3' by two pirimidines TpC or TpT. Chu et al. (1997) showed that cells from animals immunized with lysozyme in IFA together with CpG ODN produced IFNγ and the specific antibodics expressed IgG2a antibodies, whereas the cells from animals immunized with antigen in Friend's incomplete adjuvant only produced IgG1-specific antibodies.

These findings show that ISS activate the Th1 but not Th2 CD4 *T*-cells. However, it is noteworthy that the Th1 cells activated by ISS do not produce IL-2 (Klinman et al., 1997), a cytokine efficiently synthesized by most Th1 *T*-cell clones or *T*-cell hybridomas.

3.6.2. CpG ODN Induces the Secretion of IL-6 by *B*-Cells

Yi et al. (1996b) reported the CpG ODN induce *B*-cells to secrete IL-6, which in turn stimulates the secretion of IgM. Apparently, the secretion of IL-6 is dependent on the production of IFNγ. While IFNγ fails to activate *B*-cells by itself, it functions as a costimulatory molecule that augments CpG ODN-induced *B*-cell IL-6 secretion.

3.6.3. Effect of CpG ODN on Production of Cytokines by Antigen-Presenting Cells

Antigen presenting cells are able to synthesize and to secret various cytokines. IL-12 is produced within a few hours of bacterial and intracellular parasitic infections and acts as a proinflammatory cytokine. IL-12 is encoded by two genes that must function simultaneously in the same cell in order to produce active cytokine. IL-6 was discovered in human blastoid lines, and subsequent studies suggested that phagocytic cells might be the major physiological producers of IL-12 (Trinchieri, 1998). Klinman et al. (1998) demonstrated for the first time that CpG ODN increases the number of IL-12 secreting cells reaching the peak 12 hours after incubation with 1 μg of ODN. Increased secretions of IL-12 was also observed upon incubation of J774 macrophage line with ODN, as well as *in vivo* subsequent to injection with CpG ODN (Lipford et al., 1997). Anitescu et al. (1997) demonstrated that IL-10 inhibits the production of IL-12 induced by bacterial DNA. This conclusion was strengthened by experiments carried out in IL-10−/− mice, in which an increased number of IL-12 secreting cells following either single or repeated challenge with bacterial DNA were observed.

Bacterial DNA as well as CpG ODN stimulate the synthesis and secretion of TNFα by macrophages (Stacey et al., 1996; Sparwasser et al., 1997a). Increased secretion of TNFα induced by bacterial DNA injected *in vivo* may lead to lethal shock. Therefore, the ISS may exhibit double-edged sword properties. They act as strong Th1 and NK adjuvants. Both Th1 and NK cells play a determinant role in antimicrobial immunity. This is well supported by a recent demonstration that ISS triggers curative Th1 responses in lethal murine leishmaniasis (Sparwasser et al., 1997a). The ISS stimulation of synthesis of IFNγ by NK cell may be beneficial for antitumor immunity.

However, the ISS have also potentially toxic side-effect properties. The CpG ODN that increased the secretion of TNFα caused fatal shock in mice previously sensitized with D-galactose amine (Sparwasser et al., 1997a). Furthermore the CpG DNA can prime mice for Shwartzman phenomenon (Cowdery et al., 1996) and induces a dose-dependent splenomegaly. We observed that at the site of intramuscular injection with CpG ODN, but not control ODN, the mice developed a strong inflammatory reaction (Stan et al., 2000).

Figure 3.2 illustrates the strong inflammatory reaction at the site of injection of a plasmid or CpG ODN in BALB/c or BALB/c IFNγ−/− mice. This reaction, also a double-edged sword, by stimulation of secretions of IFNγ may not only upregulate the expression of MHC antigens on APC, but can also promote immunomediated processes leading to tissue damage.

3.7. MECHANISMS OF LYMPHOCYTE ACTIVATION BY CpG ODN

The mechanisms of action of CpG ODN are not completely unraveled yet. It is still unclear whether the ODN exert its stimulatory properties by binding to a membrane

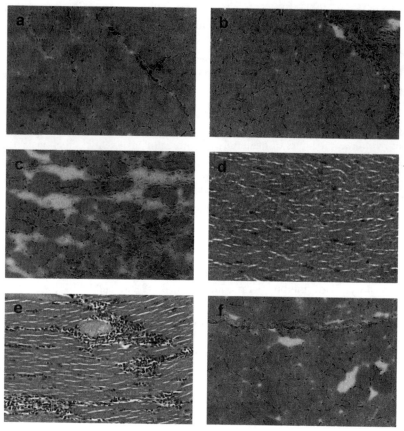

Figure 3.2. Cross sections of muscle biopsies at the site of injection stained with H&E. a) Muscle from BALB/c mice injected with saline. b) Muscles from BALB/c mice injected with a plasmid (Vh T, B plasmid described by Casares et al., 1997). c) Muscle from BALB/c injected with CpG ODN. d) Muscle from BALB/c mice injected with control ODN. e) Muscle from BALB/c IFNγ−/− mice injected with CpG ODN. f) Muscle from BALB/c IFNγ−/− mice injected with control plasmid.

receptor or, alternatively, after the uptake, interacts with regulatory proteins. There is no doubt that ODN, being soluble, small-size molecules, may be easily internalized by fluid phase pinocytosis.

However, there are studies suggesting that the internalization is mediated by receptors. Loke et al. (1989) reported the incorporation of acridine-labeled ODN by HL60 cells. While intracellular accumulation of unconjugated acridine was independent of temperature, significant intracellular accumulation of acridine-ODN was observed in a dose-effect manner at 37°C. The uptake of labeled ODN was inhibited by cold ODN, which suggested the involvement of a cell receptor in the process of internalization. A protein of 80-kDa, able to bind ODN, was isolated from the membranes of HL60 cells. This protein may be involved in the transport of ODN into the cells.

Studies carried out by Yabukov et al. (1989) on L929 mouse fibroblast and Krebs2 cells also showed that ODN bound to two surface proteins. The binding of ODN to these proteins was quite specific, since the internalization was not affected by various polyanions such as heparin, chondroitin sulfates, nor by ds, ssDNA, and tRNA. The ODN were found in both the cytoplasm and the nucleus. It is noteworthy that the internalized ODN began to be degraded 4 hours after the uptake. Benimetskaya et al. (1997) have demonstrated that ODN-bearing ISSs bind to integrin Mac-1 expressed on the surface of granulocytes and macrophages.

The scavenger macrophage receptor may also be involved in transportation of ODN across cellular membrane. There are two receptors that share similar sequences, except the C-terminal end, in which 110 amino acids of Type 1 receptor are replaced by a 6-amino acid C-terminus. Both receptors exhibit high affinity for polyanions, polysaccharides, phospholipids, and polyribonucleotides. Pearson et al. (1993) found that the ODN can bind to both Type 1 and Type 2 receptors. Taken together, these observations strongly suggest that there are several mechanisms responsible for the uptake of ODN by various cells.

ODN triggers molecular mechanisms responsible for the activation of various genes (c-myc, myn, bcl-x_1, c-jun, egr-1, bax, IL-1β, PAI-2, IL-6, TNFα, IFNγ, and IL-12). Once the CpG ODN penetrate into cells, they are found in endosomal compartments where they are probably processed. This mechanism is suggested by an observation of Yi et al. (1998) that the inhibitors of endosomal acidification specifically inhibited cytokine secretion by immature WEHI-231 B-cell line, J774 macrophage line, or spleen cells. The CpG ODN induces a rapid activation of NF kB, which is accompanied by degradation of IkBa and IkBb (Yi et al., 1998). Translocation of NFkBp65 was also demonstrated by Lipford et al. (1997). NFkB sites bind to the promoter of many genes encoding the lymphokines, including TNFα, which is activated in macrophages incubated with CpG ODN. The activation of various genes can be due to increased transcriptional activity of promoters. This is well supported by Yi et al. (1996b), who showed increased IL-6 promoter activity subsequent to incubation with CpG ODN of cells transfected with a vector in which the transcription of CAT reporter gene was driven by human IL-6 promoter. Further studies are required to determine the molecular mechanisms involved in CpG ODN gene activation.

Chapter 4

Cellular Mechanisms Involved in the Immune Response Elicited by Genetic Immunization

4.1. INTRODUCTION

The mechanisms of the induction of immune response by genetic immunization were a mystery during the five-year period when the major effort was focused to determine the immune response induced by plasmids containing genes coding for a variety of antigens. During the past two to three years, immunologists became interested in this area and achieved rapid progress with respect to characterization of cells involved in the immune response. A difficulty encountered in these studies was the utilization of various routes for administration of plasmids.

While the major players in immune responses, the lymphocytes, are the same in various tissues of the body, the initiators, the APCs, differ considerably from one tissue to another. Thus, while the muscles are easily transfected *in vivo*, the myocytes are nonprofessional APC and lack costimulatory molecules that provide a second signal required for the activation of *T*-cells. They induce tolerance rather than an immune response.

In the case of intradermal or subcutaneous immunization, the major APC is the Langerhans cell, which once activated by internalization of antigens, migrates to lymph nodes where it interacts with the lymphocytes.

In the case of oral immunization, the intestinal epithelial cells (IECs) play a key role in antigen presentation (Mayer, 1998). Class II molecules are constitutively expressed on IECs of the small bowel and, to a lesser extent, colon. Kaiserlian et al. (1989) showed that murine enterocytes can present a soluble antigen to specific class II restricted CD4 *T*-cells. Similarly, Hershberg et al. (1997) demonstrated that an IEC line transfected with DR4[b] was able to process and present antigen. Little is known about the APCs involved in the immune response following nasal or vaginal administration.

Theoretically there are several plausible mechanisms that may be responsible for the immune response elicited by genetic immunization. First, nonprofessional APCs, transfected at the site of injection of plasmid, synthesize and secrete the protein. While the native protein can be recognized directly by *B*-cells, it should be taken up by local or remote professional APCs. These cells process the protein and present the peptide to *T*-cells.

Second, nonprofessional APCs release the plasmid, which transfects the professional APCs. As an alternative variant, one may envision that the professional APCs can be transfected following phagocytosis of transfected somatic cells at the site of injection of plasmid. Third, the plasmid diffuses from the site of injection and transfects remote professional APC. Fourth, residential or circulating professional APCs are locally transfected, process endogenous proteins, and present the peptides to T-cells. Fifth, the transfection of cells at the site of injection upregulate the expression of MHC and costimulatory molecules, enabling them to present the peptides to T-cells.

4.2. CELLULAR UPTAKE OF DNA

The penetration of foreign DNA into bacterial cells was described by Avery et al. (1944). This observation, demonstrating that the DNA taken up by bacterial cells was functional (i.e., transformed the phenotype of host cell), represented a milestone discovery leading to the development of molecular biology.

Introduction of additional genes into the genome of mammalian cells, analogous to bacterial transformation, had been attempted by others. These studies took advantage of the ability of somatic cell to phagocytize particles, to pinocytize macromolecules, or to internalize ligands via receptors. Phagocytosis of DNA was demonstrated in a quite artificial system: Bensch et al. (1966) coupled on gold particles DNA with gelatin by cross-linking the protein with dialdehydes. Phagocytosis of particles by L-line (Earle) cells was observed a few minutes after incubation with L-cells. The majority of DNA particles were found in endosomes and multivesicular bodies. The presence of DNA in the vacuolar apparatus led the authors to believe that the DNA was completely degraded.

Pinocytosis of DNA by various cells was also reported. Kay (1961) showed that highly polymerized DNA was rapidly incorporated by Ehrlich–Lettre cells via fluid-phase pinocytosis. The pinocytosis of DNA is a rapid phenomenon which occurs five minutes after incubation and is energy-dependent, like the pinocytosis of various soluble macromolecules by mammalian cells (Gibb and Kay, 1962). The pinocytosis of ^{14}C-labeled DNA by Ehrlich cells was also demonstrated in vivo by Shimizu et al. (1962). The peak of incorporation was found to be at about 30–60 minutes after injection of DNA in the peritoneal cavity. Phosphodiesters, phosphorothionate, and chimeric oligodeoxynucleotides are also taken up by fluid-phase pinocytosis (Tonkinson et al., 1994; Zhao et al., 1996) and can be traced in the acid-lysosomal compartment (Tonkinson et al., 1994).

4.2.1. Receptor-Mediated Internalization of DNA

Lerner et al. (1971) showed that peripheral blood cells have DNA associated with their plasma membrane fraction. This observation raised the possibility of a receptor responsible for the binding of DNA. Studies carried out by Bennett et al. (1985) showed the existence of a DNA-binding protein receptor that mediates the internalization of DNA. This study was conducted with radiolabeled lambda phage DNA and with neutrophils, lymphocytes, and monocytes. The binding of DNA to cells was maximal after incubation for 10 minutes and was increased by Ca^{2+}, Mg^{2+}, and SO^{2-}_4 ions. The receptor displayed a high affinity (10^{-9}) for DNA binding. The DNA isolated from purified membranes had a molecular weight of 4.8×10^6. The binding of DNA to receptor was specific and not inhibited by tRNA, heparin, and mono- or polynucleotides. The protein nature of the receptor was shown in experiments in which the pretreatment of cells with trypsin, but not with neuraminidase, ablated the binding of DNA. SDS-PAGE analysis of membrane proteins of various cell types showed the binding to a single band of 30kD protein. The DNA–receptor complex is rapidly internalized and the DNA can be traced into cytoplasm. Bennett considered that DNA-binding protein may represent a scavenger-like receptor mediating the removal of circulating DNA. Apparently the function of the receptor is altered in the lymphocytes of systemic lupus erythematosus (SLE) and mixed connective tissue disease (MCTD) patients exhibiting a marked inhibition of DNA binding (Bennett et al., 1987). The internalization of oligonucleotides (ODN) is also mediated by a cellular receptor. Figure 4.1 illustrates the mechanisms of the uptake of DNA.

In summary, these observations clearly showed that exogenous or homologous, highly polymerized DNA is internalized in various cell types. Some data suggest that engulfed DNA is rapidly hydrolyzed. However, the major drawback of these studies was the lack of information regarding the expression of genes contained in highly polymerized DNA taken up by various cells.

4.3. CELLULAR MECHANISMS INVOLVED IN THE IMMUNE RESPONSE INDUCED BY INTRADERMAL GENETIC IMMUNIZATION

A large body of evidence indicates that naked DNA injected into skin is taken up by various dermal cells. In pigs and humans, the DNA is taken up mainly by epidermal cells (Hengge et al., 1996), and in mice by cells of epidermis, dermis, fat tissue, and myocytes from underlying muscles (Wolff et al., 1990).

In the skin, areas surrounding post capillary venules in the dermis contain the highest number of lymphocytes. The cellular elements of the skin immune system include lymphocytes, macrophages, mast cells, and dendritic cells (i.e., Langerhans cells). Vascular endothelium expresses adhesion molecules recruiting particular lymphocyte subsets (epidermotropic lymphocytes). The skin keratinocytes, long thought to produce only keratin, have

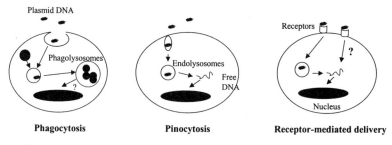

Figure 4.1. Possible mechanisms of internalization of highly polymerized DNA.

also been found to produce some lymphokines such as IL-7, which serve as a growth factor for development of epidermal *T*-cells (Matsue et al., 1993).

Our laboratory was interested in determining what cells are transfected *in vivo* following intradermal injection of plasmids. In these experiments two plasmids were used:

- pVhT,B, which contains an engineered V_H gene in which the CDR2 was replaced with a peptide of influenza hemagglutinin recognized by *B*-cells, and the CDR3 by a peptide (HA110-120) recognized by CD4 *T*-cells in association with Class II (I-E^d) molecules (Brumeanu et al., 1996).
- pNPVI, a plasmid that expresses the nucleoprotein of PR/8 influenza virus which bears the immunodominant epitope recognized by CD8 *T*-cells in association with Class I (K^d) molecules (Taylor et al., 1987).

After injection of both plasmids in the skin of mouse ears, the plasmids were detected by PCR in Class II$^+$ cells, mainly Langerhans cells, as well as in Class II$^-$ cells (Figure 4.2). PCR was also used to detect pNPVI in cells that emigrated from the skin, crawl-out cells. Figure 4.3B shows a 711 bp band corresponding to the NP insert detected with NP-specific primers and further identified by double digestion with AcsI and MlvII to yield two fragments of same molecular size as that obtained by digestion of pNPVI. These results clearly demonstrated that dermal cells were transfect *in vivo* after the injection of plasmids into the skin.

Taking into account that various dermal cells were transfected *in vivo* subsequent to intradermal injection of plasmid, it was important to determine the cell-type able to present antigen and to activate *T*-cells.

Raz et al. (1994) showed that intradermal injection of NPVI plasmid induced a long-lasting specific response. The NP was detected by anti-NP antibodies in keratinocytes, fibroblasts, and dendritic-like cells. However, in this study, the dendritic cells were charac-

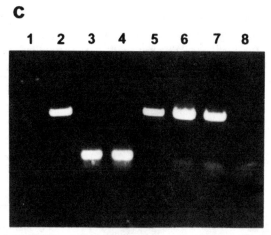

Figure 4.2. PCR analysis of pVhT,B and pC in skin of mice immunized intradermally. Lane 1, molecular markers; lane 2, pVhT,B; lane 3, pC; lane 4, crawl-out cells from mice immunized with pC; lane 5, crawl-out cells from mice injected with pVhT,B; lane 6, Class II$^+$-sorted cells from mice immunized with pVhT,B; lane 7, Class II$^-$-cells from mice injected with pVhT,B (from Casares et al., *J. Exp. Medicine* 1997, 186:1481–1486).

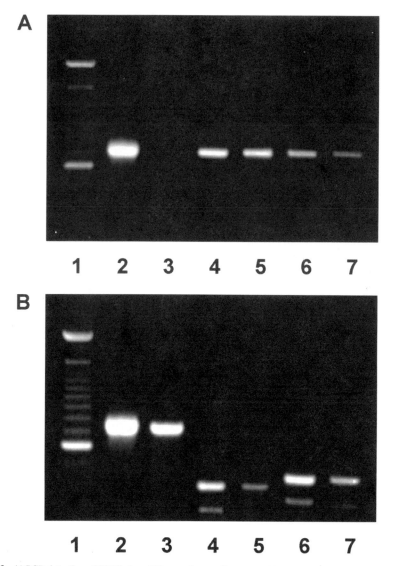

Figure 4.3. A) PCR detection of NPVI plasmid in crawl-out cells prepared from ears. Lane 1, molecular markers; lane 2, pNPVI; lane 3, pC, lane 4–7, DNA extracted from various numbers of crawl cells from mice injected with NPVI. B) Restriction digestion of *in vivo* transfected NPVI plasmid (lane 4, 6) and positive control (lane 5, 7).

terized solely by cytological criteria but not by specific cell markers. It is known that some epidermotrophic T lymphocytes also exhibit dendritic-like profiles (Mallick-Wood et al., 1998).

Condon et al. (1996) provided the first evidence that a dermal dendritic cell was transfected *in vivo* following injection into skin of a plasmid-bearing green fluorescent protein reporter gene. A dendritic cell expressing green fluorescent protein was detected in regional lymph nodes. However, because of the antigen used, this study failed to show that the transfected dendritic cells are able to activate the *T*-cells. Therefore, the crucial question was to determine the ability and the efficacy of various dermal cells to activate the *T*-cells. Casares et al. (1997b) have studied the ability of dermal cells to activate a HA110-120-specific CD4$^+$ *T*-cell hybridoma. The antigen presenting cells (APCs) from skin were separated by sorting in Class II$^+$ and Class II$^-$ cells, which then were incubated with T hybridoma cells. Activation of *T*-cells was measured by the synthesis of IFNγ and IL-4. Table 4.1 summarizes the results of this experiment. It clearly appears that while both Class II$^+$ and Class II$^-$ cells were transfected, only the Langerhans cells were able to activate the *T*-cells. However, these experiments did not rule out the possibility that Class II$^-$ cells, mainly keratinocytes and fibroblasts, synthesized the VhT,B, polypeptide that was secreted and taken up by Langerhans cells for processing and for presentation of peptide. There is a precedent for transfer of antigen from *B*-cells via exosomes (Raposo et al., 1996).

Table 4.2 illustrates the mechanisms leading to the activation of CD4 *T*-cells following intradermal injection of plasmid.

One may ask whether both dermal Class II$^+$ and Class II$^-$ cells activate the CD8 *T*-cells. Bot et al. (2000) studied the presence of influenza virus nucleoprotein in both cryostat sections of the skin as well as in crawl-out cells. Subsequent to viral infection, the nucleoprotein is synthesized in the cytoplasm and rapidly (in a few minutes) transferred into the nucleus by virtue of nuclear targeting sequences. From the nucleus, it is then translocated to cytoplasm contributing to virion assembly, with other proteins.

Ear sections from animals immunized with pNPVI were stained with labeled anti-NP and anti-Class II antibodies. As can be seen in Fig. 4.4, the nucleoprotein was found in both Class II$^+$ and Class II$^-$ cells in agreement with the Casares et al. observation. Similarly, the staining of crawl-out cells has shown cells stained with anti-NP and anti-Class II antibodies, cells stained with only anti-Class II (untransfected), and cells stained with anti-NP but not with anti-Class II antibodies. In all cases, anti-NP antibodies stained homogeneously the nuclei or the cytoplasm (Fig. 4.5) ruling out a possible uptake of NP from skin fluids, since, in that case, one should observe a granular staining of endosomes.

The ability of sorted Class II$^+$ and Class II$^-$ dermal cells to prime NP-specific CD8$^+$ CTLs was studied in transfer experiments subsequent to injection of various numbers of

Table 4.1. Activation of HA110-120-specific *T*-cell Hybridoma
by Langerhans Cells from Mice Injected with pVhT,B

APC	Origin of APC (immunization with)	*In vitro* stimulation	Activation of *T*-cells (production of)	
			IFN-γ	IL-4
Nil	Nil	Nil	—	—
Crawl-out	pControl	Nil	—	—
Crawl-out	pControl	HA110-120	+ +	+ + +
Crawl-out	pVhT,B	Nil	+	+
Crawl-out	pVhT,B	HA110-120	+ +	+ +
Class II$^+$	pVhT,B	HA110-120	+ + +	+ + +
Class II$^-$	PVhT,B	HA110-120	—	—

Table 4.2. Mechanisms of *T*-Cell Priming Following DNA Immunization

Priming of	Mechanism	Comments	References
CD8+ *T*-cells	BMD APC are crucial for CTL priming.	Not known if BMD APC take up the antigen or are directly transfected.	Corr et al., 1996; Ulmer et al., 1996; Iwasaki et al., 1997b
	Indirect priming: BMD APC that prime CTL take up the antigen released by *in vivo* transfected cells.	Argues for a "cross-priming" mechanism: antigen released by non-BMD cells and taken up by BMD APC.	Doe et al., 1996; Fu et al., 1997b
	Direct priming: BMD APC (DC) are *in vivo* transfected and directly prime CTL.	Argues for a direct priming of CTL through the classical pathway.	Porgador et al., 1998; Bot et al., 2000
		Argues against the role of *in vivo* transfected muscle cells in CTL priming.	Torres et al., 1997
CD4+ *T*-cells	Resident DCs are transfected, migrate to local lymphoid nodes, and prime CD4+ *T*-cells	Not known if release of antigen is a prerequisite.	Casares et al., 1997b

cells into spleen. Seven days after injection of cells, the frequency of CTL precursors was studied. Comparison of efficacy of Langerhans cells versus Class II$^-$ cells showed that 60,000 DC, of which only 2–3% expressed the NP, were capable of priming the CTL precursors, while three times that number of Class II$^-$ cells were required to obtain a similar effect (Table 4.3).

While the DCs express costimulatory molecules required to activate *T*-cells (Kawa-

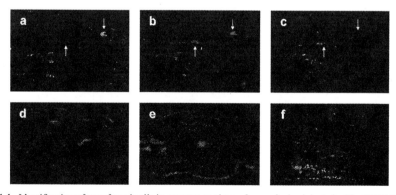

Figure 4.4. Identification of transfected cells in cryostat sections of ears of mice injected with pNPVI. The same sections were simultaneously stained with anti-class II and anti-NP antibodies, and with DAPI for nuclei. Ear sections obtained from NPVI plasmid immunized (a, b, and c) or non-immunized (d and e) mice. a: staining for NP; b and d: staining of class II; e: staining of nuclei; and f: isotype control (from Bot et al., *Int. Immunol.*, 2000, 12:825). (For a color representation of this, see figure facing page 42.)

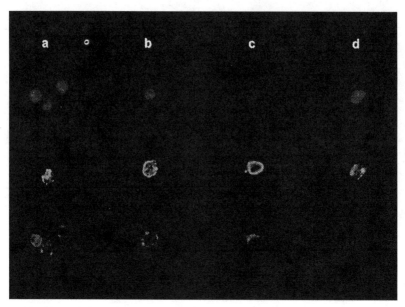

Figure 4.5. Identification of transfected crawl-out cells from ears of mice immunized with pNPVl. Cells were stained for nuclei, for class II, and anti-NP labeled antibodies. a: in a group of three class II$^+$ only a single cell expressed NP; b: a class II$^+$ cell exhibiting nuclear staining for NP; c: a class II$^+$ cell exhibiting cytoplasmic staining for NP; and d: NP$^+$/MHC class II$^-$ cell. The figure represents a composite of cells from various microscopic fields (from Bot et al., *Int. Immunol.*, 2000, 12:825). (For a color representation of this, see figure facing page 43.)

Table 4.3. CTL Response of Mice Injected with Crawl-Out Cells
Obtained from Mice Inoculated with Plasmids or Influenza Viruses

Group			PR8-specific CTLp[d]	
Crawl-out cells from mice immunized with[a]	Day of harvest[b]	Number of cells transferred[c]	Frequency^{-1}	Total number
pNPV1	1	1×10^6	1.79×10^5	558
	2	2×10^5	2.50×10^5	400
	3	1×10^5	1.72×10^5	581
pC	1	5×10^5	$>1 \times 10^6$	<100
	2	1×10^5	$>1 \times 10^6$	<100
	3	5×10^4	$>1 \times 10^6$	<100
PR8 virus	1	8×10^5	1.7×10^5	588
	1	1.6×10^5	7.7×10^5	130
B/Lee virus	1	8×10^5	$>1 \times 10^6$	<100

[a]The donor mice were inoculated into the ears (i.d.) with 30 μg of plasmids in 10 μl saline, five times; Day −2, day −1, and three times on the day of sacrifice (6, 3, and 1 hour before ear harvest).

[b]The ears were harvested at day 0 and flaps were prepared and incubated. The crawl-out cells were harvested daily for 3 days.

[c]Recipient mice were surgically opened and inoculated in the spleen with various numbers of crawl-out cells. A total of nine mice for pNPVl and pC were inoculated.

[d]The frequency of virus-specific CTLp in the spleen of recipients was estimated by limiting dilution analysis at 7 days after inoculation. The total number of splenic CTLp was estimated based on the total number of splenocytes (mean = 1×10^8 cells).

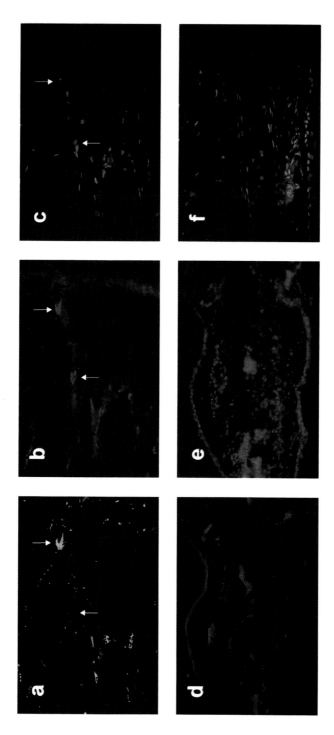

Figure 4.4. Identification of transfected cells in cryostat sections of ears of mice injected with pNPVI. The same sections were simultaneously stained with anti-class II (red) and anti-NP (green) antibodies, and with DAPI for nuclei. Ear sections obtained from NPVI plasmid immunized (a, b, and c) or non-immunized (d and e) mice. a: staining for NP; b and d: staining of class II; e: staining of nuclei; and f: isotype control (from Bot et al., *Int. Immunol.*, 2000, 12:825). (See page 41.)

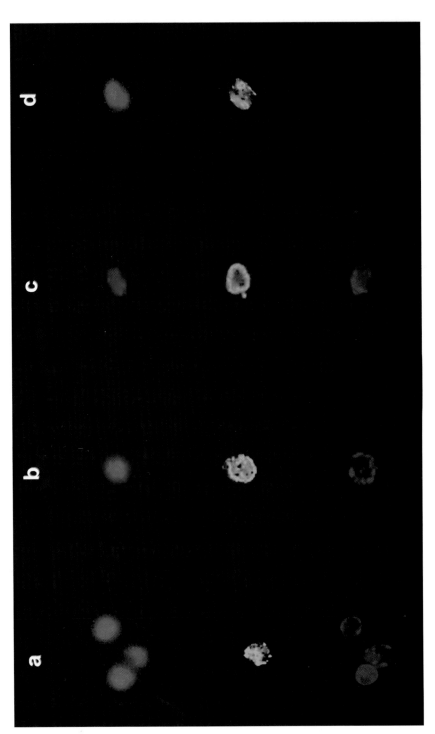

Figure 4.5. Identification of transfected crawl-out cells from ears of mice immunized with pNPVI. Cells were stained for nuclei (blue), for class II (red), and anti-NP (green) labeled antibodies. a: in a group of three class II[+] only a single cell expressed NP; b: a class II[+] cell exhibiting nuclear staining for NP; c: a class II[+] cell exhibiting cytoplasmic staining for NP; and d: NP[+]/MHC class II[−] cell. The figure represents a composite of cells from various microscopic fields (from Bot et al., *Int. Immunol.*, 2000, 12:825). (See page 42.)

mura and Furue, 1995), the keratinocytes and other dermal cells do not. The requirement of costimulatory molecules in the activation of CD8 T-cells was demonstrated in an experiment in which the CD8 T-cells were unable to produce IL-2 in response to MHC-peptide complex presented by Drosophila cells transfected with MHC genes but lacking B7 or ICAM-1 molecules (Cai et al., 1996).

Two alternative explanations can be entertained with respect to the ability of Class II$^-$ cells to activate the CTLs. First, the CD8 cells can be activated independently of costimulatory molecules in certain conditions. Goldstein et al. (1998) showed that in an APC-free system, the CD8 cells were activated by immobilized Class I-peptide complex. Alternatively, they can be activated in a bystander way, in which the costimulatory molecules are furnished by other cells (Ding and Shevach, 1994). A predominant role of DCs in the activation of CD8 compartment was also demonstrated after administration of pNPVI by gene-gun (Porgador et al., 1998). In these experiments, it was shown that directly transfected DC migrated to lymph nodes and were able to stimulate in vitro a specific T-cell response. In conclusion, intradermal injection with naked DNA causes the transfection of various dermal cells. While the DCs migrate to regional lymph nodes, where they can present the peptides and activate T-cells, Class II$^-$ cells probably can activate only epidermotrophic T-cells. Only Langerhans cells can present the peptides to CD4 T-cells, whereas both Class II$^+$ and Class II$^-$ cells are able to activate the CD8 T-cells.

4.4. CELLULAR MECHANISMS INVOLVED IN THE IMMUNE RESPONSE INDUCED BY INTRAMUSCULAR GENETIC IMMUNIZATION

Muscles are made up of myocyte fibers that contain protein filaments and hundreds of nuclei located under a plasma membrane (sarcolema). Each fiber is surrounded by endomysium composed of basal lamina and extracellular matrix. The blood supply of muscles involves endomysial capillaries. The myocytes express Class I antigens and LFA-3 but not Class II or costimulatory molecules. The major function of myocytes is to develop mechanical forces rather than to be involved in the immune response. However, they are considered nonprofessional antigen-presenting cells, since it was shown that IFNγ can induce the expression of HLA-DR on human myoblasts (Hohfeld and Engel, 1990). It is noteworthy that the myoblasts from normal subjects fail to stimulate the lymphocytes but induce tolerance (Warrens et al., 1994), whereas other investigators have shown that they may act as APCs during local immune response in autoimmune disease (i.e., myasthenia gravis) (Goebels et al., 1992).

Residential APCs can initiate an immune response. Smith and Allen (1992) showed that myosin-Class II complexes are found on residential APCs of normal mouse heart and that the expression of the Class II-myosin complex was increased in mice developing autoimmune myocarditis. Little is known about the cellular mechanisms responsible for the initiation of immune response induced by intramuscular injection of plasmid.

Antigen-specific B-cells can be stimulated by the protein secreted by transfected muscle cells, since they can recognize the epitopes on native proteins. In contrast, the CD4 or CD8 T-cells can recognize only peptides derived from the processing of exogenous or endogenous proteins, respectively.

Lack of expression of Class II molecules by myocytes led to the concept that professional APCs may be the initiators of immune response elicited by intramuscular genetic immunization. The concept that residential and/or remote APCs play an important role in immune response induced by genetic immunization derived from elegant experiments carried out by Torres et al. (1997). These authors showed that surgical excision of injected muscle within 10 minutes after DNA injection did not affect the magnitude of a T-dependent antibody response.

However, the merit of Casares et al. (1997b) studies lies in their demonstration of the role of residential APCs in the induction of immune response subsequent to intramuscular administration of plasmid. Casares et al. have studied the rate of transfection and the ability to present the peptide derived from influenza virus hemagglutin by various professional APCs purified from regional lymph nodes subsequent to injection of pVhT,B into muscles. DCs and B-cells were sorted from regional lymph nodes 24 hours after the injection of plasmid. Sorted DCs and B-cells were then used to stimulate a T-cell hybridoma specific for HA110-120 peptide recognized in association with I-E^d molecules. Only sorted DCs were able to activate the T-cells, demonstrating that the residential muscle DCs were transfected and were able to present the peptide.

Chattergoon et al. (1998) have shown that macrophages isolated from regional lymph nodes are also transfected following intramuscular administration of plasmid and are able to activate the T-cells.

Taken together, these observations clearly show that various residential APCs can be transfected in the muscles, and when they migrate to lymph nodes, can activate specific T-cells. Figure 4.6 illustrates possible cellular mechanisms mediating the activation of CD4 T-cells subsequent to intramuscular immunization. Numerous observations demonstrate

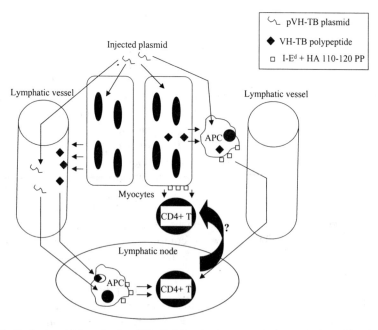

Figure 4.6. Mechanisms of the activation of T-cells following intramuscular immunization with pVhT,B plasmid.

that intramuscular genetic immunization primes CTL precursors and induces a cellular immune response.

Several mechanisms can be envisioned: First, the residential APCs are transfected, then synthesize and process the protein and present the peptide to CD8 T-cells. Second, the transfected muscle cells are lysed and the plasmid is taken up by APCs. Third, the protein secreted by myocytes is taken up by APCs, processed, and presented to CD8 T-cells. The experiments of Torres et al. (1997) suggest that the muscle cells do not play an active role in the priming of CD8 T-cells, in spite of the high rate of transfection of myocytes. This concept is supported by other experiments carried out in bone-marrow chimeric mice. Thus, Doe et al. (1994) demonstrated for the first time that bone-marrow-derived cells facilitate the induction of CTLs following intramuscular injection of plasmids. In these experiments, the CTL response was assessed in mice partially MHC-matched with the haplotype of muscles. Bone marrow cells from H-2^{bxd} F1 mice were injected into H-2^b or H-2^d SCID mice lacking mature B- and T-cells. Immunization of recipient mice with plasmids expressing HSVgD or HIV-1 gp120 glycoproteins, bearing peptides recognized in association with Class I molecules, displayed a CTL response restricted to the haplotype of bone marrow cells but not to that of myocytes of recipient. Similar results were obtained in experiments using bone-marrow chimeric mice (Corr et al., 1996; Iwasaki et al., 1997b).

The experiments of Ulmer et al. (1996) employing bone-marrow-chimeric mice also suggested that bone-marrow-derived APCs play a major role in the priming of CTLs. These authors proposed several hypotheses to explain the mechanism(s) of the activation of CD8 T-cells. They hypothesized that antigen fragments or proteins eventually complexed with heat shock protein are transferred from transfected myocytes to APCs. Several points can be entertained regarding "antigen transfer" hypothesis. First, the "transfer" can be performed by the uptake through fluid phase pinocytosis by APCs of protein secreted by myocytes, from body fluids. In this case, the protein taken up is internalized in endosomes and eventually fragmented into peptides. The endosomes do not harbor Class I molecules because there is no intersection between Class I and Class II pathways (Peters et al., 1991). Whereas Class I molecules synthesized in ER are translocated to the membrane via the Golgi secretory pathway, Class II molecules are targeted to endosomes by virtue of the associated CLIP peptide. In endosomes, they lose invariant chain, sort the peptides derived from the fragmentation of exogenous protein, and, finally, Class II-peptide complex is transferred to the membrane. There are exceptions to this rule. For example, it was shown that exogenous proteins introduced into cytoplasm of APCs by artificial procedures as osmotic shock (Carbone and Bevan, 1990), by conjugation of soluble proteins with HIV tat-derived peptide (Kim et al., 1997a), or by liposomes (Harding et al., 1991; Noguchi et al., 1991) can induce a CTL response. There are also examples of induction of a CTL response against microbial antigens (Listeriolysin of *L. monocytogenes*) (Szalay et al., 1994), an epitope expressed on *Yersinia enterolitica* (Starnbach and Bevan, 1994) or *Leishmania* (Smith et al., 1991), or *Toxoplasma gondi* (Subauste et al., 1991; Kasper et al., 1992). All these parasites are obligatory intracellular microbes. Microbial proteins or toxins can leak from vacuoles and then enter into endogenous pathways where the resulting peptides can be associated with Class I molecules required to stimulate the CD8 CTLs.

The second mechanism proposed by Ulmer et al. (1996) is an active transfer of protein synthesized by myocytes to APCs. Such transfer requires either intercellular bridges or direct contact between myocytes and APCs.

Transfer between various types of APCs was already reported. Bona et al. (1972) demonstrated that ^{14}C-labeled endotoxin was indeed identified in B-cells from macrophage–lymphocyte islands, in an experiment in which the macrophages were pulsed with radiolabeled endotoxin, washed, and then incubated with syngeneic lymphocytes (see Figures 4.7 and 4.8). The cells containing the transferred antigen were B-cells, because their membranes bound a peroxidase-labeled anti-Ig antibody. In the same way, Knight et al. (1998) showed the transfer of FITC-ovalbumin from one dendritic cell to another. However, there is no evidence of direct contact between myocytes and APC in capillaries, nor of intercellular bridges between myocytes and APC in endomysium. Thus, the most plausible explanation is that *in vivo* transfected bone-marrow-derived cells stimulate the CD8 T-cells. This concept is strongly supported by the Casares et al. (1997b) experiments demonstrating the presence of plasmid in DC isolated from regional lymph nodes at the site of intramuscular injection. Thus, apparently, the residential or circulating APCs are transfected *in vivo*, migrate into lymph nodes, where they prime the CD8 T-cells. Table 4.3 summarizes the priming mechanisms of CD4 and CD8 T-cells following injection of naked DNA.

Since it was demonstrated that the myoblasts can express Class II molecules after the stimulation with IFNγ, Stan et al. (submitted, 2000) have studied the ability of a myoblast (G7) line to activate HA110-120-specific T-cells after triple transfection with pVhT,B, and I-E^d α and β genes. The data summarized in Table 4.4 clearly demonstrated that the G7 myoblast line expressing I-E^d restriction molecules required for the recognition of HA110-120 peptide expressed in the plasmid, was able to activate HA110-120-specific T-cells. Thus, these data demonstrate for the first time that myoblasts transfected with a plasmid expressing a gene encoding a polypeptide, bearing a T-cell epitope recognized by CD4 T-cells, can activate the T-cells. These observations led to other studies aimed at investigating changes in the phenotype of myocytes at the site of injection with plasmid. These studies showed that the myocytes at the site of the injection with pVhT,B plasmid express significant level of Class II and above background level of B7.1 molecules (Stan et al., submitted, 2000). Since this effect may be related to intrinsic adjuvant properties of a plasmid, namely, CpG immunostimulatory sequences, in further experiments, the expression of Class II molecules was studied in muscles of mice injected with CpG$^+$ and CpG$^-$ ODNs. It is noteworthy that after the injection with CpG$^+$ nucleotides, a cellular infiltration associated with an increased expression of Class II was observed. This suggested that the IFNγ secreted by the inflammatory cells at the site of injection with CpG$^+$ polynucleotide was responsible for the augmented Class II expression by the myocytes. This explanation was supported by similar experiments carried out in IFNγ knockout mice. No Class II molecules were detected on the myocytes harvested from the site of injection with CpG$^+$ nucleotide from IFNγ knockout mice, in spite of the fact that these mice exhibited a strong inflammatory reaction at the site of injection (Stan et al., submitted, 2000).

These findings showed that in certain conditions, when the myocytes can express Class II and eventually B.7 molecules, they may present the antigen expressed by the plasmid and play an active role in the presentation of peptides rather to function as a simple protein factory. In light of the new observations, the picture appears more complex in the case of muscular immunization. In this case, certainly the residential APCs (i.e., DCs and macrophages) can be transfected and when migrating into regional lymph nodes may activate the T-cells. In addition, the CpG$^+$ sequences of plasmids bearing genes encoding

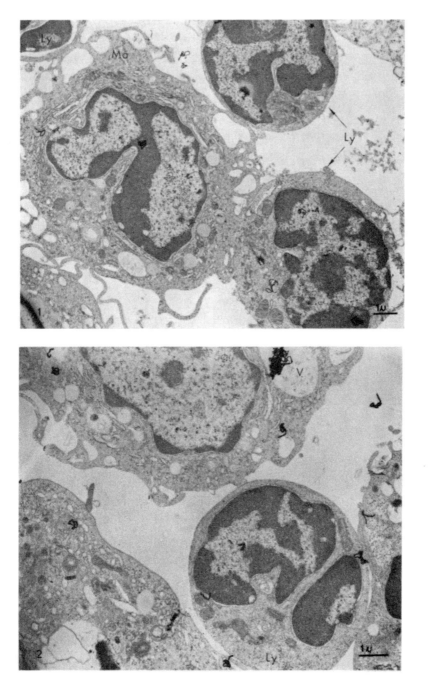

Figure 4.7. High resolution autoradiographic aspects of antigen transfer between macrophages and lymphocytes in macrophage-lymphocyte islands. Silver grains representing ^{14}C-labeled endotoxin can be observed in macrophage endosomes or lysosomes as well as in lymphocytes (from C. Bona et al., *Immunology* 1982, 23:799–816).

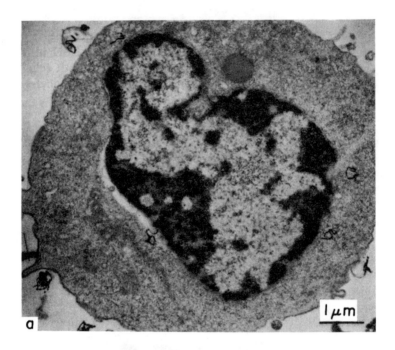

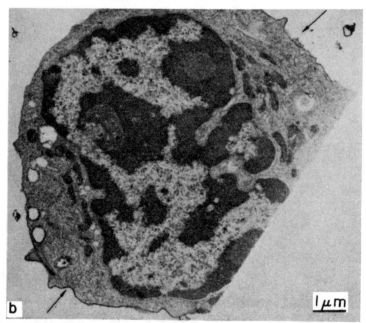

Figure 4.8. *B*-cells containing silver grains after incubation with macrophages pulsed with ^{14}C-endotoxin (from C. Bona et al., *Immunology* 1982, 23:799–816).

Table 4.4. Activation of HA110-120-Specific T-Cell
Hybridoma by G7 Myoblast Line Transfected
with pVhT,B and I-E^d α and β Genes

APC	Antigen added in culture	Percentage of activated T-cells
M12	—	0.4
M12	HA110-120	99.0
G7 (I-E^k) VhT,B	—	1.0
G7 (I-E^k) VhT,B	HA110-120	1.0
G7 I-E^d	—	2.0
G7 I-E^d	HA110-120	83.0
G7 I-E^d,pVhT,B	—	80.0
G7 I-E^d,pVhT,B	HA110-120	36.0

antigens may recruit inflammatory cells at the site of injection and, through an IFNγ-mediated process, may convert the myocytes from facultative into professional APCs. The role of APCs has also been studied after intrasplenic injection of a plasmid bearing a chimeric murine Vh gene in which a peptide of *Plasmodium* circumsporozoite protein was inserted in CDR3 (Xiong et al., 1997b). Despite the academic interest, it obviously has no or reduced interest for mass immunization of the human kingdom. In this case, it was reported that only the *B*-cells were transfected *in vivo* following the injection of the plasmid into the spleen. However the conclusion of this study is quite soft, because no attempt was carried out to characterize the transfection of splenic DCs or macrophages, nor to contrast the efficacy of various types of APCs to activate the antigen-specific lymphocytes. The expression in *B*-cells may be due to the particular nature of plasmid, which bears the promoter of the heavy chain Ig gene and a chimeric Vh gene.

In conclusion, various cells can be transfected following injection of plasmids by various routes. However, it appears that the dendritic cells are the most efficient in antigen presentation and activation of both CD4 and CD8 T-cells.

Chapter 5

Protective Immune Responses Elicited by Genetic Immunization against Viruses

5.1. INTRODUCTION

Viruses as obligatory cellular pathogens have always posed an important challenge in terms of generating effective immune responses by vaccination. Viruses enter the organism through various routes and infect certain categories of cells, borrowing the host machinery in order to replicate the genetic material and to synthesize structural and nonstructural proteins. Thus, virus infection leads to a state in which viral products that could be perceived as nonself by the immune system are mostly hidden beyond host cell membranes. The immune system evolved to recognize such products in the form of proteins or peptides of virus origin, generated through a complex intracellular machinery that samples the cytoplasmic milieu in a continuous manner. The evolution of cytotoxic T-cells is thought to be directly linked to the evolution of this intracellular sampling system, with its three main components: proteasomes, TAP, and MHC Class I molecules, whereas that of B-cells parallels the natural variation of viral proteins. Since the metabolic machines of host cell and virus are so intimately intermingled, the immune effector mechanisms evolved in such a way that either inhibits to various extent or eliminates the cells that are recognized as infected. For example, whereas cytokines such as IFN-γ inhibit viral replication, perforin released by cytotoxic cells triggers the lysis of target cells. Thus, this type of effector mechanism is brought into play whenever T-cells recognize foreign peptides on self-MHC molecules. The process of virus recognition by immune cells is more complex and is certainly not limited to the self–non-self discriminating ability of T-cells. For example, experimental models created by transgenic expression of viral antigens in certain cell types revealed that T-cells can, but do not always, react to foreign antigens (Roman et al., 1990; Oldstone et al., 1991; Ohashi et al., 1991). Two new elements of the immune system come into play at this point: innate immunity and professional APC. The current paradigm is that discrimination of nonself and sequestered self-antigens restricted to peripheral organs occurs through a process that has as central elements the employment of natural immunity and professional APC, namely, that natural immunity has the ability to rapidly detect viral infection and signal this state to other immune cells, as well as to produce effectors that limit the infection until the adaptive immunity develops. A subset of signals generated by the innate immunity activate professional APC like dendritic cells that upregulate costimulatory molecules and migrate to local lymphoid organs, where they prime specific T-cells (Steinman, 1991). Stimulatory cytokines such as IL-12 and IFN-γ, together with costimulatory molecules expressed by professional APC, such as B7.1 and B7.2, enable the naive T-cells to receive a positive signal through TCR. In contrast, TCR engagement in the absence of costimulation is thought to induce T-cell anergy (Bretscher and Cohn, 1970; Lamb and Feldman, 1984; Quill and Schwartz, 1987). Thus, this mechanism reduces the chance that certain self-antigens induce activation of autoreactive T-cells that escape thymic negative selection, while assuring a proper response against viruses. However, at least two circumstances necessitate supplementary level of regulation for the immune response. For example, during a local viral infection, there is the possibility that sequestered self-antigens are released and presented by professional APC to autoreactive T-cells. Besides this bystander mechanism of priming, some viral antigens may cross-react with self-antigens, leading to activation of autoreactive T-cells as a direct consequence of virus infection. Consequently, peripheral tolerance mechanisms should operate at the stage of mature activated and postactivated T-cells, thus allowing the occurrence of antiviral but minimizing anti-self responses. Transgenic models such as Fas and Fas-L knockout, IL-2 defective, and CTLA-4 knockout elegantly illustrated this point (Van Parijs et al., 1996; Sadlack et al., 1995; Tivol et al., 1995). It is very likely that the postactivation control of T-cells is directly determined by the quantitative level of antigen that is presented by APC, together with signals emitted by the innate immunity, namely, that a tremendous decrease in antigen level would determine a decline of the T-cell effector population, allowing instead the emergence of T memory cells that depend on the persistence of minute amounts of antigen. This is the most probable scenario during a successful response against acute viral infections that leads to the elimination of the virions from organism. If the activated T-cells are exposed in a continuous manner to a high level of antigen, as in most cases of virus-triggered autoimmune responses, T-cells are eliminated in a Fas and IL-2 dependent manner (Refaeli et al., 1998). Because this process is strictly dependent on TCR engagement in an antigen-specific manner, it may fail in certain circumstances, for example, when the self-antigen is in limited quantity and present in cells that are physiologically essential. For example, in spite of the normally operating mechanisms that maintain peripheral tolerance, transgenic mice that express viral antigen in periphery develop autoimmune diseases when infected with virus (Roman et al., 1990; Oldstone et al., 1991; Ohashi et al., 1991). Overall, the immune system has evolved such that the recognition and elimination of viruses does not frequently lead to autoimmunity.

There are two general categories of viruses based on factors related to virus biology and immune response. First are viruses that infect in a lytic manner a wide range of host cells, leading to acute syndromes. They are usually RNA viruses lacking an advanced replication machinery that undergo frequent mutations particularly in the genes encoding surface antigens, thus favoring the escape from neutralizing antibodies during subsequent infections. The T-cell response that is driven by abortively or productively infected professional APC frequently leads to prompt elimination of the virus. A classical example for this group of viruses is the family *Orthomyxoviridae*, with influenza virus as prototype. The second category of viruses is mostly represented by DNA viruses, with large genomes and restricted ability to productively infect a wide range of host cells. They frequently establish latency and avoid or downregulate the immune response through various and complex mechanisms, mediated by proteins encoded in their genome. It is possible that nonclassical pathways of antigen presentation that occur in certain professional APC evolved to deal with such viruses that avoid their infection. Examples in this category are viruses such as CMV or herpes simplex, which produce proteins that downregulate the expression of Class I molecules and, consequently, of epitope presentation to $CD8^+$ T-cells (York et al., 1994; Gilbert et al., 1996). It is noteworthy that the immune system has other effectors such as NK cells that recognize virally infected cells through other mechanisms (Yokoyama, 1998). However, numerous DNA viruses successfully avoid immune-mediated elimination and establish chronic infections. Not all viruses can be easily classified in one of these two categories. A particular exception to the rule is represented by retroviruses that establish chronic infection in lymphoid cells: Whereas latency is associated with integration of the reversely transcribed genome, the subsequent productive stage leads to the death of lymphocytes and severe immune suppression. Another exception is measles virus, an RNA virus that is a member of the family of *Paramyxoviridae*, which profoundly impairs the ability of the host to mount Th1 immune responses during certain stages of infection (Grosjean et al., 1997).

Two major strategies have been previously employed to induce protective immunity against viruses. First is inoculation of killed microbes that, in spite of good humoral responses, display poor ability to induce protective T-cell responses. In particular, killed vaccines do not generate virus-specific CTL that plays crucial roles during recovery from infection or protection against reinfection with variant strains. In the same category are subunit and peptide-based vaccines. The lower efficiency of these types of vaccines is mainly due to the absence of nucleic acids that play adjuvant roles and to a more limited number of epitopes.

Live attenuated vaccines have the advantage of inducing good CTL responses, as well as humoral and Th responses. This is due to the fact that attenuated microbes are still capable of infecting certain host cells including APC, a process that is followed by the generation of peptide—Class I complexes as well as Th1-inducing signals. Significant side effects can occur in immune depressed individuals such as children and aged. The process of virus attenuation is therefore central to producing such vaccines.

The continuous search for a new generation of vaccines against viruses is fueled by certain factors: (1) the lack of effective vaccines against certain viruses (i.e., retroviruses, herpes viruses); (2) the limited performance of licensed vaccines (i.e., influenza virus); (3) the potential limited performance or expected side effects of candidate vaccines based on conventional strategies (i.e., live-attenuated HIV vaccine; live-attenuated influenza virus vaccine). Plasmid-based expression vectors display a few characteristics that have made them attractive as a new candidate strategy for designing antiviral vaccines. First, DNA vaccines are able to elicit significant CTL responses that are important for recovery from viral infections, being superior in this concern over the killed vaccines. The ability of a vaccine to trigger both antibodies and CTL is very likely to enhance dramatically its protective effects. Furthermore, CTL induction occurs in the absence of vector replication, as is usually the case with live attenuated vectors. Sometimes even limited replication of attenuated viruses may lead to side effects or serious disease if virulent strains emerge. Furthermore, the construction of plasmid-based vaccines should be faster compared to generation of attenuated virus strains that usually require multiple cell culture passages. A potential advantage of DNA vaccines may be the poor negative interference of preformed antibodies that may seriously affect the boosting performance of T-cell response in the case of live, attenuated vaccines, or the immunogenicity of vaccines given to neonates born of immune mothers. Another characteristic that makes DNA vaccines good candidates for antiviral vaccines is their ability to trigger Th1 responses based on the adjuvant ability of unmethylated CpG motifs or immune stimulatory sequences. It is widely thought that whereas Th1 immunity favors protective cellular responses against viruses, Th2 responses are detrimental. Published and emerging studies pinpointed the species-specific, strong adjuvant effect of unmethylated CpG motifs, manifested through enhancement of antibody response and IFN-γ production by specific *T*-cells primed by simultaneous injection of protein antigens (Klinman et al., 1999a). The effects of CpG motifs on natural immunity are persistent, thus justifying a certain interest in using these immune stimulatory elements as "broad vaccines" that arm the innate response against virulent microbes (Klinman et al., 1999b). The characterization of primate-specific immune stimulatory CpG motifs is a subject of interest for multiple groups. Two features of DNA vaccines await further characterization or improvement: first, potential side effects due to the injection of recombinant DNA, namely, mutagenesis or autoimmunity; and second, the modest magnitude of immune response requiring multiple boosts, high plasmid doses, or alternative strategies of inoculation.

During the past years, following the demonstration that inoculation of plasmid-based expression vectors leads to transgene expression as well as immunity (Tang et al., 1992), many studies have addressed the potential of this new vaccination technique to generate protective immunity in animal models of virus infection. At the present, immune response and/or protection elicited by plasmid-expressing antigens from more than thirty viruses have been studied (Table 5.1). For the sake of clarity, we have used the genetic classification of viruses in order to approach in a more detailed manner the characterization of immunity induced by DNA vaccination. Each section begins with a brief introduction regarding the biological and clinical significance of a particular category of viruses, immune responses, followed by presentation of DNA vaccination approaches in experimental models and conclusions or perspectives in context of alternative immunization strategies.

5.2. IMMUNE RESPONSES AGAINST RNA VIRUSES ELICITED BY GENETIC IMMUNIZATION

We approach the issue of DNA vaccination against RNA viruses taking into consideration the genetic classification of RNA viruses: (1) the single-stranded, negative-sense RNA viruses (important pathogens: influenza virus, measles virus, rabies virus, Ebola virus); (2) the single-stranded, positive-sense RNA viruses (important pathogens: encephalitis viruses, hepatitis C and E viruses); (3) the double-stranded RNA viruses (i.e., rotaviruses); and (4) the retroviruses.

5.2.1. Negative-Sense, Single-Stranded RNA Viruses

This category of RNA viruses contains important human and animal pathogens. Members of the family of *Orthomyxoviridae*, such as influenza virus, or *Paramyxoviridae*, such as measles, parainfluenza, mumps and respiratory syncytial virus, are responsible for common illnesses throughout the world. Usually, these infections are transmitted via

Table 5.1. Experimental Models for Genetic Immunization against Viral Infectious Diseases

RNA viruses	Single-stranged and negative sense	
	Orthomyxoviridae	Influenza virus
	Paramyxoviridae	Measles virus
		Newcastle disease virus[a]
		Sendai virus[a]
		Bovine RSV[a]
	Rhabdoviridae	Rabies virus
		Infectious hematopoietic necrosis virus[a]
	Arenaviridae	LCMV
	Filoviridae	Ebola virus
	Single-stranded and positive sense	
	Flaviviridae	Hepatitis C virus
		St. Louis encephalitis virus
		Dengue virus
		Tick-borne encephalitis virus[a]
		Japanese encephalitis virus[a]
		Russian spring to summer encephalitis virus
		Bovine viral diarrhea virus[a]
	Picornaviridae	Encephalomyocarditis virus[a]
		Foot-and-mouth disease virus[a]
	Coronaviridae	Infectious bronchitis virus*[a]
	Unclassified[b]	Hepatitis E virus
	Double-stranded	
	Reoviridae	Rotaviruses
	Retroviruses	
	Retroviridae	HIV
		SIV*
		FIV*
		HTLV
		Cas-Br-M murine leukemia virus
DNA viruses	*Hepadnaviridae*	HBV
		Duck HBV[a]
	Herpesviridae	Bovine herpes virus[a]
		Herpex simplex virus
		Cytomegalovirus
		Pseudorabies[a]
	Papovaviridae	Papilloma virus
Subviral agents		Prions

[a]Presently not associated with human disease but pathogenic for certain species.
[b]Formerly classified in the family of *Caliciviridae*.

aerosols, have acute evolution, are self-limited, and do not lead to life-threatening diseases. However, some populations such as infants and aged individuals, are prone to develop serious syndromes and, in certain conditions, lethal complications. Other families that contain important animal pathogens are the *Rhabdoviridae, Filoviridae, Bunyaviridae,* and *Arenaviridae*. Occasionally, transmission to humans of viruses that are members of these families, such as rabies, Marburg, Ebola, or Hantaan virus, is followed by dramatic clinical syndromes and even epidemics associated with high morbidity and mortality. Thus, in general, the development of effective vaccines against single-stranded RNA viruses of negative sense has threefold importance, according to the pathogen that is addressed: (1) It may prevent epidemics (i.e., influenza virus); (2) it protects animals against widespread zoonotic infections (i.e., rabies virus); and (3) it protects humans against rare but lethal infections due to accidental exposure to animal viruses (i.e., Ebola virus, rabies virus).

5.2.1.1. Genetic Immunization against Influenza Virus

Influenza virus continues to represent a serious health problem throughout the world. The segmented RNA genome of influenza virus allows an exquisite mechanism of generation of new strains that avoid or delay immune recognition by virtue of antigen variation. Animal reservoirs such as pigs and birds are sources of influenza virus strains that can exchange gene segments with human adapted strains during coinfection of the same organism, leading to shift variants of the original strains. Usually, the emergent shift variants that are able to infect humans carry new envelope genes of a distinct subtype, avoiding the immune recognition by preformed antibodies. Most frequently, internal proteins are highly conserved, assuring recognition and virus elimination by CTL. However, since new shift variants bear modified B-cell and Th epitopes, the human population is highly susceptible to infection and the accompanying respiratory disease. The ability of influenza virus to propagate via aerosols enhances the probability of pandemics due to shift variants. In rare instances, the emergence of new strains with unusually high virulence leads to increased morbidity and mortality, the first segment of population affected being young and aged humans.

Since orthomyxoviruses and, in general, the RNA viruses lack advanced genetic proofreading mechanisms, the rate of point mutations is relatively high, on the order of 10^{-4}. This facilitates selection of new drift variants that bear mutated B-cell epitopes and are responsible for endemic perpetuation. The pneumonia that accompanies influenza virus infection is dependent on the virulence of that particular strain and on both the kinetics and magnitude of the immune response. For example, highly virulent strains with increased ability of replication in a wider range of host cells lead to a more rapid virus spread and host cell destruction. The kinetics and magnitude of immune response directly depend on the frequency of specific B- and T-cell precursors as well as their type. For example, T-cell memory subsets are thought to comprise expanded populations of T-cells, independent of antigen-persistence, as well as T-cells dependent on continuous antigen stimulation. Whereas the first type of T-cells resemble the naive population, the second type is endowed with higher ability to respond to antigens, including lower activation threshold and faster differentiation to effector cells. Since the T-cell compartment plays a crucial role in the response against influenza viruses by allowing the induction of neutralizing antibodies as well as contributing directly to the formation of CTL and cytokine-producing cells, an important component of anti-influenza vaccines should be the T-cell epitopes. T-cell epitopes, especially CTL epitopes, are important from another point of view: Whereas the major Class I restricted epitopes are encoded by internal proteins and are therefore conserved among different subtypes, the neutralizing B-cell epitopes, as well as dominant Th epitopes, are expressed by hemagglutinin (HA) and neuraminidase (NA), and are therefore subject to drift and shift variation. Consequently, anti-influenza vaccines that do not elicit CTL memory have limited protectivity against certain strains or close variants.

This is indeed the case with the killed influenza vaccine or subunit vaccine that require periodic administration in anticipatory manner. Importantly, even in the absence of B-cell responses, the T-cell immunity is able to mediate protective responses to influenza virus (Bot et al., 1996b). In spite of the fact that T-cell immunity by itself is not able to prevent the infection, which is the attribute of preformed neutralizing antibodies, it limits the virus replication and mediates its elimination. Thus, vaccines that induce memory CTL, as well as Th and B-cells, display increased protection against homologous virus. Also, and more importantly, they show enhanced protection against drift and shift variants that may lead to decreased morbidity and mortality, circumventing the obvious limitation of prediction accuracy as well as the natural drift variation during pandemics. These are among the most important reasons for promoting the study of DNA and live attenuated vaccines as immunization strategies against influenza virus, alternative to conventional killed or subunit vaccines.

The first published study on DNA immunization in influenza virus (Ulmer et al., 1993) was important in two ways. First, it was the first report that showed protection ability in an infectious model of a vaccine prototype entirely based on DNA. Second, the expression vector encoded nucleoprotein (NP) of influenza virus that primed CTL immunity against a heterologous strain. Subsequent studies confirmed the generation of CTL as well as antibody immunity following intramuscular inoculation of plasmid DNA expressing NP (Yankauckas et al., 1993; Montgomery et al., 1993). Furthermore, it was shown that protection in mice is mediated by CD8+ T-cells and the immunity persists at least 1 year postvaccination (Yankauckas et al., 1993). Subsequent studies showed that CTL priming followed NP delivery in mice by alternative strategies: administration of Semliki Forest virus based RNA vaccine (Zhou et al., 1994); and intradermal or gene-gun immunization with plasmids expressing NP (Raz et al., 1994; Pertmer et al., 1995). These studies showed that the dermal route seems to be roughly ten times more effective based on the dose–response profile in generating protective immune responses following DNA inoculation.

Subsequent studies employing DNA immunization with plasmids expressing NP of influenza virus were used to answer important questions regarding this vaccination strategy (Table 5.2). Thus, is was shown that different means of plasmid delivery lead to nonidentical Th profiles. Whereas intramuscular inoculation of DNA leads to Th1 responses, intradermal administration leads to mixed Th1/Th2 responses (Pertmer et al., 1996). More recent studies addressed the mechanism of CTL priming in mice inoculated with plasmids expressing NP: Independent groups showed that bone-marrow-derived cells are crucial for priming NP-specific CTL (Corr et al., 1996; Fu et al., 1997b). An NP-expressing plasmid was used for the first time to demonstrate that neonatal immunization with DNA induces protective responses against a virus (Bot et al., 1996a). In an effort to address the role of dominant CTL epitopes in the protection conferred by plasmids expressing NP, novel immunorecessive CTL epitopes were defined by mutating anchor residues of a major Class I epitope (Fu et al., 1997a). Recently, DNA immunization of IFN-γ deficient mice revealed a protective role for this cytokine during the recall response against influenza virus (Bot et al., 1998b). All these studies underlined the versatility of the NP-based experimental system in addressing a large spectrum of fundamental questions.

Parallel with the studies addressing immune responses to plasmids expressing NP, there was tremendous interest in describing the immune response following administration of DNA-based expression vectors encoding HA of influenza virus. First attempts to

Table 5.2. Immune Responses and Protection against Infection Subsequent
to Genetic Immunization with Plasmids Expressing Influenza Virus Antigens

Species	Antigen	Immunity	Protection	Reference
Mice	Nucleoprotein	Abs, CTL	Yes	Ulmer et al., 1993
		Abs, Th	ND	Pertmer et al., 1996
	Hemagglutinin	Abs	Yes	Montgomery et al., 1993
		Abs, Th	ND	Feltquate et al., 1997
	Plasmid mixture (HA + NP)	Abs, Th, CTL	Yes	Bot et al., 1998a
Chickens	Hemagglutinin	Abs	Yes	Robinson et al., 1993
Ferrets	Hemagglutinin	Abs	Yes	Donnelly et al., 1995
	Plasmid mixture (MI + HA + NP)	Abs	Yes	Donnelly et al., 1995
Nonhuman primates	Plasmid mixture (MI + HA + NP)	Abs	ND	Donnelly et al., 1995
Pigs	HA + NP	Abs	Yes	Macklin et al., 1998

ND, not determined.

immunize with plasmids expressing HA were carried out in chickens, using an antigen from an H7 avian strain (Robinson et al., 1993; Fynan et al., 1993b). The intramuscular immunization was followed by induction of small antibody titers but significant protection after infectious challenge with the homologous strain. The proof of concept regarding effectiveness of plasmids expressing HA was simultaneously obtained in mice (Montgomery et al., 1993). A subsequent study showed that protective immunity against homologous challenge in the avian experimental system can be obtained by delivering the plasmid intramuscularly, intravenously, intratracheally or intradermally, by gene-gun (Fynan et al., 1993b). Gene-gun-based inoculation of plasmid expressing HA into chickens, led to B-cell memory cells that persisted for over a year in the spleen and bone marrow (Justewicz and Webster, 1996). More recently, it was shown in avian (Kodihalli et al., 1997) as well as mouse models (Bot et al., 1997a) that genetic immunization with HA induces protective immunity against drift variants. The mechanism of protection most likely involves the priming of Th cells against major Class II epitopes as well as antibodies against few conserved B-cell epitopes. However, as expected, HA immunization constantly failed to prime protective responses against shift variants. Intramuscular inoculation of HA plasmid was shown to induce a Th1-biased response (Deck et al., 1997; Bot et al., 1997b). In contrast, gene-gun inoculation in the skin or muscle of HA-expressing plasmid was followed by responses characterized by a Th2 profile (Feltquate et al., 1997).

Compared to live virus immunization, DNA immunization with HA-expressing plasmids leads to lower antibody titers (Boyle et al., 1996; Bot et al., 1997b). However, the efficacy of HA-expressing plasmids compared to the killed virus seems to be equal or superior, particularly in newborn mice (Deck et al., 1997; Antohi et al., 1998). Furthermore, although NP has the advantage of generating cross-reactive immunity against shift variants, HA-expressing plasmids were found to give higher protective levels (Robinson et al., 1997; Macklin et al., 1998). Besides questions related to the immunogenicity of HA-based DNA vaccination in newborns (Antohi et al., 1998; Bot et al., 1999), we have employed studies aimed at characterizing the responsiveness of aged mice (Radu et al., 1999). Despite the well-documented defective response of aged organisms to conventional influenza virus vaccines, DNA vaccination with HA of 2-year-old mice resulted in protective immunity, similar to the DNA vaccination of young mice. Not taking into account the advent of gene-gun delivery, there have been attempts to improve the effectiveness of DNA vaccines against influenza virus in three ways: (1) mucosal administration of DNA based on the assumption that a local immune response is more effective (Ban et al., 1997; Macklin et al., 1998); (2) coadministration of HA-expressing plasmid with a plasmid encoding IL-6 as costimulatory cytokine (Larsen et al., 1998); and (3) coadministration of plasmid-expressing HA and internal proteins (Donnelly et al., 1995, 1997; Bot et al., 1998a). The latter strategy was shown to induce significant responses in nonhuman primates as well as to protect against heterologous challenge in ferrets (Donnelly et al., 1995). A DNA-based prototype vaccine eliciting HA-specific neutralizing antibodies, as well as CTL against M1 and NP proteins, was found to be more effective than the licensed vaccine, against challenge with a drift variant, and as effective against homologous virus (Donnelly et al., 1997).

In spite of the continuous accumulation of information regarding safety and immunogenicity of DNA-based vaccines in preclinical models, the transition to clinical trials may pose a few problems, particularly regarding the case of influenza virus: First, the risk/benefit ratio may not yet be favorable for a rapid implementation of plasmid vaccines against influenza virus; second, the design of human clinical trials should take into account the noise level due to previous natural exposure to virus; and third, the delivery strategy and formulation should minimize the quantity of administered DNA while optimizing the response.

5.2.1.2. Genetic Immunization against *Paramyxoviridae*

Members of this family are grouped in two subfamilies, *Paramyxovirinae* and *Pneumovirinae*, based on morphological criteria, genome organization, and biological role of the proteins. *Paramyxovirinae* contain three genera, depending on the presence of hemagglutinin and neuraminidase: *Paramyxovirus*, *Rubulavirus*, and *Morbilivirus*. In each genus of *Paramyxovirinae* there are important human pathogens that affect especially infants and children.

Parainfluenza viruses (genus *Paramyxovirus*), which are very heterogenous from an immunological point of view, are responsible for 30–40% of all acute respiratory infections in infants and children. However, the clinical syndromes associated with parainfluenza infection are usually mild. The protective immunity is thought to comprise IgA local antibodies that do not usually persist more than three months postinfection, allowing for reinfections with similar or different strains. Sendai virus, the mouse parainfluenza virus Type 1, is widely used as an experimental model for studying the immune response to this category of viruses.

Mumps virus, a member of the genus *Rubulavirus*, displays tropism for salivary glands and epithelioid cells, leading to a common and self-limited childhood disease. Virus-specific IgG antibodies are thought to provide lifelong protection, although reinfections may occur. Active vaccination is recommended for all children at fifteen months of age and is provided by one of the components in the currently employed trivalent vaccine (against mumps, measles, and rubella). This live attenuated vaccine obtained by tissue culture passage provides protection from disease but does not prevent infection, due to the suboptimal antibody titers that are elicited. Newcastle disease virus is a member of the genus *Rubulavirus* and is a known avian pathogen.

The most prominent human pathogen of the genus *Morbilivirus* is measles virus, which leads to a childhood infection manifested by affliction of respiratory tract, lymphoid system, skin, and sometimes the central nervous system. There are two particularities of measles virus: First, following the binding to CD46 antigen on professional APC, measles induces acute immune depression associated with Th2-type cytokines, leading to increased susceptibility to secondary but sometimes lethal infections (Grosjean et al., 1997); second, in rare circumstances, defective measles virus persists a long time in the central nervous system, leading to a severe syndrome called subacute sclerosing panencephalitis. In spite of the availability of a live attenuated vaccine that markedly diminished the incidence of measles infection in developed countries, measles remains an important health problem in developing countries, due especially to the associated immune depression that predispose infected children to secondary infections. The live vaccine elicits effective immunity by inducing antibody titers that persist more than 18 years in most of the recipients. However, since the response in 5% of the vaccinated children is suboptimal, a boost at ages of 4–6 years is recommended. Cellular immunity is probably involved in the recovery from primary infection and may confer resistance at the port of entry.

Pneumovirinae, composed of a single genus, the *Pneumoviruses*, differ from *Paramyxovirinae* regarding both the number of proteins and the attachment protein. They contain a prominent human pathogen, namely, respiratory syncytial virus, which is a leading cause of severe respiratory infections in newborns and infants. Vaccination against respiratory syncytial virus poses an important challenge, since even natural infection does not confer protective immunity. Moreover, there is some evidence that immune pathology may participate in the disease. The role of cellular immunity is still poorly understood. In spite of the occurrence of secretory and serum antibody responses, as well as cellular immunity, reinfection is still possible. Based on the empirical observation that the magnitude of disease upon reinfection is lower when secretory antibody titers are higher, there are attempts to generate vaccines. Ongoing effort is aimed at generating attenuated virus strains by introducing mutations in genes responsible for virulence, using reverse genetics. The same genus contains viruses that affect other species in a related manner, for example, the bovine respiratory syncytial virus.

Regarding the viruses from the family *Paramyxoviridae*, DNA vaccination efforts at preclinical levels focused mostly on immunization against measles virus (Table 5.3). One driving force behind the creation of a new vaccine against measles virus is the low availability of the licensed live, attenuated vaccine in countries that cannot afford proper cold-chains. An early study attempted to generate protective immunity against measles virus by DNA immunization of mice with a plasmid-encoding NP. However, in spite of the significant titers of NP-specific IgG antibodies generated by DNA immunization, no significant protection against a mouse-adapted measles virus strain was noted (Fooks et al., 1996). Another study showed the induction of specific antibodies as well as CTL after mouse immunization with plasmids expressing HA or NP of measles virus (Cardoso et al., 1996). The immunogenicity of DNA vaccines in terms of neutralizing antibodies was soon extended to the fusion glycoprotein of measles virus (Yang et al., 1997). More importantly,

Table 5.3. Immune Response against Plasmids Expressing Antigens of *Paramyxoviridae*

Virus	Antigen	Species	Immunity	Reference
Measles virus	NP	Mice	Abs	Fooks et al., 1996
	NP or HA	Mice	Abs or CTL	Cardoso et al., 1996
	HA or fusion glycoprotein	Mice and rabbits	Abs	Yang et al., 1997
Newcastle disease virus	F protein	Chicken	Abs	Sakaguchi et al., 1996
Bovine respiratory syncytial virus	G protein	Calves	Protective[a]	Schrijver et al., 1997
Sendai virus	NP	Mice	Abs, Th, and CTL	Martinez et al., 1997

[a]Read out by assessing protective ability of immunization against infectious challenge.

this study showed that rabbits immunized with plasmids expressing HA or fusion proteins developed significant titers of virus-neutralizing antibodies. A recent report described the profile of Th cells induced in mice by vaccination with a plasmid-expressing HA of measles virus, at various stages during ontogeny (Martinez et al., 1997). There were attempts to induce local immunity by mucosal administration of a plasmid-expressing measles HA. Thus, intranasal or buccal administration of plasmid induced significant systemic CTL activity (Etchart et al., 1997).

A vaccine against Newcastle disease virus has potential veterinary implications. One study demonstrated that immunization of one-week-old chickens with plasmid expressing the F protein of Newcastle disease virus led to antibody induction and a degree of protection that was evident only two months later (Sakaguchi et al., 1996). However, interestingly, only the linear plasmid was immunogenic and the immune response was increased by a formulation containing Lipofectin, a substance that facilitates transfection.

Another vaccine of veterinary use is that against bovine respiratory syncytial virus (BRSV). A recent study aiming to characterize the protective efficiency of a plasmid-expressing G protein of BRSV showed that whereas DNA immunization significantly lowered the virus shedding after challenge of calves with BRSV, the degree of protection was lower than that afforded by a live recombinant vaccine (Schrijver et al., 1997). This report may be considered a prelude to future studies that will probably address the problem of effective immunization against human respiratory syncytial virus, from the point of view of DNA vaccination.

The experimental model of Sendai virus, albeit of low practical significance, was employed to answer some general questions regarding DNA immunization. First, a study addressed the dependency of immune response generated by a plasmid expressing NP of Sendai virus, on the age of inoculation. It was shown that DNA vaccination of mice with NP can induce CTL, antibodies, and Th cells even if applied during the earliest stages of postnatal development (Martinez et al., 1997). A more recent study confirmed the immunogenicity of DNA vaccination with NP of Sendai virus and demonstrated a significant protection against lethal challenge (Chen et al., 1998). This study suggested that there are no apparent differences between CTL generated by DNA immunization or nasal infection with Sendai virus, regarding the precursor frequency and the fine specificity for dominant and subdominant epitopes.

5.2.1.3. Genetic Immunization against Other Single-Stranded RNA Viruses of Negative Sense

Rhabdoviruses are probably the most widespread viruses in nature, infecting plants as well as invertebrate and vertebrate species. Rabies virus (*Lyssavirus* genus) infects wild carnivores and occasionally dogs, cats, cattle, and humans. Since the clinical syndrome associated with rabies infection is frequently dramatic, with affliction of central nervous system and increased lethality, effective vaccination against this particular pathogen is important especially in the individuals that may come in contact with the virus. The correlation between virus-specific IgG antibodies and protection is known. However, virus exposure usually requires passive administration of immune globulin, since active immunization with the rabies virus vaccine grown in human cells is limited to risk categories.

The rabies virus was among the first microbes studied from the point of view of immunogenicity and protection ability of DNA vaccines (Table 5.4). An early study showed the induction of cellular and humoral responses after immunization of mice with a plasmid expressing the rabies virus glycoprotein (Xiang et al., 1994). Furthermore, the same study reported that DNA vaccination was protective against challenge with rabies virus. A second report from the same group showed that the immunity after DNA immunization was long-lasting and side effects such as tolerance or autoimmunity were not apparent (Xiang et al., 1995a). An independent group recently reported similar results that confirm the immunogenicity and protection ability of plasmid vaccines expressing the rabies virus glycoprotein (Ray et al., 1997). As a new element, intradermal inoculation of plasmid was at least ten times more effective than intramuscular administration, based on the dose–effect relationship (Ray et al., 1997). Taking advantage of the rabies virus experimental model, Xiang and Ertl (1995b) were among the first to demonstrate that coinoculation of plasmids expressing virus antigens and cytokines augments the immune responses. Thus, whereas coinoculation of plasmids expressing rabies glycoprotein and GM-CSF led

Table 5.4. Genetic Immunization against Viruses
from the Families of *Rhabdoviridae*, *Arenaviridae*, and *Filoviridae*

Virus (Family)	Antigen	Species	Immunity	Reference
Rabies virus (*Rhabdoviridae*)	GP	Mice	Abs, Th, CTL	Xiang et al., 1994
Infectious hematopoietic necrosis virus (*Rhabdoviridae*)	GP or GP + NP	Rainbow trout	Abs	Anderson et al., 1996a
LCMV (*Arenaviridae*)	NP or GP	Mice	Abs, CTL	Yokoyama et al., 1995 Martins et al., 1995 Zarozinski et al., 1995
Ebola virus (*Filiviridae*)	NP or GP	Guinea pig	Abs, *T*-cells	Xu et al., 1998

to enhanced *T*- and *B*-cell immunity, coadministration of a plasmid expressing IFN-γ unexpectedly resulted in a decrease of the immune response.

Another member of the family of *Rhabdoviruses* is the infectious hematopoietic necrosis virus that infects fish and sometimes causes important economical problems. The study of gene expression and immunogenicity of plasmids in fish led to remarkable results, showing that inoculation of the firefly luciferase gene under fish or virus promoters into the skeletal muscle of rainbow trout led to local protein expression for at least three months (Anderson et al., 1996b). The initial early promoter of CMV was more effective than fish promoters in driving the gene expression. Furthermore, inoculation of plasmids that express the glycoprotein and nucleoprotein of infectious hematopoietic necrosis virus led to antibody responses and, importantly, to protection of fish against virus challenge (Anderson et al., 1996a).

The family *Arenaviridae* contains human pathogens such as Lassa, Junin, Machupo, and Guanarito viruses that often cause fatal infections. The spread from rodents probably occurs via aerosols. Infection generates antibodies and memory *T*-cells that effectively protect against reinfections. Based on this observation, a live attenuated vaccine against Junin virus has been obtained and successfully tested. In the case of Lassa fever, transfer of antibodies obtained from late-convalescent humans protect laboratory animals against disease. Lymphocytic choriomeningitis virus (LCMV), a member of the *Arenaviridae* family, has been studied for more than a half a century in infected mice. Cellular-mediated immunity plays an important role in the recovery from LCMV infection of laboratory animals. Accidental LCMV transmission to humans may cause from very mild flu-like symptoms to severe disease associated with meningitis. Although studies are still scarce regarding DNA vaccination against arenaviruses that are significant pathogens for humans, immunization against LCMV was very thoroughly investigated (Table 5.4). Early reports showed the immunogenicity in terms of antibodies and CTL of plasmids expressing viral glycoprotein or nucleoprotein of LCMV (Yokoyama et al., 1995; Zarozinski et al., 1995). Furthermore, plasmid vaccination allowed significant protection against subsequent challenge with LCMV. Another study explored the ability of DNA immunization with a plasmid-expressing nucleoprotein of LCMV to confer protection against virus strains of LCMV that infect mice in a persistent manner (Martins et al., 1995). In spite of the fact that a significant percentage of the immunized mice displayed reduced titers and eventual clearance of virus, the immune responses were not detectable before infection, suggesting that DNA immunization is weaker compared to live virus immunization. In an effort to improve the immunogenicity of DNA immunization with NP of LCMV, it was more recently shown that fusing the NP gene to an ubiquitin motif enhanced the generation of Class I epitope complexes and thus the CTL response (Rodriguez et al., 1997). The study of DNA immunization of mice with plasmids expressing NP of LCMV led to two other important observations: First, DNA inoculation is generally followed by a significant but localized inflammatory response (Yokoyama et al., 1997); second, the priming of CTL by neonatal DNA vaccination is not necessarily inhibited by maternal antibodies (Hassett et al., 1997).

The family *Filoviridae* contains two extremely virulent viruses that cause lethal infections in humans, namely, Marburg and Ebola virus. These viruses only accidentally infect human hosts and rapidly lead to widespread organ damage associated with external and internal bleeding due to intravascular disseminated coagulation. There is ongoing effort in delineating the mechanisms of protective immunity against these viruses and designing effective vaccines for high-risk individuals. Recently, a study carried out in guinea pigs showed that plasmids expressing viral nucleoprotein or glycoprotein of Ebola virus elicited significant titers of antibodies (Xu et al., 1998). Furthermore, the immunized animals were protected against challenge in a manner dependent on the glycoprotein-specific humoral and cellular response.

5.2.2. Genetic Vaccination against Single-Stranded RNA Viruses of Positive Sense

This category of RNA viruses contains important human pathogens: encephalitis viruses (Flaviviruses), hepatitis viruses (hepatitis C and E viruses), and viruses from the family of *Picornaviridae*.

5.2.2.1. Genetic Immunization against *Flaviviridae*

The family *Flaviviridae* contains two genera: *Flavivirus* and *Pestivirus*. The first genus contains human and animal pathogens, and the second contains animal pathogens. Besides these two genera, hepatitis C virus (unnamed genus), an important human pathogen, is part of the family *Flaviviridae*. Flaviviruses, like dengue viruses, St. Louis encephalitis virus, tick-borne encephalitis viruses, and Japanese encephalitis virus, are transmitted between vertebrates by insect vectors. The cytolytic replication of encephalitis viruses in the local lymph nodes may be followed in certain circumstances by central nervous system invasion, replication in neurons and glial cells, and severe associated inflammation. Pestiviruses (i.e., Bovine viral, diarrhea virus) infect only animals, are transmitted by direct or indirect contact, and lead to mucosal replication and associated disease. Hepatitis C virus, a human pathogen that is transmitted via blood or bodily secretions, is responsible for acute as well as chronic hepatic infectious disease.

In spite of the wide spectrum of antibodies generated following infection with a particular flavivirus, only certain epitopes on E protein may confer protection. Consequently, acquired immunity does not mediate heterologous protection. However, cellular immunity, together with antibody-mediated cellular cytotoxicity directed against NS-1, may help during the recovery phase. Killed vaccines are available against Japanese encephalitis and tick-borne encephalitis in endemic regions. In the case of yellow fever, there is a highly effective live-attenuated vaccine (strain 17D). One of the major targets for the development of vaccines is dengue fever: Both live attenuated and recombinant subunit vaccines are explored in laboratories. No vaccine is available in the case of St. Louis encephalitis, although the disease is being addressed by controlling the vector.

Because of the clinical implications, the effectiveness of genetic immunization against hepatitis C virus generated an increased interest. Another factor that complicates the development of vaccines is the high variability of the envelope epitopes, focusing the immunization efforts to internal proteins. Finally, predicting the protective ability of vaccines against hepatitis C virus is a difficult task, since the only reliable experimental model is the chimpanzee. Early studies reported the immunogenicity of plasmids expressing the core antigen (Lagging et al., 1995) or nucleocapsid (Major et al., 1995), when

Table 5.5. Genetic Immunization against *Flaviviridae*

Virus	Antigen	Species	Immunity	References
Hepatitis C virus[a]	Core protein	Mice	Abs, Th, CTL	Lagging et al., 1995 Chen et al., 1995
	Nucleocapside	Mice	Abs	Major et al., 1995
	E2 glycoprotein	Mice	Abs	Tedeschi et al., 1997
	E1, E2, and core protein	Mice	Abs, CTL	Saito et al., 1997
St. Louis encephalitis virus[b]	prM/E	Mice	Abs	Phillpotts et al., 1996
Dengue virus[b]	PreM and E protein	Mice	Abs	Kochel et al., 1997
Tick-borne encephalitis virus[b]	Nonstructural proteins	Mice	Protective immunity	Mitrofanova et al., 1997
	prM and E proteins	Mice	Abs	Schmaljohn et al., 1997
Japanese encephalitis virus[b]	prM + E or NS1 proteins	Mice	Abs	Lin et al., 1998
Bovine viral diarrhea virus[c]	gp53 (E2)	Mice	Abs	Harpin et al., 1997

[a]Unnamed genus.
[b]Genus *Flavivirus*.
[c]Genus *Pestivirus*.

inoculated into mice (Table 5.5). However, whereas the core antigen-expressing plasmid generated antibodies, Th and CTL, the nucleocapsid was immunogenic only when administered as a fused construct with hepatitis B virus antigens. A subsequent report confirmed the strong CTL response to the core antigen when administered in the form of DNA vaccine, using an *in vivo* tumor challenge strategy (Tokushige et al., 1996). Further work focused on testing plasmids that express envelope antigens. Thus, mouse immunization with a plasmid encoding the E3 protein led to antibody priming (Tedeschi et al., 1997). However, the fine specificity of these antibodies excluded the hypervariable region that is thought to carry protective epitopes.

A subsequent study, while confirming the immunogenicity of envelope antigens, underlined a dominant role for the core protein in generating CTL immunity by DNA immunization (Saito et al., 1997). A recent study attempted manipulation of the immune response to a plasmid expressing the core antigen by coadministration of cytokine-expressing plasmids (Geissler et al., 1997a). Thus, while IL-2 and GM-CSF significantly increased the humoral and cellular responses, IL-4 displayed a suppressor effect on CTL generation. Since a significant drawback of experimental analysis of protection afforded by DNA vaccination against HCV is the lack of small animal models of infection, recently, an HLA-A2.1-transgenic mouse model has been developed (Arichi et al., 2000). DNA vaccination with the core antigen of such transgenic mice bearing the aforementioned human HLA allele resulted in long-lasting CTL immunity, able to mediate significant but not sterile protection against a recombinant vaccinia virus expressing the core antigen of HCV.

A few studies explored the possibility of inducing immunity against tick-borne encephalitis viruses by DNA immunization. A carefully designed study demonstrated that gene-gun immunization of mice with plasmids expressing the prM and E antigens of two different strains of tick-borne flavivirus, namely, Russian spring–summer encephalitis or

Central European encephalitis virus, generated protective humoral immunity against homologous and heterologous challenge (Schmaljohn et al., 1997). Another study demonstrated the protective ability of plasmids expressing nonstructural proteins of tick-borne encephalitis viruses when inoculated into BALB/c mice (Mitrofanova et al., 1997).

A recent report describes the immunogenicity of plasmids expressing structural or nonstructural antigens of Japanese encephalitis virus, that is, a mosquito-borne flavivirus (Lin et al., 1998). When inoculated into mice, plasmids expressing prM and E proteins induced neutralizing antibodies that afforded a certain level of protection. Surprisingly, a plasmid that expressed the nonstructural protein NS1 conferred significant protection against challenge that was associated with antibody-dependent cellular cytotoxicity.

Another study showed that immunization of young mice with a plasmid expressing the prM/E protein of St. Louis encephalitis virus, mounted specific antibodies and were protected against virus challenge (Phillpotts et al., 1996). One report examined the generation of immune responses against dengue virus by genetic immunization of mice (Kochel et al., 1997). Intradermal immunization with plasmids expressing preM or E proteins of dengue Type-2 virus was followed by induction of *in vitro* neutralizing antibodies. Finally, another report addressed the generation of immunity by genetic vaccination against an animal pathogen that was recently classified in this family, namely, bovine viral diarrhea virus (BVDV). Inoculation into mice of a plasmid expressing the major glycoprotein (E2) of BVDV induced cross-reactive antibodies against multiple virus strains (Harpin et al., 1997).

5.2.2.2. Genetic Immunization against Other Single-Stranded RNA Viruses of Positive Sense

An important family of RNA viruses with extensive pathogenic implications for the human population is *Picornaviridae*. Usually, these viruses that replicate in the epithelial cells of the nasopharynx and digestive tract lead to inapparent or mild disease, but occasionally replication in lymphatic nodes is followed by viremia and infection of the central nervous system or other internal organs. Genus *Enterovirus* contains the polioviruses, Coxsackie viruses, echoviruses, and new enteroviruses that are implicated in various syndromes such as meningitis, encephalitis, enteritis, and respiratory and skin infections. Genus *Rhinovirus* contains agents that are responsible for mild, common upper respiratory infections, and rarely, lower respiratory infections, in neonates. Genus *Hepatovirus* includes a single agent, namely, hepatitis A virus. Other genera include important animal pathogens: *Cardiovirus* (encephalomiocarditis virus) and *Aphtovirus* (foot-and-mouth disease viruses). Immunity comprises neutralizing IgA and IgG antibodies as well as cellular response. However, protection from infection is mediated by strain-specific neutralizing antibodies. Effective vaccines are available only in the case of poliovirus (killed or live attenuated vaccine).

An original attempt to create a DNA vaccine against foot-and-mouth disease, a well-characterized veterinary problem, comprised the generation of plasmid-based vectors that encompassed the microbial genome (Ward et al., 1997) (Table 5.6). Cell transfection or *in vivo* inoculation of such vectors led to production of virus particles endowed with low replication ability. Administration of such plasmids to pigs was followed by generation of neutralizing antibodies and slight protection against virus challenge. Thus, direct manipula-

Table 5.6. Immune Response against Plasmids Expressing Antigens
of Single-Stranded RNA Viruses of Positive Sense

Virus (*Family*)	Antigen	Species	Immunity	Reference
Picornaviridae				
Encephalomyocarditis virus	VP1	Mice	Abs	Sin et al., 1997
Foot-and-mouth disease virus	All antigens (genome-length)	Pigs Mice	Abs	Ward et al., 1997
Coronaviridae				
Infectious bronchitis virus	Nucleocapsid	Chicken	CTL	Seo et al., 1997
Unclassified[a]				
Hepatitis E. virus	ORF-2 structural protein	Mice	Abs	He et al., 1997

[a]Previously classified in the family of *Caliciviridae*.

tion of the genome of positive-sense RNA viruses at the level of DNA may prove a powerful and rapid means to obtain attenuated vaccines.

Another report examined the response of mice inoculated with a plasmid expressing the VP1 antigen of encephalomyocarditis virus (Sin et al., 1997). The immunization was followed by induction of antibodies and protection against virus challenge, enhanced by coadministration of a plasmid expressing GM-CSF.

The family *Coronaviridae* contains two genera: *Coronaviruses*, responsible for the common cold in humans and respiratory infections in animals (infectious bronchitis virus), for which no vaccines are available; and *Torovirus*, which contains agents responsible for poorly described respiratory and enteric infections in humans and animals.

Inoculation of chickens with a plasmid expressing the nucleocapsid protein of infectious bronchitis virus (IBV) led to induction of CTL responses that were cross-reactive against multiple virus strains (Seo et al., 1997). The authors took advantage of this experimental setup in order to characterize IBV-specific CTL epitopes in chickens.

The hepatitis E virus, previously classified as a member of caliciviridae, displays particularities that resulted in its placement in a separate, unclassified taxon. It infects humans and is transmitted via the fecal–oral route. Large epidemics in developing countries are associated with significant morbidity and mortality in pregnant women.

A single study showed that inoculation of a plasmid expressing ORF-2 structural protein of hepatitis E virus into BALB/c mice was followed by induction of specific antibodies, as revealed by ELISA and Western Blot (He et al., 1997) (Table 5.6).

5.2.3. Genetic Immunization against Rotaviruses

Rotaviruses, a genus of the family *Reoviridae*, consist of double-stranded RNA viruses. Besides rotaviruses that are important human pathogens, the family *Reoviridae* contains other genera, among them the *Reoviruses* and *Orbiviruses* that are responsible for heterogenous, poorly characterized syndromes, or febrile encephalitis conditions, respectively.

Rotaviruses are classified according to antigenic specificity into groups, subgroups and serotypes. Group A and B rotaviruses are responsible for enteric disease in infants and children, associated with diarrhea, vomiting, and fever. The underlying mechanism is represented by lytic replication in mucosal cells of the proximal small intestine. Transmission occurs via fecal–oral route and is increased in developing countries. Severe dehydration due to rotavirus-induced diarrhea may lead to serious morbidity and mortality in the young segment of the population. Worldwide, rotavirus infection of infants and children poses a tremendous medical challenge, since it causes from 30% to 50% of all cases of severe childhood diarrhea. Interestingly, rotaviruses from other serologic groups are cause of similar syndromes in animals: groups C and E (pigs), group D (fowl), and group F (birds). Based on the correlation between antibody titers and the gravity of disease, it is currently thought that serum and secretory antibodies bear neutralizing ability in a serotype-specific manner. Vaccines based on attenuated strains of rotavirus are under development.

Because of the numerous clinical implications, the evaluation of DNA vaccines against rotaviruses in preclinical models has been a subject of investigation. The first reports described the humoral (Herrmann et al., 1996a) and CTL responses (Herrmann et al., 1996b) following DNA immunization of mice with plasmids expressing VP4, VP6, or VP7 proteins of rotavirus. Whereas DNA immunization with VP4 and VP7 led to induction of virus-neutralizing antibodies, all antigens primed significant CTL immunity. Interestingly, any of the three plasmids tested conferred significant protection in mice against rotavirus challenge, as assessed by reduction of virus titers. A subsequent study showed that the protection was limited to homologous challenge and that secretory IgA might have been responsible for it (Chen et al., 1997). The highest titers of secretory IgA antibodies were found in mice immunized with a plasmid expressing VP6. This protein is a good candidate for a subunit vaccine, since it encompasses cross-reactive epitopes. However, a study carried out by an independent group showed that in spite of presence of IgG antibodies after DNA immunization of mice with VP6, no IgA titers or protection against infectious challenge were evident (Choi et al., 1997). Thus, raising effective immunity against rotaviruses by DNA immunization requires answers to two questions: What is the mechanism of protective immunity against rotaviruses? Which are the cross-reactive epitopes that have the ability to confer protection?

5.2.4. Genetic Immunization against Retroviruses

The family *Retroviridae* is characterized by its peculiar mechanism of replication that involves reverse transcription of viral RNA into linear, double-stranded DNA that oligomerizes, circularizes, and integrates into host genome. Transcription of the resulting DNA insert produces a few species of mRNA as well as full-length viral RNA. An mRNA spanning the whole genome results in polypeptides that, upon cleavage, lead to structural proteins, protease, reverse transcriptase, and integrase. Other mRNA species lead, by translation, to regulatory proteins. A few genes are relatively common in all retroviruses: *env* encodes two envelope proteins, *gag* encodes up to six nonglycosylated proteins, *pro* encodes the protease, and *pol* encodes the reverse transcriptase and integrase. Endogenous proviruses are ancient retroviruses that, inserted into genome, lost one or a few elements crucial for replication, leading to vertical transmission. The pathology induced by retroviruses results from the fact that insertion into host DNA may induce cell transformation due to inactivation of antioncogenes. Alternatively, some retroviruses may express their own oncogenes. Extensive virus replication leads to host cell lysis and/or syncytial formation that result in loss of function at the level of cell populations. There are at least four mechanisms that act to a different extent under different circumstances and are responsible for the remarkable ability of retroviruses to escape from immune responses: Certain retroviruses (such as HIV and HTLV) infect and replicate in *T*-cells, leading to immunodeficiency; the reverse transcription introduces mutations that, under immune selection, lead to variants that are not recognized by memory *T*-cells or antibodies; certain virus proteins directly inhibit the immune function; and, finally, virus integration associated with reduced or no transcription leads to virus persistence in a stealthy manner and vertical transmission to daughter cells.

Two genera are particularly important regarding human pathology. Genus *Lentivirus* includes human immunodeficiency viruses (HIV) 1 and 2 that cause the acquired immune deficiency syndrome, a global health threat due to lack of effective treatment and fatal outcome. The disease is thought to be the consequence of *T*-cell deficiency that leads to severe infections and malignancies. Regarding the immunity, it is still uncertain if a completely protective response can be elicited. Ongoing studies address potential effective immune responses consequent to natural exposure. First, they are based on a few observations that humans exposed to HIV display specific antibodies but no infectious virus. There is laboratory evidence that *env*-specific antibodies exert neutralizing activity, although their *in vivo* role is still controversial. Second, virus-specific CTL may play a role not only by killing the infected cells, but also indirectly, by producing certain poorly known cytokines that suppress the virus replication. Consequently, the present paradigm is that an eventual protective response requires broad humoral as well as cellular immunity. Candidate recombinant subunit or live attenuated vaccines (in the form of recombinant retroviruses such as SIV) are being developed and are undergoing preclinical and clinical trials. However, each of these two strategies has drawbacks: Recombinant subunit vaccines do not elicit significant CTL, whereas live attenuated viruses may still pose serious infectious hazards. For example, attenuated SIV vaccines based on mutated Nef, a gene that is considered essential for virus replication, cause disease when injected into young monkeys.

HIV is the most extensively studied virus regarding immunization via DNA-based vectors (Table 5.7). Initial attempts were carried out to generate immune responses in mice inoculated with plasmids expressing envelope protein of HIV-1. Thus, administration of a plasmid expressing gp160 was followed by induction of antibodies endowed with *in vitro* neutralizing ability, as well as specific *T*-cells that proliferated upon *in vitro* stimulation (Wang et al., 1993a). The proof of concept regarding the immunogenicity of gp160-expressing plasmid was soon extended to nonhuman primates (Wang et al., 1993a). Furthermore, it was shown that plasmid inoculation of nonhuman primates was followed by induction of neutralizing antibodies against the homologous laboratory strain. Subsequent studies defined more precisely the immunity induced by DNA vaccination of mice with envelope-derived antigens. Thus, it was shown that administration of envelope-expressing plasmids induces, besides antibodies, specific CTL as well as Th cells (Fuller and Haynes, 1994; Lu et al., 1995; Wang et al., 1995). Various strains of mice responded to a similar extent regarding the antibody production upon DNA immunization with env-expressing plasmid (Ishii et al., 1997b). A comparison between the immunogenicity of plasmid DNA

Table 5.7. Immune Response to Plasmids Expressing HIV Antigens

Species	Antigen	Immune response	Reference
Rodents	Env (gp 160)	Abs, Th	Wang et al., 1993
	Env (gp 120)	Abs, CTL, Th	Fuller and Haynes, 1994
	Gag/p24 together with env	Abs, CTL	Lu et al., 1995
	Rev; env	Abs, Th, CTL	Shiver et al., 1996
	Nef	CTL	Asakura et al., 1996
	Nef; Rev; Tat; p37; evn	Abs, Th	Hinkula et al., 1997a, 1997b
	Env-2	Abs, Th	Agadjanyan et al., 1997
	Env (gp-120)	Abs, CTL	Barnett et al., 1997[a]
	Allogeneic MHC	Abs, CTL	Dela Cruz et al., 1999
Rabbit	Env	Abs	Okuda et al., 1997
			Richmond et al., 1997
Monkeys	Env	Abs	Wang et al., 1993b
	Env	Abs, CTL, Th	Wang et al., 1995
			Lekutis et al., 1997
			Shiver et al., 1997
	Rev; env (gp 120)	Abs, Th	Shiver et al., 1996
	Gag, env	Abs	Fuller et al., 1996
	Env; Rev; gag-pol	Abs, CTL, Th	Boyer et al., 1996, 1997a, 1997b[b]
Humans	Nef, Rev, Tat	CTL	Calarota et al., 1998
		Abs, Th	Calarota et al., 1999
	Env, Rev	Abs, CTL, Th	MacGregor et al., 1998
			Boyer et al., 1999

[a]Study carried out in mice and guinea pigs.
[b]Studies showing protection against infectious challenge.

expressing gp120 and the recombinant protein obtained in baculovirus infected cells and formulated in various adjuvants showed that whereas the titers of antibodies elicited by DNA immunization were lower, the specificity profile resembled the one following natural infection in humans (Peet et al., 1997). Another study showed for the first time the induction of neutralizing antibodies and CTL that were active against diverse HIV-1 isolates, following the inoculation in nonhuman primates of a plasmid expressing gp160 (Wang et al., 1995). A subsequent study showed *in vivo* protection of nonhuman primates conferred by a plasmid-expressing envelope protein against challenge with a SIV/HIV-env recombinant virus (Boyer et al., 1996). Independent groups confirmed the immunogenicity of plasmids expressing envelope protein administered in nonhuman primates by intramuscular injection (Shiver et al., 1996; Liu et al., 1996) or gene-gun immunization (Fuller et al., 1996).

Subsequent to the demonstration that plasmids expressing envelope protein are immunogenic, many groups focused their research on the characterization of the immune responses to internal or regulatory proteins, in an effort to improve the cellular immune response thought to be essential for both cross-reactivity as well as potency of the vaccine. Thus, it was shown that inoculation of plasmids expressing Rev, Nef, or Tat into mice is followed by induction of CTL and Th cells (Shiver et al., 1996; Asakura et al., 1996; Hinkula et al., 1997a). In parallel, there was a continuous interest in improving the immunogenicity of DNA-based vaccines against HIV in both rodents and nonhuman primates. One obvious strategy that fit well with the paradigm that protective immunity against HIV requires a broad humoral and cellular immune response was to coinoculate plasmids that express different HIV proteins. Thus, it was demonstrated that inoculation in mice of combinations of plasmids expressing the regulatory proteins Tat, Rev, and Nef, together with the structural proteins env and gag, led to broad immunity in terms of antibodies and CTL, without detectable negative interference among antigens (Hinkula et al., 1997a, 1997b). This principle, applied in a small preclinical trial in chimpanzees, showed protection against heterologous challenge with a particular HIV-1 strain following immunization with plasmids expressing env, rev, and gag/pol (Boyer et al., 1997b). Interestingly, inoculation of HIV-infected chimpanzees with a plasmid expressing both env and Rev of the HIV-1MN isolate led to the decrease of virus load to background levels (Boyer et al., 1997a). This particular result raised expectancies regarding a potential role for DNA immunization as therapeutic vaccine in HIV-infected individuals (Ugen et al., 1997a). The principle of multiantigenic vaccines was even extended to antigens from different viruses; thus, immunization of mice and rhesus monkeys with a plasmid expressing an HIV epitope fused with hepatitis B surface antigen resulted in a broad immunity against both microbes (Le Borgne et al., 1998).

An interesting approach to raise immunity against HIV virions has been recently investigated (Dela Cruz et al., 1999). It consists of immunization against allogeneic histocompatibility leukocyte antigens (HLA), based on previous studies that showed the presence of "donor" MHC molecules in the envelope of infectious virions. DNA vaccination with foreign MHC Class I and II molecules in a mouse model resulted in antibody responses and CTL responses directed to MHC epitopes. Antibodies induced by such MHC-based vaccines (either conventional or DNA vaccine) may bind to infectious virions, thus protecting against infection in a manner dependent on the titer at mucosal surfaces and recognition of shared epitopes.

Alternative strategies were employed to enhance or modulate the immune response to plasmids expressing HIV antigens. Earlier studies showed that whereas intramuscular injection of plasmids expressing env led to Th1 responses (Shiver et al., 1997), gene-gun immunization or intradermal injection, although more effective from a dose–response point of view, induced more Th2-biased responses (Fuller and Haynes, 1994). One way to increase or modulate the cellular responses after DNA immunization with plasmids encoding HIV antigens was to coadminister cytokines or costimulatory molecules. For example, repeated gene-gun-mediated codelivery of plasmids expressing gp120 and IL-2, IL-7, or IL-12 led to enhancement of Th1 and suppressed Th2 responses (Prayaga et al., 1997). Intradermal inoculation of Nef-expressing plasmid, together with a plasmid expressing GM-CSF, increased the antibody and Th response to Nef (Svanholm et al., 1997). Two different groups reported enhanced CTL and Th1 immunity following coinoculation of plasmids expressing HIV antigens and IL-12 (Tsuji et al., 1997b; Kim et al., 1997a). An extensive study addressing the effect of various cytokine-expressing plasmids on the immune responses generated by inoculation of HIV antigen-expressing DNA vectors was recently published (Kim et al., 1998). The humoral response was increased by coinoculation of IL-4-, IL-5-, IL-10-, IL-2-, and IL-18-expressing plasmids. The Th proliferation was increased following coinoculation of IL-2 or TNF-α genes. The CTL response was enhanced following coinoculation of TNF-α and IL-15 genes. Furthermore, coinoculation of CD86- and IL-12-expressing plasmids significantly enhanced the CTL immunity primed by DNA-based HIV vaccine (Kim et al., 1997a), presumably by providing critical costimulation for CTL precursors. Independent work established that whereas B7.2-expressing plasmid enhanced CTL responses to env- or rev-expressing vectors, B7.1 did not (Tsuji et al., 1997c). The study suggested that the increase of CTL response was mediated by direct B7.2–CD28 interaction, since it was inhibited by CTLA-4Ig. Another recent study showed that coinoculation of plasmids expressing env/rev and TCA3 cytokine was followed by enhanced CTL and Th1 responses associated with increased local inflammation at the site of inoculation (Tsuji et al., 1997a). Altogether, these studies indicate that a promising means to enhance the protective ability of plasmids expressing HIV antigens is by coadministration of cytokines and costimulatory molecules.

Another avenue employed to enhance the immunogenicity of plasmids expressing HIV antigens consisted in formulation of DNA in various adjuvants. Adjuvants such as mannan-coated liposomes (Toda et al., 1997), monophosphoryl lipid A (Sasaki et al., 1997), cationic liposomes (Ishii ct al., 1997a) or Ubenimex (Sasaki et al., 1998b) increased the T-cell responses and, in some circumstances, the humoral responses primed by env- and rev-expressing plasmids. However, the mechanism associated with the enhanced response in the presence of such lipid-based adjuvants is still controversial, since it did not necessarily lead to increased *in vivo* transfection (Sasaki et al., 1997). One possibility may be the direct effect of adjuvants on professional APC. At least in the case of mannan-coated lipid vesicles, the mechanism may involve preferential mannose-receptor-mediated uptake by professional APC-like dendritic cells.

Alternative routes of vaccine administration against HIV, like mucosal immunization, raised tremendous interest, since immunity at the port of entry can play important protective roles. Intranasal administration in mice of a plasmid expressing gp160 and rev was followed by induction of local antibody response and systemic humoral and cellular immunity (Okada et al., 1997; Asakura et al., 1997). Addition of plasmids that express IL-12 or GM-CSF significantly enhanced the induction of CTL (Okada et al., 1997). The observation that mucosal immunization with DNA vaccines against HIV is immunogenic was extended to plasmids expressing regulatory proteins (Hinkula et al., 1997a), or to alternative delivery sites, namely, vaginal mucosa (Wang et al., 1997a). A recently published comparison between the immunogenicity of muscular versus mucosal administration of plasmids showed similar T-cell immunity but a higher IgA response in the case of mucosal immunization (Sasaki et al., 1998b). Furthermore, there is some interest in enhancing the mucosal immunity by formulating the plasmids in lipid-based adjuvants (Okada et al., 1997; Sasaki et al., 1998b).

Other ways to increase the immunogenicity of plasmids expressing HIV antigens were recently reported. Replacing certain codons of wild-type gp120 with sequences from highly expressed human genes led to increased expression and immunogenicity of DNA vaccine (Andre et al., 1998). Another study showed that by redirecting a secreted HIV antigen to cytoplasm, the induction of CTL was enhanced (Tobery et al., 1997).

Advantages of DNA immunization such as Th1 and CTL response can be combined with advantages of protein immunization such as higher antibody titers. A few reports showed significant immune responses after immunization with DNA boosted by various HIV proteins (Fuller et al., 1997a; Barnett et al., 1997; Okuda et al., 1997). More recently, it was shown that a combination regimen comprising DNA priming followed by boost with recombinant fowl pox virus resulted in significant containment of infection with immunodeficiency virus in rhesus macaques (Robinson et al., 1999).

Based on preclinical results, recent clinical trials with DNA vaccines against HIV have been started. The first two clinical trials employed HIV-positive individuals and were aimed at assessing the safety and immunogenicity of plasmid cocktails expressing Nef, Rev and Tat (Calarota et al., 1998), or env and Rev (MacGregor et al., 1998). Generally, the inoculation of plasmids was well tolerated. Furthermore, the results suggested that inoculation of plasmids expressing regulatory proteins boosted the CTL response (Calarota et al., 1998). Inoculation of structural genes was shown to increase the level of antibodies as well as to boost CTL and Th immunity in a dose-related manner (MacGregor et al., 1998). There has been no evidence until now that plasmid immunization in these HIV-infected individuals led to a significant decrease of viral titers. In these lines, DNA vaccination of asymptomatic-infected individuals with constructs bearing *Nef*, *Rev*, or *Tat* did not reduce by itself the viral load, despite the detectable, long-lasting *T*-cell response (Calarota et al., 1999). A follow-up with highly active antiretroviral treatment (HAART regimen) in these patients contributed to *de novo* induction of HIV-specific CTL, probably due to an improvement of CD4$^+$-assisted *T*-cell help. Another recent clinical study on nine asymptomatic-infected individuals showed strong correlation between the *T*-cell response triggered and dose of DNA vaccine bearing *env* and *Rev* elements (Boyer et al., 1999). The induction of specific CTL was somewhat disappointing, but in the group immunized three times with 300 μg of plasmid/inoculation, the antigen-specific *T*-cell proliferation and the serum levels of MIP-1α, a chemokine thought to activate dendritic cells, were enhanced. These preliminary results set the stage for future clinical trials, including those in noninfected individuals.

Genus *Lentivirus* includes a few related viruses that infect various species of non-human primates (simian immunodeficiency viruses) as well as other species (feline immunodeficiency virus, bovine immunodeficiency virus), leading to similar immune deficiency syndromes eventually associated with autoimmunity and tumors. An unnamed genus includes human *T*-cell lymphotropic virus (HTLV) viruses that infect the *T*-cells, leading to adult *T*-cell leukemia by inducing *tax*-mediated cell transformation. Rarely, HTLV infection leads to tropical spastic paraparesis, which is a poorly understood neurological disease.

Different genera contain animal pathogens that cause leukemias, lymphomas, sarcomas, or carcinomas: murine leukemia viruses, feline leukemia and sarcoma viruses (genus unnamed, mammalian and reptilian Type C retroviruses); Rous sarcoma virus, avian leukosis viruses (genus unnamed, avian Type C retroviruses); mouse mammary tumor virus (Type D retroviruses); and genus *Spumavirus*, with poorly known disease association.

Some groups studied the response of DNA vaccines against simian immunodeficiency virus (SIV) as a model for immunization against HIV (Table 5.8). This model has an advantage in that it affords the evaluation of protection against SIV in their natural hosts, namely, nonhuman primates. Immunization of rhesus monkeys with plasmids expressing env and gag of a SIV isolate generated Class I restricted CTL responses (Yasutomi et al., 1996). Rhesus macaques immunized with plasmids expressing various SIV proteins mounted transient humoral but more persistent cellular responses (Lu et al., 1996). However, DNA vaccination did not prevent persistent infection or decrease of CD4$^+$ *T*-cell number after intravenous challenge with SIV (Lu et al., 1996). Similar results were obtained by gene-gun vaccination of rhesus monkeys with plasmids expressing envelope proteins (Fuller et al., 1997b), except that a transient protective effect was more evident in this study. Interestingly, the protective effect, consisting in decreased viral loads and enhanced num-

Table 5.8. Immune Response to Plasmids Expressing Antigens of Retroviruses

Virus	Antigen	Species	Immunity	Reference
Simian immunodeficiency virus	Env	Monkeys	Abs, CTL	Lu et al., 1996
	Env, gag	Monkeys	Abs, CTL	Yasutomi et al., 1996
	Env, gag	Mice	Abs	Indraccolo et al., 1998
Feline immunodeficiency virus	Full-length genome	Cats	Abs	Rigby et al., 1997
	gp120; p10	Cats	Abs	Cuisinier et al., 1997
Human T lymphotropic virus	Env	Mice	Abs	Grange et al., 1997
	Env	Rats	CTL	Kazanji et al., 1997
Cas-Br-M murine leukemia virus	Full-length genome; env	Mice	CTL	Sarzotti et al., 1997

ber of CD4$^+$ *T*-cells, did not correlate with the antibody titers, underlining the role of cellular immunity.

Regarding DNA immunization against HTLV-1, recent studies show that inoculation of mice or rats with plasmids encoding env and Rev primed *B*-cell and CTL responses (Kazanji et al., 1997; Grange et al., 1997; Agadjanyan et al., 1998). The humoral responses were suboptimal, but after boost with proteins or recombinant viruses, the antibody titers were significantly enhanced. No data are available yet in nonhuman primate models.

A few attempts were made to induce immunity against other animal retroviruses by DNA immunization. Whereas the inoculation in cats of a plasmid-expressing gp120 of feline immunodeficiency virus (FIV) was followed by induction of antibodies, the slight protective effect against FIV challenge noted in some of the vaccinated cats did not correlate well with their titer (Cuisinier et al., 1997). Expression of viral proteins following DNA immunization was elegantly illustrated by successful infection with FIV consequent to inoculation of a plasmid encompassing the entire virus genome (Rigby et al., 1997). In a different experimental model, namely, Cas-Br-M murine leukemia virus, inoculation of plasmids expressing virus antigens was followed by induction of protective CTL even at the earliest stages of life (Sarzotti et al., 1997).

Thus, a lot of studies have already demonstrated that genetic vaccination with plasmids expressing retrovirus antigens is immunogenic, with the cellular response usually being more prominent than the humoral one (Tables 5.7 and 5.8). These studies facilitated the transition to clinical trials with DNA-based vaccines against HIV. However, studies reporting protective immunity are still rare, a situation that has stimulated the research for overall improvement of the efficacy of DNA vaccines.

5.3. IMMUNE RESPONSES AGAINST DNA VIRUSES ELICITED BY GENETIC IMMUNIZATION

DNA viruses have elicited considerable interest from the point of view of genetic immunization, due to reasons that are dependent on the targeted virus. Thus, in spite of the existence of a recombinant subunit vaccine against hepatitis B virus, there is tremendous effort going on toward the development of a DNA-based vaccine against this important human pathogen. This is particularly due to the putative advantages in terms of efficacy afforded by genetic immunization, as well as to reduced costs. In contrast, the effort to develop DNA-based vaccines against herpesviruses and papillomaviruses is based on both their importance for human pathology and the lack of effective vaccines.

5.3.1. Genetic Vaccination against *Hepadnaviridae*

The family *Hepadnaviridae* contains two genera: *Orthohepadnavirus* (including the human pathogen hepatitis B virus, as well as viruses that infect other mammals) and *Avihepadnavirus* (including duck hepatitis virus).

Hepatitis B virus, a major human pathogen, is widely distributed throughout the world, particularly in Southeast Asia, where between 8% and 20% of the population carry the virus and 70–95% have been previously exposed to it. It causes an acute inflammatory disease of the liver that is followed in approximately 10% of infected individuals by chronic infection. About 25% of individuals with chronic infection develop a serious syndrome, chronic active hepatitis, that leads to liver fibrosis and failure. The virus is transmitted via blood or body fluids and actively replicates in hepatocytes. It is thought that part of the pathology associated with active and chronic hepatitis is due to immune-mediated cell destruction. The hepatitis B virus is an enveloped virus with a circular, mainly double-stranded DNA genome that is associated with an endogenous DNA-dependent DNA polymerase. Interestingly, the replication of hepatitis B virus involves an RNA intermediate that is reverse-transcribed by the virus polymerase. The envelop proteins are of three antigenically distinct species: S-proteins, M-proteins, and L-proteins. The defective virus particles associated with HBsAg are mainly composed of S-proteins. The core is mainly composed of HBcAg. Another antigen that is shed in soluble form is HBeAg, bearing diagnostic significance. During acute infection, both humoral and cell-mediated responses are elicited against the three major antigens: HBsAg, HBcAg, and HBeAg. However, only the antibody response against HBsAg is thought to protect against acute infection. Based on this empirical observation, two successive generations of vaccines were previously developed: HBsAg in the form of particles purified from the blood of carriers and, more recently, a recombinant HBsAg vaccine obtained in yeast. These vaccines are endowed with low ability to induce cellular responses, particularly CTL. Since an effective cellular immunity mediates the recovery from acute infection, potential vaccines that stimulate CTL responses are of interest. Even more importantly, enhancing cellular immunity in chronic carriers may lead to elimination of virus. However, there is a fine balance between positive and negative consequences of boosting the cellular immunity in chronic carriers, since a suboptimal response may only exacerbate the disease but not clear the virus.

Together with genetic immunization against influenza virus (Ulmer et al., 1993) and HIV (Wang et al., 1993b), HBV was one of the first experimental models that was addressed from this point of view (Davis et al., 1993a) (Table 5.9). Inoculation of a plasmid-expressing HBsAg into regenerating muscles of mice was followed by antigen production and secretion, as well as priming of antibodies in all the immunized animals (Davis et al.,

Table 5.9. Immune Response Raised by Plasmids Expressing Hepatitis B Virus Antigens

Virus strain	Antigen	Species	Immunity	Reference
Hepatitis B virus	Envelope proteins	Mice	Abs	Davis et al., 1993 Michel et al., 1995 Major et al., 1995
	Envelope proteins	Mice	CTL	Davis et al., 1995 Schirmbeck et al., 1995
	Core proteins	Mice	Abs, CTL	Kuhrober et al., 1997
	Envelope proteins	Monkeys	Abs	Davis et al., 1996
	Envelope or core proteins	Mice	Abs, Th, CTL	Geissler et al., 1997b Kuhrober et al., 1997
	Envelope proteins	Monkeys	Abs, CTL	Le Borgne et al., 1998
	HBs Ag	Humans	Abs	Tacket et al., 1999
Duck hepatitis B virus	Pre-S/S or S envelope protein	Ducks	Abs	Triyatni et al., 1998

1993a). A subsequent study pinpointed the beneficial role regarding immunogenicity, of delivering the DNA into regenerating muscles by needles or jet injection (Davis et al., 1994). The observation regarding immunogenicity of HBsAg-expressing plasmids was soon extended to the other envelope proteins (Michel et al., 1995). Furthermore, this study suggested a similarity concerning the fine specificity of antibodies induced by genetic immunization with envelope antigen and those noted in infected humans. Another study advanced the hypothesis that upon *in vivo* production following DNA immunization, surface antigen assembles into defective particles that are immunogenic (Mancini et al., 1996a). Subsequent studies established that DNA vaccination with plasmids expressing HBsAg primed significant Class I restricted CTL responses that were evident even in low responder strains of mice (Davis et al., 1995; Schirmbeck et al., 1995). Based on the detection of virus antigen in circulation, it was speculated that CTL priming following DNA immunization occurs via a nonclassical exogenous pathway (Davis et al., 1995). The effectiveness of antibody and CTL priming by genetic immunization with HBsAg greatly depended on the vector, the most effective regulatory element being the initial, early promoter of CMV (Bohm et al., 1996). An important advance was made when it was demonstrated that plasmid-based intramuscular immunization with the major and middle envelope proteins induced specific antibodies in chimpanzees (Davis et al., 1996). The response was dose-dependent and predominantly consisted of IgG1 isotypes. Interestingly, in a subsequent study (Prince et al., 1997), a similar observation was made in infant chimpanzees. This study showed that two infant chimps immunized with a plasmid-expressing surface antigen not only developed antibodies but were also protected against HBV challenge, as assessed by the lack of HBsAg and core-specific antibodies. Finally, a recent study carried out in rhesus macaques showed that plasmids expressing HBV envelope antigens elicited both antibody and CTL responses (Le Gorgne et al., 1998). Furthermore, inoculation of a plasmid expressing a chimeric HBV/HIV antigen induced immunity against both viruses in that species of nonhuman primates.

Of particular importance is the potential ability of DNA vaccination to facilitate the clearance of virus in chronically infected individuals, since the recombinant vaccine is ineffective in this concern. This aspect was initially studied in transgenic mice that express envelope antigen in hepatocytes, that is released in circulation, as a model of chronic infection with HBV (Mancini et al., 1996b). Interestingly and somewhat unexpectedly relative to the paradigm of tolerance to self-antigens, transgenic mice immunized with DNA-expressing HBsAg not only mounted humoral responses but also displayed a significant reduction in the circulating antigen as well as specific RNA message in hepatocytes, without evidence for hepatic toxicity. A subsequent study suggested that use of adjuvants or cytokines may increase the ability of DNA vaccination to overcome nonresponsiveness due to chronic persistence of HBV antigens (Davis et al., 1997).

Other groups focused their efforts toward the design of vectors expressing internal antigens and characterizing the immune response in animal models. An early study showed that inoculation of a plasmid expressing the core antigen into mice determined a humoral and CTL response (Kuhrober et al., 1997). An interesting subsequent study showed that mice immunized with plasmids expressing either the intracellular (HBcAg) or secreted (HBeAg) form of the core antigen, mounted CTL responses in two distinct haplotypes (Kuhrober et al., 1997). An independent group confirmed the immunogenicity in terms of antibodies and CTL, of plasmids expressing envelope and nucleocapsid proteins (Geissler et al., 1997a). Plasmids expressing internal antigens may prove useful especially as a component of therapeutic vaccines in chronically infected individuals.

Clinical trials regarding DNA vaccination against HBV were recently started by a few different groups. Some data were released on a Phase I safety/immune response study comprising DNA vaccination by gene-gun of seven healthy volunteers, with the HBs antigen (Tacket et al., 1999). Despite the fact that the vaccine was well tolerated, this preliminary report showed only a very modest effect regarding the humoral response. However, the studied protocol comprised only two administrations at submicron doses, so that upcoming data are expected to broaden our knowledge concerning the relationship between the dose, route, and regimen of vaccination, and the magnitude of immune response.

A recent report described the immunogenicity of plasmids expressing the pre-S/S or S proteins of duck hepatitis B virus (Triyatni et al., 1998). This study showed that in spite of the fact that both plasmids induced high antibody titers in Pekin ducks, the neutralization efficiency and mechanism was dependent on immunogen. The precursor (pre-S/S) was unexpectedly endowed with lower ability to induce antibodies that neutralized the virus in a rapid manner, pinpointing the importance of carefully designing the expressed component of DNA-based vaccines.

5.3.2. Genetic Vaccination against *Herpesviridae*

Herpesviruses have a complex structure: an envelope, tegument, nucleocapsid, and a core associated with the linear, double-stranded DNA genome. Virions have approximately 30 different structural proteins and their genome expresses a similar number of nonstructural proteins. Following cell infection, transcription and translation are regulated in a cascading manner, controlled by key proteins. Immediate early genes encode factors that turn on early genes involved in the replication of viral DNA. Late genes are mostly translated into structural proteins. Herpesviruses are responsible for heterogenous syndromes following transmission by contact. Most of the infections are lifelong and, in certain cases, lead to neoplasia.

The herpesviruses are classified into three subfamilies: *Alphaherpesvirinae, Betaherpesvirinae*, and *Gammaherpesvirinae*. In the subfamily *Alphaherpesvirinae*, there are three important human pathogens: human herpesviruses 1 and 2 (from genus *Simplexvirus*) and varicella-zoster virus (genus *Varicellovirus*). The subfamily *Betaherpesvirinae* contains human cytomegalovirus and human herpesviruses 6A, 6B, and 7, responsible for a pediatric syndrome manifested by rash and fever. The subfamily *Gammaherpesvirinae* includes Epstein–Barr virus, responsible for an acute infectious disease (mononucleosis) and, in certain cases, *B*-cell lymphomas.

Herpes simplex viruses 1 and 2 infect the epithelial cells at the port of entry, producing a characteristic vesicular lesion. Following local replication, the virus ascends the local sensory nerves to the corresponding dorsal root ganglia, where it establishes latency. During reactivation, the virus spreads distally to generate vesicular lesions on skin or mucosa. The infection is very serious in immune-compromised hosts. Candidate subunit and live attenuated vaccines are in development phase.

Varicella-zoster virus (VZV) is responsible for a common childhood infectious syndrome manifested by a characteristic rash and fever. In adults, the reactivation of latent virus leads to shingles, a vesicular rash with dermatomal distribution. A live attenuated vaccine against VZV has recently been licensed.

Cytomegalovirus (CMV) is responsible for a serious syndrome in congenitally infected neonates. In immune-competent individuals, the primary infection leads to mononucleosis. In immune-deficient individuals, infection with cytomegalovirus often leads to life-threatening, generalized infection. Vaccines against CMV are in the developmental stage.

A tremendous number of herpesviruses are responsible for animal diseases. Most often, they have very narrow host ranges. For example, bovine herpesviruses and pseudorabies virus are included in the subfamily *Alphaherpesvirinae*. They are responsible for characteristic diseases in bovines (mamillitis, skin disease, rhinotracheitis) or pigs (Aujeszky's disease), respectively.

A plasmid expressing the gIV protein of bovine herpes virus 1 was among the first DNA vaccine prototypes tested in preclinical models (Cox et al., 1993). Inoculation of mice with gIV-expressing plasmids resulted in specific antibody response. Furthermore, cattle injected with the same plasmid displayed protective antibodies as well as decreased virus titers after infectious challenge. This preliminary report was followed by other, numerous reports regarding DNA vaccination against herpes simplex virus types 1 and 2, cytomegalovirus, and pseudorabies (Table 5.10).

An early study showed that DNA vaccination of mice with a plasmid expressing the glycoprotein B (gB) of HSV-1 induced protective immunity in a zosteriform murine model (Manickan et al., 1995). The protection was apparently mediated by CD4$^+$ *T*-cells, as

Table 5.10. Immune Response against Plasmids Expressing Herpes Virus Antigens

Virus	Antigen	Species	Immunity	Reference
Bovine herpesvirus	gIV	Mice, cattle	Abs	Cox et al., 1993
Herpes simplex virus	HSV-1			
1 and 2	ICP27; gB	Mice	CTL[a]	Rouse et al., 1994
	gB	Mice	Abs, Th	Manickan et al., 1995
	gD	Mice	Abs	Ghiasi et al., 1995
	HSV-2			
	gB, gD	Mice, guinea pigs	Abs	McClements et al., 1996 Kriesel et al., 1996 Bourne et al., 1996
	gB, gD	Mice	Abs, T-cells	Manning et al., 1997 Pachuk et al., 1998
Pseudorabies	gD	Pigs	Abs	Monteil et al., 1996
Cytomegalovirus	Human CMV			
	pp65	Mice	Abs	Pande et al., 1995
	Mouse CMV			
	pp89	Mice	CTL	Gonzales Armas et al., 1996

[a]*In vitro* only.

revealed by adoptive transfer experiments. The level of neutralizing antibodies was low and the overall Th profile was switched toward Th1 immunity. Specific $CD8^+$ T-cells were not readily detectable. However, a previously published report by the same group showed that macrophages or dendritic cells *in vitro* pulsed under different conditions with plasmids expressing gB or ICP27 proteins of HSV-1 were able to induce specific CTL from naive precursors (Rouse et al., 1994). Interestingly, in contrast to dendritic cells, the macrophages were able to prime CTL after being pulsed with DNA devoid of cationic lipid. A recent report compared the abilities of *in vitro* transfected dendritic cells and macrophages to induce protective immunity against HSV-1 when injected into muscles of mice (Manickan et al., 1997a). The results showed that only transfected dendritic cells could induce protective immunity, pinpointing the potential importance of these cells in the priming of immunity subsequent to DNA vaccination. The same group took advantage of their experimental model to address another important point regarding DNA vaccination, namely, the immunogenicity of plasmids in neonates, in the presence or absence of maternal antibodies (Manickan et al., 1997b and Chapter 9).

Another study investigated the effectiveness of a different HSV-1 antigen, namely, gD. In spite of the detectable titer of specific antibodies, there was no detectable T-cell immunity primed by a plasmid-expressing gD (Ghiasi et al,. 1995). Furthermore, although it was significantly protective against infectious challenge in a mouse model, the level of protection was low. Since the recombinant gD protein affords a higher level of protection in the same model, it was concluded that DNA vaccination is a suboptimal method of immunization. An interesting, recently published study described the immunogenicity and protection ability of a gB-expressing plasmid when administered intranasally (Kuklin et al.,

1997). This study showed that mucosal administration of DNA led to significant IgA responses associated with systemic *T*-cell immunity. However, surprisingly, intramuscular immunization was at least as efficient as the intranasal route in inducing protective antibodies at distal mucosal sites (Kuklin et al., 1997). Overall, these results indicating moderate immune responses following DNA vaccination against HSV-1 are likely to fuel new studies aimed at optimizing the efficiency of genetic immunization. Thus, a more recent report described a Sindbis virus–based vector expressing gB of HSV-1 that primed antibodies and *T*-cell immunity in mice, with increased dose-related efficiency as compared to plasmid DNA (Hariharan et al., 1998).

Another herpesvirus studied from the point of view of genetic immunization was HSV-2, mostly responsible for the genital herpes. An early report described the ability of two plasmids expressing gD or gB antigens of HSV-2 to induce humoral response and protection of mice against lethal challenge (McClements et al., 1996). The observation was extended by the same study to guinea pigs. Independently, another group reported that a plasmid expressing gD2 of HSV-2 induced significant antibody response as well as protection against disease elicited by virus infection, particularly when the plasmid was coinoculated with D_3 vitamin (Kriesel et al., 1996). Another report extended this observation to guinea pigs and, most importantly, showed that DNA vaccination protected against not only primary disease but also recurrent disease (Bourne et al., 1996). Similar conclusions were subsequently reported by another group that pinpointed the beneficial effect of coadministrating plasmids that express gD and gB of HSV-2 (McClements et al., 1997). A recent study characterized in more detail the cellular response to gD-expressing plasmid inoculated in mice (Pachuk et al., 1998). Interestingly, another study, aimed at assessing the efficiency of different forms of vaccines against HSV-2, found that delivery of gB and gD antigens by adeno-associated virus led to increased humoral responses compared to plasmid-based or recombinant protein immunization (Manning et al., 1997). Probably, the viral vector mediates more effectively the cellular internalization of vaccine, leading to increased antigen expression.

Few reports described the immunogenicity of plasmids expressing CMV antigens. One study showed that plasmids expressing pp65 of the human CMV, a tegument protein, induced humoral response when inoculated into mice (Pande et al., 1995). A more recent study examined the response of BALB/c mice to a plasmid expressing protein, pp89, of murine CMV, known to express protective epitopes (Gonzales Armas et al., 1996). In spite of the low levels of specific antibodies elicited by DNA immunization, the significant CTL response very probably was responsible for the decreased virus titers in the immunized mice.

Pseudorabies, a virus with certain veterinary importance, was approached by two groups from the point of view of DNA immunization. In a study among the first to approach the issue of neonatal DNA immunization, piglets immunized at Day 1 and boosted at Day 42 after birth with a plasmid expressing gD protein of pseudorabies showed moderate antibody responses that were insufficient to protect against infectious challenge (Monteil et al., 1996). Interestingly, piglets immunized with DNA born from immune dams failed to mount antibody responses in that study. However, in a more recent study, the delivery of gD antigen by a replication-defective adenovirus vector circumvented the inhibition of immune response by maternal antibodies (Le Potier et al., 1997). An independent study showed that DNA vaccination of pigs against pseudorabies confers protection against the disease caused by virus replication (Gerdts et al., 1997).

5.3.3. Genetic Vaccination against Papillomavirus

The family *Papovaviridae* contains two genera: *Papillomavirus* and *Polyomavirus.* The genome is double-stranded DNA that may persist in an integrated form in infected cells in the case of polyomaviruses, or in episomal form in the case of papillomaviruses. Whereas polyomaviruses are associated with rare urinary and central nervous system diseases, particularly in immune-compromised subjects, papillomaviruses are significantly associated with premalignant and malignant lesions of epithelial origin (warts, papillomas, carcinomas). Often, the virus DNA is integrated in the genome of malignant cells. Papillomaviruses have a narrow host range. Interestingly, different papillomaviruses cause distinct lesions. Notably, human papillomaviruses 16 and 18 are significantly associated with premalignant and malignant genital lesions. Various strains of papillomavirus cause benign lesions of the skin and mucosa in other species, such as rabbits, dogs, and cows. The immunity against papillomaviruses is poorly understood, although it is thought that cellular immunity plays an important role in the remission of papillomas. Antibodies against conformational epitopes on capsid proteins assembled in viral particles are thought to exert protection against virus infection.

An early report examined the immune response of animals to a plasmid expressing the L1 capsid protein in a cottontail rabbit papillomavirus model (Donnelly et al., 1996). The authors found that immunized rabbits mounted significant titers of neutralizing antibodies that mediated protection against virus challenge. An independent study confirmed this observation subsequent to employing gene-gun-mediated delivery of L1-expressing plasmid in the same experimental model (Sundaram et al., 1997). Again, the protection of immunized animals against formation of papilloma subsequent to infection was significant.

5.4. IMMUNE RESPONSE TRIGGERED BY DNA IMMUNIZATION AGAINST NONCONVENTIONAL VIRUSES

Nonconventional viruses, or prions, are small infectious particles of proteic structure that lack nucleic acids. They are transmissible among certain species and induce fatal neurological diseases: kuru, Creutzfeldt–Jakob disease in humans and scrapie in animals. Interestingly, prion infection is associated with posttranslational modification of a host protein PrP^c to a pathogenic isoform, PrP^{Sc}. Prion-associated diseases are induced by two mechanisms: horizontal transmission among individuals of a species (e.g., cannibalism or iatrogenesis), or mutations that affect PrP^c and are transmitted vertically. The immune response against prions is virtually unknown. The immune system seems to be tolerant to PrP^c, so that PrP^c-deficient mice were excellent tools for investigating the immunity against PrP^c, but more importantly, for obtaining antibody reagents that can be used in research and clinics. Mice deficient in PrP^c were immunized with plasmids expressing different human prion proteins (Krasemann et al., 1996). The immunized knockout mice mounted vigorous polyclonal responses against the human isoforms of prion protein. In contrast, the PrP^{c+} wild-type mice were not responsive. Antibodies raised by genetic immunization of $PrP^c-/-$ mice with plasmids expressing human PrP^c were mostly directed to the octapeptide repeat region, rather than to the neurotoxic domain or GPI anchor. Such PrP^c-specific reagents were invaluable for the recent advances in this field, such as characterization of PrP^c expression in nervous and nonnervous tissues (Mabbott et al., 1998).

5.5. CONCLUSIONS AND PERSPECTIVES

By now, a tremendous number of viruses have been explored in preclinical models from the perspective of genetic immunization. The most intensively investigated viruses are either pathogens with large human circulation, such as influenza virus, herpes simplex viruses, and hepatitis B virus, or pathogens that are responsible for lethal syndromes in humans, such as HIV. From a different point of view, three main reasons justified the research and development of prototype DNA vaccines in these cases: first, the lack of effective vaccines (HIV, herpes viruses); second, the limited efficacy of currently available vaccines (influenza virus and hepatitis B virus, particularly in chronic carriers); and third, the increased cost of production and/or distribution of licensed vaccines (hepatitis B virus).

Regarding the immunogenicity, plasmids expressing antigens from virtually all viruses that were investigated from the perspective of genetic immunization elicited humoral and/or cellular responses. The most effective routes of delivery regarding the dose–effect relationship were intradermally by gene-gun and, to a lesser extent, intramuscularly. As a rule, the effectiveness of *T*-cell priming was higher than that of *B*-cell priming, as revealed by studies that addressed this aspect. Generally, the magnitudes of the immune responses were similar or lower compared to those elicited by live viruses. However, an obvious advantage of DNA immunization is the broad response elicited that spanned CTL, Th, and humoral immunity in the absence of vector replication.

Studying the protection afforded by DNA immunization against viruses in preclinical models proved to be a serious challenge for the groups involved in the field. The reasons were twofold: First, the response elicited by plasmids was not always appropriate from a qualitative point of view; and second, the magnitude of immune responses was not always sufficient. These aspects were more recently addressed in a conjugated effort of the scientific community to improve the protection ability of DNA vaccines in rodent and nonhuman primate models. For example, intradermal administration of plasmids, particularly by gene-gun, was shown to improve the dose–effect profiles. Coadministration of plasmids expressing different antigens, or antigens and cytokines, was another means to improve the efficacy of DNA-based vaccines. Administration of DNA vaccines via alternative routes and adjuvant formulation provides still other avenues that are being actively explored. Still, it might be the case that other vectors that bear antigen genes endowed with higher ability to transfect cells *in vivo*, but devoid of replication as well as antigenicity, may be a better solution for the future.

Two previous stages in the research and development of genetic vaccines against the aforementioned viruses that are the most important for human pathology were essentially completed or will be soon completed: a first stage that allowed the demonstration of the proof of concept, namely, immunogenicity and protective ability in rodent models; and a second stage that demonstrated immunogenicity, protection ability, and safety of DNA vaccines in nonhuman primate models. Based on these results in preclinical trials, clinical trials with DNA vaccines against major virus pathogens have already begun or will begin in the near future. In the case of HIV, where community pressure is so intense, the results of the first two clinical trials carried out in infected individuals, assessing immunogenicity and safety, are already available. In spite of the good safety profile showed by these Phase I trials, DNA vaccines have not displayed excellent immunogenicity, fueling continuous research at preclinical level for their improvement. However, the clinical data do not yet allow a statistically significant analysis in terms of protection, and the results of the upcoming clinical trials are expected with great interest.

Chapter 6

Immune Responses Elicited by Genetic Immunization with Bacterial, Fungal, or Parasitic Antigens

Genetic vaccination has been investigated to varying extents in models that study immunity against bacteria and parasites. For reasons detailed here, two major potential targets were extensively studied: *Mycobacterium tuberculosis* and *Plasmodia*.

6.1. DNA-BASED IMMUNIZATION WITH BACTERIAL OR FUNGAL ANTIGENS

Since most bacteria grow in bodily fluids, it is thought that the humoral response plays the critical role in the protection. In contrast, cellular immune responses play a major role in infections caused by obligatory intracellular microbes and parasites. The moderate ability of DNA vaccines to elicit strong humoral responses may explain why most of the studies were focused on immunity against viruses. In addition, the transcription of bacterial open reading frames and translation of resulting mRNAs in a eukaryotic environment are not always facile tasks.

Thus, genetic immunization has been studied in models that mostly comprise obligatory intracellular bacteria. In these cases, cellular immunity plays a critical role in protection, and the ability of DNA vaccines to induce the Th1 arm that regulates cellular and humoral responses may be beneficial for vaccination against these types of pathogens. While it is unlikely in the near future that DNA vaccines will replace effective toxoids, for certain bacteria, highly efficient vaccines are still unavailable. A major human pathogen, *Mycobacterium tuberculosis*, still represents a significant medical threat throughout the world and will be discussed separately, since it is the focus of most of the research regarding DNA vaccines against bacteria.

6.1.1. Immunization with Plasmids Expressing Mycobacteria Antigens

In spite of the abrupt decrease of tuberculosis due to antibiotic therapy, because of the following factors, tuberculosis is still a leading cause of morbidity and mortality throughout the world: limited effectiveness of the live attenuated *M. bovis* (BCG) vaccine; limited availability in certain geographical areas of the BCG vaccine or therapeutic means; and the emergence of drug-resistant strains of *M. tuberculosis*.

The primary infection occurs following airborne transmission. The bacteria enter the lung macrophages and, instead of being destroyed, multiply and spread to regional lymph nodes as well as other organs. Interestingly, in 98% of individuals infected with *M. tuberculosis*, the emerging cellular response, consisting of CTL and *T*-cells secreting gamma-interferon, limits the spread of bacteria. However, the bacteria persist in a dormant state in primary lesions, and, in approximately 2% of infected individuals, they reactivate, leading to secondary disease. The reactivation is frequently associated with compromised immunity due to age, improper alimentation, or disease. Microbes disseminate systemically via blood, reseed the lungs, and spread to other organs. Tissue lesions are caused by DTH reactions associated with a delayed and ineffective cellular response. It is still unclear if protection and DTH are mediated by similar or distinct subsets of *T*-cells. However, it appears that specific *T*-cells recognize immunodominant epitopes derived from the big family of stress proteins shared by numerous bacteria. The control of tuberculosis in developing countries has been attempted through vaccination with an attenuated strain of *M. bovis*, namely, bacillus Calmette–Guérin (BCG). However, clinical trials with BCG have displayed tremendous variability in terms of protection against infection or various forms of disease.

The first report in a preclinical model of a DNA-based vaccine against *M. tuberculosis* (Lowrie et al., 1994) showed that *in vivo* expression of hsp65 from *M. leprae*, obtained by various means, including inoculation of plasmid, led to the priming of specific CD4$^+$ and CD8$^+$ *T*-cells that could transfer resistance against challenge with *M. tuberculosis*. Subsequent studies were seminal in delineating the mechanism of protection conferred by DNA immunization with hsp65 in the murine model of *M. tuberculosis* (Table 6.1). Thus, the ability to confer protection upon adoptive transfer was higher in the case of CD8$^+$ *T*-cells able to lyse infected macrophages and to produce IFN-γ (Silva, 1995; Lowrie et al., 1997b). Strikingly, upon murine infection with *M. tuberculosis*, and in contrast to DNA immunized mice, most of the specific *T*-cells were CD44^{low}, secreted IL-4 rather than IFN-γ, and were endowed with low protection ability upon adoptive transfer (Bonato et al., 1998). These findings are important in three ways: First, a single antigen that is not specific for *M. tuberculosis* confers protection upon DNA immunization; second, the protective cells are CD8$^+$ CTL; and third, DNA immunization can circumvent the poor immune response associated with this type of infection. Other heat shock proteins produced by mycobacteria, such as hsp70, 36- and 6kDa, were found to be immunogenic and induced various degrees of protection when expressed in plasmids used to immunize mice (Lowrie et al., 1997a).

Effective immunity was more recently demonstrated against other mycobacteria antigens. For example, mouse immunization with a plasmid expressing a secreted protein, Ag85A, was followed by induction of humoral and cellular immune responses that were

Table 6.1. Genetic Immunization with Bacterial Antigens

Bacteria	Antigen	Immunity	Reference
Mycobacterium tuberculosis	hsp 65,70, 30, 6 kDa	Th, CTL	Lowrie et al., 1994 Lowrie et al., 1997b
	Ag 85A,B	B, Th, CTL	Huygen et al., 1996 Lozes et al., 1997
	38 kDa antigen	Th, CTL	Zhu et al., 1997a, 1997b
	19 kDa, AhpC antigens	Abs	Erb et al., 1998
Mycoplasma pulmonis	Expression library	Abs, Th	Barry et al., 1995 Lai et al., 1995
	A7-1, A7-2 antigens	Abs, Th	Lai et al., 1997
Clostridium tetanii	Fragment C protein	Abs, Th	Anderson et al., 1996
Borrelia burgdorferi	OspA antigen	Abs, Th	Simon et al., 1996
Staphylococcus aureus	PBP2' antigen	Abs	Ohwada et al., 1999
Streptococcus pneumoniae	PspA antigen	Protection	McDaniel et al., 1997
Brucella abortus	L7/12 antigen	Abs, Th	Kurar and Splitter, 1997
Cowdria ruminantium	MAP1 antigen	Abs, Th	Nyika et al., 1998
Chlamydia trachomatis	MOMP, CTP antigens	Abs, *T*-cells	Zhang et al., 1997

equally protective against challenge with *M. tuberculosis* or *M. bovis* (Huygen et al., 1996). Subsequently, the same group demonstrated effective DNA immunization against another component of the antigen 85 complex, namely, Ag85B (Lozes et al., 1997). Inoculation of plasmids expressing Ag85A or Ag85B led to induction of CTL as well as Th1 cells. Interestingly, plasmids expressing secreted or nonsecreted forms of Ag85A elicited similar humoral and cellular responses (Ulmer et al., 1997). Recently, epitope mapping of the *T*-cell response subsequent to DNA immunization with Ag85A or to *M. tuberculosis* infection showed that the plasmid elicited a broader response in terms of specific *T*-cells secreting IL-2 and IFN-γ (Denis et al., 1998). Furthermore, DNA immunization, but not *M. tuberculosis* infection, elicited CTL response. Thus, the observation that DNA immunization may circumvent the low immunogenicity of the whole microbe seems to hold true in different antigenic systems (Bonato et al., 1998; Denis et al., 1998). A potential cause for this phenomenon may be the absence of immune suppressive factors of bacterial origin from the DNA vaccine formulation. While showing the immunogenicity of a plasmid expressing the 38 kDa protein of *M. tuberculosis*, strengthened the observation that DNA immunization induces a broader *T*-cell response compared to infection (Zhu et al., 1997a). DNA immunization against the 38 kDa protein primed Th1 and strong Tc1 responses endowed with protective ability (Zhu et al., 1997b). Finally, another recent study explored the immunogenicity of plasmids expressing different mycobacteria antigens, namely, the 19 kDa and AhpC proteins (Erb et al., 1998). In spite of the humoral response that was readily detectable in mice immunized with these plasmids, no CTL and no protection against infectious challenge were demonstrated (Erb et al., 1998).

A recent exciting study addressed the potential therapeutic value of DNA vaccination against *Mycobacteria tuberculosis* in an animal model. It was found that DNA vaccination of infected animals can switch an ongoing ineffective immune response to one that kills the bacterium and promotes its clearance (Lowrie et al., 1999). This observation may open an avenue for the prevention of disease in infected individuals and even for immunotherapy in combination with chemotherapy of patients presenting with disease.

Thus, DNA vaccines against *M. tuberculosis* that employ the stress protein hsp65 or the secreted protein Ag85 are promising vaccination alternatives for at least two reasons: First, they might circumvent the apparently low protective ability of the conventional BCG vaccine, and second, they do not interfere with the monitoring of infection as measured by DTH reaction to tuberculin.

6.1.2. Immunization with Plasmids Expressing Antigens from Other Bacteria or Fungi

Mycoplasma pulmonis (*M. pulmonis*) is the smallest bacterium, having only between 500 and 1000 genes. It is responsible for certain atypical respiratory syndromes. The availability of animal models for infection greatly facilitated its study from multiple points of view.

Two interesting advances in DNA vaccination have been made in this experimental system. An early report showed for the first time that immunization of mice with total or partial expression libraries from *M. pulmonis* conferred protection against infectious challenge (Barry et al., 1995). Expression libraries were obtained by inserting cloned DNA (cDNA) pieces into mammalian expression vectors, under strong promoters. The implications of this technique may be far reaching, since, first, it provides a shortcut for designing protective vaccines even in the absence of knowledge about protective epitopes, and second, it offers a relatively rapid means to define protective antigens using sequential immunizations with progressively restricted partial libraries. There is a potential drawback to this method, particularly in the case of complex microbes, namely, the likelihood of administering genes that express proteins with toxic or immunosuppressive effects.

The second interesting observation in this experimental system described the ability of a DNA vaccine expressing defined *M. pulmonis* proteins (A7-1 and A8-1) to promote the clearance of pneumonia even when administered 1 week after infection (Lai et al., 1997). Very likely, this prototypical therapeutic vaccine enhanced humoral and cellular responses to protective epitopes, circumventing their limited immunogenicity in the context of infection.

Borrelia burgdorferi is responsible for Lyme disease, a chronic syndrome that affects various organs, particularly the joints. *Borrelia*, a Gram-negative spirochete with internal flagella, is transmitted to humans by tick bites. Characteristically, following the infection, there is relapsing fever associated with bacteremia. During remissions, the bacterium is sequestered in the tissues where it can change its surface antigenic structure, presumably leading to escape from neutralizing antibodies. Infection with *Borrelia* leads to arthritis, carditis, and neuritis. The pathogenesis of the syndrome is poorly understood. The recombinant outer-surface lipoprotein was shown to be protective in experimental models.

Immunization of mice with a plasmid expressing the outer surface lipoprotein (pOspA) of *Borrelia* was followed by induction of specific antibodies as well as *T*-cells (Zhong et al., 1996). Interestingly, whereas the *T*-cell response was dominated by CD4[+]

Th1 cells specific for a dominant Class II restricted epitope, the prominent isotype of the induced antibodies was IgG1, which is thought to be associated with Th2 responses. The same authors reported a surprising finding, namely, that immunization of mice with DNA expressing pOspA under its own prokaryotic promoter was followed by induction of Th1 cells, protective antibodies, and increased resistance against spirochete challenge (Simon et al., 1996). Naturally, this discovery may have implications reaching beyond the issue of DNA immunization, to the field of prokaryotic gene regulation in a eukaryotic environment. The same study reported that passive antibody transfer from DNA-immunized animals to severe combined immunodeficiency (SCID) mice led to increased protection against *Borrelia* challenge. A more recent study showed that immunization of mice with a plasmid expressing OspA of the B31 strain of *Borrelia burgdorferi* induced protective humoral immunity against two other strains, N40 and Sh-2-82 (Luke et al., 1997). This recent observation is particularly significant in the light of surface antigenic variation of *Borrelia burgdorferi* that poses a challenge to efforts to develop cross-protective vaccines.

Plasmids expressing other bacterial antigens were studied as well. *Clostridium tetani* is a Gram-positive anaerobic bacterium that multiplies and produces exotoxins in contaminated wounds. The tetanus toxin binds to neuronal gangliosides, blocks glycine release, and induces sustained contraction of antagonistic muscles. Vaccination with tetanus toxoid is followed by active immunity. Recently, it was shown that immunization of mice with a plasmid expressing the nontoxic C terminal part of tetanus toxin primed *T*- and *B*-cell responses (E.D. Anderson et al., 1996a; R. Anderson et al., 1997). The titer of IgG2a antibodies was sufficient to confer significant protection against infectious challenge.

Other recent reports showed immunization of mice with plasmids expressing antigens from *Streptococcus pneumoniae*, *Brucella abortus*, *Cowdria ruminantium*, and *Chlamydia trachomatis*. For example, a single report described the immunity primed by inoculation of a plasmid expressing the pneumococcal surface protein A (PspA) of the extracellular pathogen *S. pneumoniae* (McDaniel et al., 1997). Interestingly, there was a moderate but significant effect of DNA immunization in terms of protection. While similar results were obtained in the case of DNA vaccination with *B. abortus* antigen L7/12 expressed from CMV promoter, the expression vector bearing the bovine MHC Class I promoter was less effective (Kurar and Splitter, 1997). Another study investigated the effect of a prototypical DNA vaccine against the intracellular bacteria *C. trachomatis*, a relatively common cause of blindness. DNA immunization with a surface antigen (major outer-membrane protein) but not an internal antigen (cytosine triphosphate synthetase) induced humoral and cellular responses, as well as significant protection (Zhang et al., 1997). A recent report examined the cellular and humoral response triggered by immunization of mice with a plasmid expressing the major antigenic protein 1 (MAP1) of *C. ruminantium*, a rickettsial agent with veterinary importance (Nyika et al., 1998). Again, moderate but statistically significant protection against infectious challenge was seen in the mice immunized with MAP1-expressing plasmid compared with the group injected with control vector. An interesting experimental approach was employed against methicillin-resistant *Staphylococcus aureus* by DNA vaccination with the penicillin-binding protein (PBP2′) (Ohwada et al., 1999a). This study showed significant efficiency of such an antivirulence-factor vaccine, resulting in growth inhibition of the penicillin-resistant strain of bacteria.

In a recent study, potential applications for DNA vaccines in the area of antifungal protection were suggested. Immunization of BALB/c mice with a plasmid coexpressing

IL-12 and the fungal antigen 'Ag2' of *Coccidioides immitis* resulted in induction of strong antibody and Th1-biased response, with limited but significant protective effects against infectious respiratory challenge (Jiang et al., 1999).

Thus, in spite of the relatively limited extent to which DNA immunization with bacterial or fungal antigens was explored, certain conclusions can be drawn. First, DNA immunization is a promising strategy to induce protective immunity in the case of obligatory intracellular bacteria such as *M. tuberculosis*, mediated by CTL and Th1 CD4+ cells. Second, immunity against microbes, at least in experimental models, can be induced in the case of extracellular bacteria such as *M. pulmonis*, *S. pneumoniae*, or against the toxin produced by *Clostridium tetanii*. This underscores again the broad response elicited by DNA vaccines, since, in these last cases, opsonins or antitoxin antibodies, rather than cellular response, play the major protective role.

6.2. DNA-BASED IMMUNIZATION WITH PARASITIC ANTIGENS

Vaccination against parasites is an emerging and exciting field of genetic immunization. Parasites pose interesting and difficult problems in terms of protective vaccination, due to their enormous complexity as well as mechanisms of escaping immune surveillance. Some parasites exhibit high ability to vary their antigens during certain development stages (*Plasmodium*, *Giardia*, African trypanosomes). Others evade the immune system by entering host cells (*Plasmodium*, *Leishmania*, *Toxoplasma*, American trypanosomes). Other parasites share antigens with host cells or produce immune suppressor factors (African and American trypanosomes). Defining protective mechanisms and the corresponding antigens proves to be the most challenging step toward developing vaccines against parasites.

Most of the efforts regarding antiparasite vaccines are focused on *Plasmodium*, because malaria causes millions of deaths yearly. Compared to classical vaccines such as recombinant protein or peptides, DNA vaccination displays the advantage of inducing significant CTL responses against pre-erythrocytic forms, without the use of adjuvants. Ideally, an effective vaccine against malaria should be specific for sporozoites or hepatic pre-erythrocytic forms that do not exhibit antigenic variability. In addition, the plasmid DNA is endowed with adjuvant activity that may be particularly important for priming Th1 responses and inhibiting Th2 responses. However, the differential role of Th1 and Th2 responses may vary with the parasite. For example, whereas the Th1 cellular responses may be important for protective immunity against certain intracellular parasites such as *Leishmania major*, Th2-assisted immunity may be of particular importance during the defense against multicellular parasites, especially worms. Based on this observation, it is expected that DNA-based immunization would display variable protective ability depending on the targeted parasite.

6.2.1. Immunization with Plasmids Expressing Antigens from the Genus *Plasmodium*

Malaria is a disease caused by species of the genus *Plasmodium*, which are protozoa transmitted to humans by infected mosquitoes. *P. falciparum* is the cause of severe malaria, as well as cerebral complications and black fever. The sporozoites in the salivary gland of mosquitoes are inoculated into human hosts and infect the hepatocytes. At that stage, while the parasites mature to liver-stage schizonts, the hepatocytes express *Plasmodium*-derived epitopes that may be recognized by specific CTLs. The infected hepatocytes release merozoites that infect red blood cells. Maturation of the parasites inside red blood cells leads to either gametocytes or merozoites that can infect more red blood cells. Mosquitoes, upon feeding, are infected with gametocytes that undergo fertilization in stomach and maturation to sporozoites that are infectious for humans, in the mosquito salivary glands. The rupture of erythrocyte schizonts is responsible for fever and chills. Infected erythrocytes may obstruct the capillaries or venules in vital organs such as the brain, leading to the severe complications specific for advanced malaria.

Interestingly, in spite of the fact that infected individuals mount humoral and cellular responses against different *Plasmodium* antigens expressed at various stages during life cycle, the passive or acquired immunity does not protect against reinfections. However, illness associated with reinfection is less severe. Of particular importance are antibodies against the erythrocyte-stage parasites that interfere with the pathogenesis of the most serious complications of the infection. Antibodies against gametocytes negatively interfere with the infectious potential of the blood. Most interestingly, cellular immunity against the hepatic stage of the parasite may be involved in early interruption of the biological cycle. Because of the enormous incidence of infection, the associated morbidity and mortality, especially throughout developing countries, and the difficulty in eradicating the insect vector, effective vaccines against *P. falciparum* are acutely needed.

An effective vaccine against malaria raises a significant challenge because of the remarkable ability of the parasite at various stages to modify critical epitopes, thus escaping protective responses. Consequently, vaccines that protect against parasite forms at early stages of biological cycle are preferred. As noted previously in animal models, irradiated sporozoites induce protective responses. Prototypical vaccines, composed of recombinant proteins or peptides representing antigens or epitopes expressed by the parasite at various developmental stages, failed to demonstrate a significant protective capacity (reviewed by Kwiatkowski and Marsh, 1997). Thus, the evaluation in clinical trials of peptide-based vaccines was not encouraging. This can be related to the low immunogenicity and MHC restriction of peptides, as well as to natural genetic variation of *Plasmodium* antigens.

Since there are no current reliable vaccines against malaria, the assessment of DNA vaccination strategy in experimental models raised tremendous interest (Table 6.2). In particular, the concept that DNA immunization, by promoting intracellular expression of antigens, may be a good CTL inducer was convincing enough to stimulate the study of protection against the early liver stage of the disease. A first, seminal report showed that intramuscular inoculation into mice of a plasmid expressing the circumsporozoite protein (CSP) of *P. yoelii* leads to induction of specific antibodies and CTL (Sedegah et al., 1994). This study produced two notable conclusions: first, that DNA immunization actually induced higher levels of antibodies and CTL compared to irradiated sporozoites; and second, that the protection conferred by DNA immunization against challenge with sporozoites was dependent on CD8$^+$ T-cells. However, only approximately half of the DNA-immunized mice were protected against the challenge with 10^2 sporozoites, indicating that the immunity was not optimal from a qualitative and/or quantitative point of view (Sedegah et al., 1994; Hoffman et al., 1994). Since immunization with irradiated sporozoites induces optimal protection, it was speculated that epitopes not found on CSP might exert significant

Table 6.2. Immunity-Induced by DNA-Based Vaccines Expressing *Plasmodium* Antigens

Antigen	Model	Immunity	Reference
CSP of *P. yoelii*	Mice	Abs, Th, CTL	Sedegah et al., 1994
			Mor et al., 1995
CSP, HEP 17 of *P. yoelii*	Mice	CTL	Doolan et al., 1996
SSP2 of *P. yoelii*	Mice	Protection	Hoffman et al., 1997a, 1997b
CSP of *P. berghei*	Mice	Abs	Leitner et al., 1997
CTL epitopes of *P. falciparum*	Mice	CTL	Hanke et al., 1998
CSP of *P. yoelii*	Nonhuman primates	Abs	Gardner et al., 1996
			Gramzinski et al., 1997
CSP of *P. falciparum*	Humans	CTL	Hoffman et al., 1997a
			Wang et al., 1998a

protective roles (Hoffman et al., 1994). A subsequent report from the same group actually showed increased protection, close to 100%, in BALB/c mice immunized with a combination of plasmids expressing CSP and another hepatic-stage antigen, PyHEP17 (Doolan et al., 1996). The same study addressed the problem of genetic restriction of protection and showed, as expected, that the combination of plasmids expressing different antigens leads to significant protection in multiple mouse strains. Recently, it was reported that DNA vaccination against still another *P. yoelii* sporozoite antigen (PySSP2) induced protection in mice (Hoffman et al., 1997a). Most interestingly, the protection conferred by these pre-erythrocytic DNA vaccines was totally dependent on CD8$^+$ T-cells, IFN-γ, and nitric oxide (Sedegah et al., 1994; Doolan et al., 1996). This result strongly argues that Tc1 cells specific for hepatic-stage antigens either directly and/or through the employment of additional effectors, such as activated macrophages, clear the parasite from the infected hepatocytes. The question—whether actual lysis of infected hepatocytes is necessary for the clearance—is still not answered. However, it seems clear that the different mechanisms of protection mediated by CD4$^+$ versus CD8$^+$ T-cells are MHC restricted (Doolen and Hoffman, 1997).

The profile of the Th response subsequent to DNA immunization of mice with a plasmid expressing the CSP of *P. yoelii* was analyzed in detail from the point of view of cytokine secretion and isotypes of specific antibodies (Mor et al., 1995). Surprisingly, intramuscular inoculation of this plasmid was followed by priming of CSP-specific Th2 responses, including IgG1 antibodies. Only after the boost was there a significant shift toward a Th1-type immune response, which may indirectly suggest an explanation for the interesting result obtained with CSP-expressing plasmids in newborn mice, namely, that single inoculation induced long-term *B*- and *T*-cell unresponsiveness (Mor et al., 1996). CSP, as delivered by plasmid-based expression vectors, may be endowed with low ability to prime highly-proliferating Th1-dependent immune cells, at least in certain mouse strains. Follow-up studies addressed the unusual observation of tolerance induction by neonatal DNA vaccination of mice with CSP. The window associated with tolerance induction was only 1 week following birth, but the unresponsiveness persisted for approximately 1 year (Ichino et al., 1999). Interestingly, although the direct dependence of unresponsiveness on the dose of plasmid suggested "high-zone tolerance" mediated by deletion/anergy, CD8$^+$ T-cells could transfer the unresponsive state (Ichino et al., 1999) and coimmunization with

GM-CSF-expressing plasmid prevented the tolerance (N. Ishii et al., 1999b). Thus, the data imply generation by neonatal DNA vaccination with CSP of unusual, long-lived CD8[+] T-suppressor cells. An interesting question—both from the point of view of potential side effects of neonatal DNA vaccination and applications in autoimmunity areas—that remains to be answered is the antigen-dependency of this phenomenon.

Immunization of mice with different *Plasmodium* antigens or different forms of antigen produced interesting observations. For example, DNA immunization of BALB/c mice with plasmids expressing CSP of *P. berghei* showed, first, that the highest antibody response was obtained by intradermal immunization and multiple boosts; second, that repeated intradermal administration of DNA led to polarization from Th2 toward Th1 response; and third, that immunization with irradiated sporozoites induced comparable humoral responses (Leitner et al., 1997). A recent report in a similar experimental model showed that whereas DNA priming and subsequent boost with recombinant vaccinia virus was followed by increased protection against infectious challenge, priming with vaccinia and boost with DNA were not effective (Schneider et al., 1998). Follow-up studies strengthened the idea that priming with DNA and boosting with conventional-type vectors affords inherent advantages regarding the quality and magnitude of immune response (Degano et al., 1999). Other recent reports showed immunogenicity in mice with plasmids expressing tandem repeat epitopes of *P. falciparum* (Gerloni et al., 1997; Hanke et al., 1998).

Subsequent to the demonstration of efficacy for DNA vaccines against malaria in rodents, efforts were aimed at characterizing and optimizing the immune response in non-human primates. Relatively recent studies reported successful priming of CSP-specific antibodies in Aotus monkeys inoculated intradermally with a plasmid expressing CSP of *P. yoelii* (Gardner et al., 1996; Gramzinski et al., 1997). Noteworthy is that these studies showed the efficacy of DNA immunization in priming humoral response to be similar to that of peptide/adjuvant-based immunization (Gramzinski et al., 1997).

Recently, the first initiated clinical trial was aimed at assessing the safety and immunogenicity of a plasmid expressing CSP of *P. falciparum* (Hoffman et al., 1997b; Doolan et al., 1997b). A particularly important endpoint of this Phase I/II clinical trial was the ability of DNA vaccines to induce specific CD8[+] T-cells. Recently reported results of this trial show the safety of DNA vaccines up to doses of 2.5 mg/inoculation, administered to healthy volunteers, and induction of CSP-specific CTL restricted by multiple HLA Class I alleles (Wang et al., 1998a). Taking into consideration the positive results of this preliminary trial, a new clinical trial will probably be initiated. This time, the vaccine will consist of multiple plasmids expressing CSP, HEP17, SSP2, and possibly other hepatic-stage antigens of *P. falciparum* (Hoffman et al., 1997b; Hedstrom et al., 1997). Volunteers will be challenged with sporozoites, and the protection conferred by multiple-gene vaccination will be thus evaluated (Hoffman et al., 1997b). Recently, some data were released from a Phase I safety and tolerability clinical trial addressing vaccination with various doses (20–2,500 µg/three times, intramuscular) of Pf-CSP-expressing plasmid (Le et al., 2000). Importantly, only a few mild side effects confined to the injection site were noted in the 20 volunteers that were vaccinated. Despite the significant CTL immunity induced by this CSP-expressing DNA vaccine, no antigen-specific antibodies were detected in the immunized volunteers. Protection data will certainly be very important in evaluating the efficacy of antimalaria DNA vaccines in humans.

In conclusion, prototypical DNA vaccines studied, particularly in the model of

P. yoelii, proved to be immunogenic. Their protection ability depended on priming of CD8$^+$ T-cells as well as simultaneous expression of multiple antigens that could circumvent both the genetic variability of the recipients and the antigen variation of the parasite. In fact, the efforts of DNA vaccination against malaria are focused on developing vectors that express hepatic-stage antigens, with the hope of preventing early cycles of the parasite. Based on these considerations, a potentially more optimal DNA vaccine comprising multiple antigens is to be tested in humans.

6.2.2. DNA Vaccination against Other Parasites

Leishmania major, together with *Plasmodium yoelii*, was one of the first parasites evaluated from the point of view of DNA immunization. Various *Leishmania* species cause mucocutaneous (*L. major*) or visceral lesions (*L. donovani*). The parasite is transmitted from infected sand flies in the form of promastigotes that infect and proliferate in phagolysosomes of macrophages and other cells of the reticuloendothelial system. In the extracellular space, the parasite evades the immune response by bearing self-HLA antigens on the membrane that are picked up from the host cells.

BALB/c mice infected with *L. major* develop a Th2-mediated disease. Early reports showed that immunization of BALB/c mice with a plasmid expressing the gp63 antigen of *L. major* was followed by induction of Th1 responses that protected susceptible mice against infectious challenge (Xu and Liew, 1994, 1995). In contrast, BALB/c mice injected with only the control vector did not display any protection. DNA immunization of BALB/c mice with a different antigen, namely, LACK, was followed by induction of Th1 immunity and protection against infectious challenge with promastigotes. The protection correlated with the production of IFN-γ and was dependent on CD8$^+$ T-cells (Gurunathan et al., 1997). The immune response primed by DNA vaccine mimicked the response elicited by the recombinant LACK protein plus IL-12 and was superior to the response triggered by recombinant protein alone. Further work in a different antigenic system showed that DNA immunization of mice with the surface Ag-2 of *L. major* primed a protective Th1 response (Sjolander et al., 1998). In stark contrast, immunization with immune stimulatory complexes (ISCOMs) containing Ag-2 led to mixed Th1/Th2 responses that were nonprotective. Another recent study underscored the tremendous importance of the Th profile during the immune response of BALB/c mice to *L. major*. Intriguingly, administration of synthetic oligodeoxynucleotides containing CpG motifs (CpG-ODN) to BALB/c mice previously infected with *L. major* induced reversion of the ongoing Th2 response as well as recovery from disease (Zimmermann et al., 1998). This study elegantly illustrates the beneficial role as adjuvant for the plasmid-based expression vectors, particularly in such instances of Th2-driven infectious diseases, but at the same time calls for more careful dissection of antigen-specific and nonspecific consequences of DNA inoculation. A very recent study approached DNA vaccination from a different perspective by using "expression library"-based immunization against multiple antigens of *L. major* (Piedrafita et al., 1999). Using the BALB/c model of selecting sublibraries associated with protection against infection with *L. major*, the authors could narrow down a protective sublibrary from 10^5 to 10^3 clones after two rounds of partition and selection.

Other investigators have studied the effect of DNA immunization against different unicellular parasites (Table 6.3). Thus, the immunization of BALB/c mice with a plasmid expressing the p30 protein of *Toxoplasma gondii* or an expression genomic library of *Trypanosoma cruzi* led to the generation of specific humoral responses (Angus et al., 1996; Alberti et al., 1998). An independent group showed that DNA immunization of calves with two allelic forms (Tams1-1 and Tams1-2) of the major merozoite surface antigen of *Theileria annulata* induced a degree of protection against infectious challenge in the absence of detectable titers of antibodies (d'Oliveira et al., 1997). It is noteworthy that calves vaccinated with ISCOMs containing Tams-recombinant proteins displayed a similar effect, namely, enhanced protection associated with detectable titers of specific antibodies. More recently, BALB/c mice were successfully immunized via intranasal instillation with a DNA vaccine expressing the 15-kDa antigen of *Cryptosporidium parvum*, a protozoan parasite infecting the enterocytes of immune-suppressed individuals (Sagodira et al., 1999). The immunization resulted in induction of specific IgA in the gastrointestinal tract, systemic IgG, and local and systemic T-cell responses.

One of the most intriguing potential applications for DNA immunization is vaccination against multicellular parasites. An early report showed that inoculation of BALB/c mice with a plasmid expressing the paramyosin (Sj97) of *Schistosoma japonicum*, a trematode worm, was followed by priming of specific antibodies (Yang et al., 1995). However, mouse inoculation of a plasmid expressing another *S. japonicum* antigen, Sj26, was not followed by antibody induction. A subsequent study, while confirming the immunogenicity of paramyosin, or paramyosin fragments when delivered by plasmid expression vectors, showed lack of antibody responses against other antigens of *S. japonicum*: glutathione-S-transferases, calreticulin, glyceraldehyde-3-phosphate dehydrogenase, a 22.6 kDa membrane associated antigen, and a 14 kDa fatty-acid-binding protein (Waine et al., 1997). Most importantly, the antiparamyosin antibodies elicited by DNA immunization failed to protect the mice against challenge with cercariae of *S. japonicum*. This result illustrates the difficulties in mounting protective immune responses against trematode worms (Waine et al., 1997). Another recent study addressed the potential application of DNA immunization for the vaccination against *S. mansoni* (Dupre et al., 1997). Inoculation of rats with a

Table 6.3. DNA Immunization against Other Parasites

Parasite	Antigen	Species	Immunity	Reference
Leishmania major	gp63 antigen	Mice	*T*-cells	Xu and Liew, 1994
	LACK antigen	Mice	CTL	Gurunathan et al., 1997
	Ag-2	Mice	Th	Sjolander et al., 1998
	Expression library	Mice	Abs, Th	Piedrafita et al., 1999
Trypanosoma cruzi	Expression library	Mice	Abs	Alberti et al., 1998
Cryptosporidium parvum	15 kDa Ag	Mice	Abs, Th	Sagodira et al., 1999
Toxoplasma gondii	p30 protein	Mice	Abs	Angus et al., 1996
Schistosoma japonicum (Sj)	Sj 96, 26 antigens	Mice	Abs	Yang et al., 1995
and *S. mansoni* (Sm)	Various Sj antigens	Mice	Abs	Waine et al., 1997
	Sm 28GST antigen	Rats	Abs	Dupre et la., 1997
Theileria annulata	Tams1 antigen	Calves	Protection	d'Oliveira et al., 1997
Taenia ovis	45W antigen	Sheep	Abs	Rothel et al., 1997

plasmid expressing the 28 kDa glutathione-S-transferase antigen of *S. mansoni* was followed by the priming of long-lasting IgG antibodies. Importantly, these antibodies were able to mediate *in vitro* antibody-dependent cellular cytotoxicity against the parasite larvae (Dupre et al., 1997). In spite of the demonstration of *in vivo* priming by this DNA vaccine in rats subsequently challenged with parasites, no conclusive evidence regarding *in vivo* protection is available yet.

The immune response against *Taenia ovis* antigen 45W was recently examined in sheep immunized with a plasmid-based or recombinant vaccine (Rothel et al., 1997). The specific antibody response triggered by genetic immunization, although present, was relatively modest and not significantly enhanced by boosting. In contrast, priming with the plasmid-based vaccine and boosting with the recombinant protein with adjuvant led to significantly enhanced antibody titers. However, only animals immunized with DNA and boosted with recombinant adenovirus or protein mounted protective responses.

Thus, except for the cases of *Plasmodium* and *Leishmania*, the study of DNA vaccination against parasites is only beginning. Work still needs to be carried out regarding more profound assessment of DNA vaccines against other uni- and multicellular parasites. The work should be directed at both defining the protective mechanisms and antigens, and understanding if and how the strategy of genetic immunization can help in that concern.

6.3. CONCLUSIONS AND PERSPECTIVES

During the last few years, major advances were made in the field of DNA vaccination against two leading pathogens, a bacterium and a parasite, namely, *M. tuberculosis* and *Plasmodium*, respectively.

Two categories of *Mycobacterium* antigens, stress and secreted proteins, were shown to be immunogenic and protective in rodent models. Both categories of antigens exert their protective effects through the induction of Th1-assisted CTL immunity. Most importantly, while such antigens still induce protective immunity, they allow independent testing for infection through classical means, namely, the tuberculin reaction. However, rarely have such new DNA vaccines displayed higher protection ability compared to conventional live attenuated BCG vaccine in preclinical models. Probably, a future prototype vaccine against *M. tuberculosis* would contain combinations of antigens, both stress and secreted, thus ensuring a broader and increased immunity.

The accumulated experience in the field of DNA immunization against malaria offers clues as to how an ideal vaccination strategy should be designed. First, there is a tremendous consensus in the scientific community that the target should be the hepatic-stage antigens, since they are expressed relatively early during the biological cycle and are recognized by CTL, and readily induced by genetic immunization. Second, combinations of antigens may not only enhance the overall immunity but also may circumvent the genetic restriction of the immune response as well as antigenic variability of the parasite. Third, very recent developments in the field suggest that a vaccination protocol of priming with DNA and boosting with more classical vectors, such as recombinant viruses, would result in enhanced immunity (Schneider et al., 1998; Sedegah et al., 1998). Studies in nonhuman primates led to subsequent initiation of clinical trials that are currently ongoing or recently reported (Wang et al., 1998a).

While the studies regarding DNA immunization against other bacterial or parasitic pathogens are not so advanced, they have already generated some important knowledge. One of the most exciting new strategies of vaccination, the expression library immunization, was successfully applied in preclinical models and may have potential applications in rapidly designing protective vaccines against poorly described pathogens, as well as circumventing antigen variation of certain parasites. The study of DNA vaccine against bacteria led to a deeper understanding of the factors that regulate the transcription and translation of bacterial open reading frames in mammalian context (Strugnell et al., 1997). Another interesting advance in the field of DNA vaccines came with the understanding of the molecular basis of the adjuvant activity of plasmids. DNA immunization against *Leishmania major* elegantly illustrates this aspect.

During the next few years, more information will emerge regarding the safety and efficiency of malaria vaccines in humans and perhaps we will witness the first clinical trial of a DNA vaccine against tuberculosis. Possibly, methods to modify the magnitude and quality of immune responses primed by DNA vaccines will offer new solutions for vaccination against various bacteria or parasites.

Chapter 7

Autoimmunity, Allergy, and Genetic Vaccines

7.1. BACTERIAL DNA: ANTIGEN AND IMMUNE MODULATOR

Three parameters of the plasmid-based expression vectors may interfere with the homeo-stasis of the immune system, responsible for self–nonself discrimination and regulation of response to nonself. First, the presence of immune stimulatory unmethylated CpG motifs in bacterial DNA (Krieg, 1996; Tighe et al., 1998) is responsible for the Th1-promoting adjuvant activity. Second, the plasmid DNA itself acts like an antigen and may trigger the generation or enhancement of anti-DNA antibodies above pathological thresholds. Third, the antigens expressed by plasmid-based vectors may cross-react to a certain extent with self-antigens. These three properties, together with factors such as route, frequency, and dose of inoculation may be exploited, with the aim of preventing or suppressing auto-immune and allergic conditions. Furthermore, understanding the interplay among these factors will eventually allow for minimizing unwanted side effects of DNA-based vaccines.

Beforehand, based on the known characteristics of DNA vaccines, one may expect certain applications in the area of allergy and a few concerns regarding potential triggering or exacerbation of autoimmunity. First, because the allergic phenomena are mediated by Th2 cells, the strong Th1 stimulatory activity of bacterial plasmids may be exploited with some benefits. In contrast, Th1-mediated immune pathology, as well as anti-DNA antibody-mediated disease, may be enhanced by genetic vaccination. However, our data showed that administration of plasmids to mice or baboons did not result in induction of anti-ds DNA antibodies (Bot et al., 2000, submitted) that spontaneously occur in SLE. If these general examples are the somewhat expected situations that are consistent with current paradigms in immunity, there are intriguing potential applications of genetic vaccines in this area. For example, plasmid-based vectors may be used actually to deliver Th2-promoting cytokines that can prevent or interrupt Th1-mediated pathological processes. Furthermore, antigen delivery via plasmid-based expression vectors may be used to downregulate antiself-immune responses. We provide specific examples for the aforementioned cases. However, the area of DNA vaccines in autoimmunity and allergy is relatively new, and there are still numerous unanswered questions that obviously restrict our ability to confidently apply them in this concern.

7.2. DNA VACCINES IN ALLERGIC CONDITIONS

Allergy is an immune-mediated pathological process caused by IgE antibodies and associated inflammation triggered by allergen-specific Th2 cells that have escaped from normal immune homeostasis.

Earlier attempts to use DNA-based vaccines for suppressing allergic responses originated from the empirical observation that inoculation of plasmid expression vectors was associated with Th1 rather than Th2 immune responses. Induction of Th1 memory cells specific for allergens may downregulate the subsequent priming of pathogenic Th2 cells, thus preventing allergic reactions. Hsu et al. (1996b) reported that intramuscular inoculation of rats with a plasmid expressing a common allergen, Der p5, of the house dust mite, prevented the induction of specific IgE antibodies as well as asthma subsequent to aerosol sensitization. Furthermore, immunization of mice with this allergen-expressing plasmid, despite induction of humoral and cellular immune responses, greatly prevented the generation of specific IgE antibodies subsequent to intraperitoneal (i.p.) challenge with recombinant protein (Hsu et al., 1996a). One of the most interesting conclusions of these reports is that allergen-specific $CD8^+$ T-cells seem to be associated with the beneficial antiallergic effects. Whereas it is relatively straightforward to explain their induction following DNA immunization, it is more difficult to explain their stimulation during allergen challenge without accepting a role for nonclassical pathways of processing and presentation in the context of MHC Class I molecules.

Using a different experimental system, an independent group showed similar results: namely, inoculation of DNA expressing bacterial β-galactosidase (β-gal) induced T-cells that produced IFN-γ and IgG2a-specific antibodies, and largely prevented the induction of specific IgE antibodies subsequent to inoculation of recombinant protein in alum (Raz et al., 1996). However, there are three significant differences regarding the approach or the results: first, despite intradermal administration of the β-gal-expressing plasmid, the T-cell response was strongly biased toward Th1. Second, DNA immunization significantly suppressed the IgE antibodies and induced Th1 cells even in mice primed with recombinant β-gal in alum, which triggers strong Th2 responses. Third, $CD4^+$ as well as $CD8^+$ T-cells from plasmid-immunized mice were able to suppress the onset of IgE response upon subsequent inoculation of recombinant protein (Lee et al., 1997). Most interestingly, the suppression of IgE antibodies by previous DNA immunization was significantly impaired in β2-microglobulin-deficient mice (Lee et al., 1997), underscoring again the unexpected role for $CD8^+$ T-cells. Since the suppression of IgE antibodies occurred in a specific manner, namely, being restricted to the original antigen (Raz et al., 1996; Hsu et al., 1996b), it is more probable that specific $CD8^+$ T-cells primed by DNA vaccine are restimulated by protein or allergen. Moreover, this observation underscores the important role of the bacterial plasmid as expression vector for the allergen, a conclusion that is coherent with the inability of control plasmids to induce similar effects (Hsu et al., 1996a; Raz et al., 1996). A more recent follow-up report underscored the potential of DNA expression vectors to promote Th1 immunity simultaneously with the downregulation of a preexisting Th2-controlled IgE response to LacZ or OVA in a BALB/c mouse model (Raz and Spiegelberg, 1999). The effect could be reproduced by adoptive transfer of either $CD4^+$ or $CD8^+$ antigen-specific T-cells and correlated with the induction of Th1-promoting cytokines in antigen-presenting cells. In a mouse model of food allergy to the peanut antigen (Arah2), mucosal immunization with a DNA expression vector resulted in decreased levels of anaphylaxis-inducing IgE antibodies (Roy et al., 1999). Interestingly, the formulation of DNA in chitosan nanoparticles led to a more pronounced effect, probably due to protection of plasmid and enhanced expression in the intestinal epithelium.

Due to the more recent identification of bacterial CpG motifs that stimulate the innate immunity and Th1 responses, there has been a justified interest in understanding the contribution, and perhaps defining the therapeutic benefit, of such oligodeoxynucleotides (ODN). Two directions were followed: first, use of CpG ODN to enhance the immunogenicity of protein-based vaccines; and second, use of the ODN to suppress allergic reactions. Coinoculation of HBsAg/alum, together with CpG ODN in mice, was followed by a significant increase of specific antibody response, a strong Th1 response, but most intriguingly, by the generation of specific CTL (Davis et al., 1998). This observation shows that the effect of DNA immunization including CTL induction can be entirely reproduced by immunization with protein in adjuvant plus CpG ODN. Another recent study, directly relevant for the potential of CpG ODN to suppress pathogenic Th2 responses, showed that coinoculation of ODNs with allergen (*Schistosoma mansoni* eggs) prevented specific symptoms in a murine model for asthma (Kline et al., 1998). The effect was associated with decrease of lung eosinophilia and prevention of IgE, Th2 responses, as well as bronchial hyperreactivity subsequent to local challenge with allergen. Thus, priming with the allergen in presence of CpG ODN largely prevented a subsequent Th2 pathogenic response. Data are not yet available and it would be interesting to know the effect of ODN-based therapy on sensitization of animals with allergen. Such information may lead to new prophylactic approaches in individuals prone to allergy. A significant clue regarding the role of immune-stimulatory CpG motifs was provided by a more recent analysis of the Th profile of immune response elicited by Bet v1, a major allergen of birch pollen, delivered as protein via recombinant DNA, with or without addition of CpG motifs (Hartl et al., 1999). The contrasting Th1 response elicited by DNA vaccine in this BALB/c model was more pronounced upon addition of stimulatory CpG motifs.

This information indicates that (1) DNA-based expression of allergen can prevent Th2 pathogenic responses; (2) CpG ODN may reproduce the effects of plasmids when administered together with the allergen; (3) except for few data (Raz et al., 1996), it is not generally known to what extent DNA-based immunization can be used to ameliorate Th2 responses in previously sensitized organisms.

7.3. DNA VACCINATION AGAINST AUTOIMMUNE DISEASES

Autoimmune diseases are mediated by *T*-cells and/or antibodies that recognize self-epitopes. Through various mechanisms, autoreactive lymphocytes escape central and peripheral tolerance and in certain conditions are activated, inflicting disease. Depending on the disease or experimental model, genetic and environmental factors are involved to a different extent. For example, whereas non-obese diabetic (NOD) mice develop diabetes independently of exposure to environmental antigens, some transgenic mice that express viral antigens in the pancreas develop diabetes through cross-reaction with nonself antigens. Designing strategies to suppress autoimmunity should take into consideration such points. For example, inducing antigen-dependent mediated cell death by frequent inoculation of soluble antigen might be very difficult in individuals that are genetically defective in the Fas-mediated cell-death pathway. As an alternative approach, one may want to try switching the pathogenic phenotype of the autoreactive *T*-cells toward nonpathogenic or suppressor cells. In contrast, the antigen-activated cell-death strategy may work better in the case of autoimmune diseases triggered by cross-reaction with nonself antigens. It is very important to stress that since autoimmune diseases usually occur in individuals with one or more affected tolerance checkpoints, selective immune therapeutic strategies are effective only if they address or circumvent these defects.

A few studies approached gene delivery of antigens as a means to prevent the onset of autoimmunity in animal models (Table 7.1). An initial report described the effect of immunization of Lewis rats with a plasmid expressing hsp65 (heat shock protein) on the induction of adjuvant arthritis (Ragno et al., 1997). Interestingly, despite the fact that rats preinoculated with plasmid displayed increased hsp65-specific antibody and *T*-cell responses even after adjuvant injection, they were clinically protected against arthritis. Possibly, genetic immunization induced suppressor cells or, alternatively, directly downregulated a subset of precursors of pathogenic *T*-cells. A subsequent interesting report studied the effect of genetic immunization of Lewis rats on the susceptibility to experimental allergic encephalomyelitis (EAE) triggered by immunization with guinea pig myelin basic protein (MBP) 68-85 peptide in complete Freund's adjuvant (CFA) (Lobell et al., 1998). The plasmid used for immunization expressed the similar peptide as well as a microbial motif responsible for the binding to Fc of IgG. Genetic immunization with this construct

Table 7.1. DNA Vaccines in Preclinical Models of Autoimmunity and Allergy

Disease category	Experimental model	Reference
Allergy (Th2-mediated pathology)	House dust mite allergy (Der p5 allergen)	Hsu et al., 1996a, 1996b
	Immune response to LacZ	Raz et al., 1996
		Lee et al., 1997
	Latex allergy (Hev b5 allergen)	Slater and Colberg-Poley, 1997
	Murine asthma (CpG-ODN)	Kline et al., 1998
	Peanut allergy (Arah2 allergen)	Roy et al., 1999
Immune-mediated pathology (Th1-dependent)	Herpetic stromal keratitis (plasmid-mediated delivery of cytokines)	Daheshia et al., 1997
	Theiler's virus encephalomyelitis (VP2 and VP3 antigens)	Tolley et al., 1999
Autoimmunity		
Plasmid-mediated antigen delivery	Adjuvant arthritis (hsp65 antigen)	Ragno et al., 1997
	EAE (MBP 68-85)	Lobell et al., 1998
	EAE (PLP 139–151)	Ruiz et al., 1999
	Autoimmune diabetes (insulin B chain)	Coon et al., 1999
Plasmid-mediated idiotype delivery	TCR of *T*-cells from rheumatoid arthritis	Williams et al., 1994
	Vβ8.2 of MBP-specific *T*-cells	Waisman et al., 1996
Plasmid-mediated cytokine delivery or modulation	TGFβ in MRL/lpr/lpr mice	Raz et al., 1995
	TNF-α in EAE model	Wildbaum and Karin, 1999

largely prevented the induction of EAE. However, there are three notable particularities of this study. First, the dose of plasmid used for immunization was approximately 10–100 times higher than minimal doses that elicit immune responses. Second, there was no significant Th switch caused by genetic immunization in this model. Third, the IgG binding ability of the expressed construct was required, suggesting that endogenous internalization via Fcγ receptors facilitated the suppressor effect of the peptide. This interesting and somewhat surprising result may be explained by one or both of the following mechanisms: FcγR-mediated targeting of antigen to professional APC (Zaghouani et al., 1993a), followed by more effective antigen-induced T-cell death and/or FcγR-mediated triggering of suppressor cytokines such as IL-10 (Sutterwala et al., 1998) that might facilitate T-cell anergy induction. Follow-up studies, while shedding some light on the mechanisms of suppression, certainly underlined an interesting characteristic of the EAE model, namely, the pleiotropic effect of IFN-γ. Thus, surprisingly, the elimination of immune stimulatory CpG motifs from the MBP-expressing vector abolished its suppressing effect (Lobell et al., 1999). Independently, another group showed that IFN-γ induction by noncoding bacterial DNA contributes to disease suppression (Boccaccio et al., 1999). These results are still at odds with a report demonstrating exacerbation of disease by preinjection of CpG motifs in SJL/J mice infected with Theiler's murine encephalomyelitis virus or inoculated with proteolipid protein (PLP) peptides (Tsunoda et al., 1999).

Such discrepancies stemming from mechanistic differences may reveal potentially important issues that have to be considered before employing large-scale antigen-based immune therapy via genetic expression vectors: (1) the level of understanding the mechanism of disease in various clinical subpopulations; (2) the possibility of designing vectors that, irrespective of the disease stage and variability of pathogenic factors, are devoid of aggravating effects. Three subsequent studies complicated the emerging model regarding the mechanism of suppressive DNA vaccines: for example, one study suggested that DNA vaccination with an encephalitogenic PLP epitope suppresses the disease via anergy due to reduced costimulation, leading to decreased production of Th1 cytokines (including IFN-γ) in the brain (Ruiz et al., 1999). In the Lewis rat model, it was shown that DNA vaccination with one MBP epitope could not suppress the disease triggered by another MBP encephalitogenic epitope (Weissert et al., 2000), arguing against a bystander suppression mechanism. In sharp contrast, in a transgenic model of autoimmune diabetes based on epitope mimicry, vaccination with DNA expressing the insulin B chain resulted in induction of regulatory CD4$^+$ T-cells that migrated to the local lymph nodes and downregulated the activity of antiself CD8$^+$ T-cells, probably via IL-4 production (Coon et al., 1999).

Thus, these recent studies led to surprising results, because the plasmid-based vectors display intrinsic Th1 adjuvant properties as well as limited expression level of antigens, making them poor candidates for either Th2 switch or antigen-induced T-cell death on these theoretical grounds. However, it is not yet clear what immune mechanisms operate in the cases mentioned earlier and to what extent different mechanisms may operate in different models.

Another strategy for suppressing autoimmune responses is by indirectly targeting the autoreactive T-cells through the idiotypic network. The principle consists in generating T-cells that recognize epitopes in the variable region of TCR from autoreactive T-cells. These anti-idiotypic T-cells would turn off the pathogenic T-cells. Furthermore, genetic immunization displays the advantage of CTL priming that may mediate deletion of idiotypic autoreactive T-cells. The limitation of this strategy stems from the frequent polyclonal character of the autoreactive T-cells, particularly during later stages of disease, when epitope spreading is involved. An early report described the cloning of several full-length TCR from T-cells infiltrating the synovial tissue of patients with rheumatoid arthritis (Williams et al., 1994). Inoculation of plasmids expressing such TCR into mice was followed by induction of TCR-specific immune responses that were tested against TCR-α/β negative murine T-cell hybridoma transfected with human TCR. A more recent study took advantage of the restricted utilization of V_β on MBP-reactive pathogenic T-cells from H-2^u mice with EAE (Waisman et al., 1996). Vaccination of the mice with a plasmid-expressing V_β8.2 protected them against MBP-induced EAE. However, the apparent shift toward a Th2 profile of MBP-reactive T-cells in the mice vaccinated with plasmid was rather unexpected. This observation raises two issues: First, what is the mechanism responsible for this shift? Second, can such a mechanism be used to induce bystander suppressor T-cells? Possibly, V_β8.2-specific T-cells raised by genetic immunization might have selectively suppressed precursors of pathogenic T-cells or, alternatively, might have shifted the differentiation of Th0 precursors toward Th2 phenotype. Recently, independent support for this type of approach has been generated in a model of autoimmune-induced neuritis, largely mediated by T-cells bearing V_β5 and V_β8.2 elements (Matsumoto et al., 2000). Vaccination with an expression vector encoding V_β5 resulted in attenuated autoimmune disease, confirming the role of this subset of T cells in the pathogeny and further pinpointing this interesting therapeutic strategy.

Another strategy to control autoimmune diseases is by cytokine-mediated immune modulation. An early report showed that monthly inoculation of plasmid-expressing TGF-β into MLR/lpr/lpr mice significantly delayed the onset and progression to SLE (Raz et al., 1995). Presumably, increased levels of systemic TGF-β directly suppressed pathogenic T-cells, slowing down the synthesis of IgG antibodies specific for chromatin or Fc. In contrast, monthly inoculation of a plasmid-expressing IL-2 had opposite effects, speeding up the onset of lupus in this experimental model. Together, these results suggest that plasmid-mediated cytokine delivery can be used for the purpose of immune modulation in autoimmune conditions. More details about this strategy of immune modulation are provided in the context of models for immune-mediated pathology during antimicrobial responses. More recently, two reports described successful modulation of EAE using an indirect approach based on DNA vaccination, namely, raising immunity against proinflammatory cytokines or chemokines. Thus, DNA vaccination with a TNF-α expression vector raised anti-TNF-α antibodies capable of inhibiting the disease (Wildbaum and Karin, 1999). In a similar experimental model, DNA vaccination with vectors expressing MIP-1α or MCP-1—known to be maximally expressed in the brain after the onset of disease—suppressed the disease (Youssef et al., 1999). It is interesting to notice, beyond the fact that some details of the mechanism remain elusive, that such a strategy comprises generation of immune responses by DNA vaccination against self-epitopes on regulatory molecules (i.e., cytokines or chemokines).

In conclusion, three plasmid-based strategies have been tested in preliminary experimental models of autoimmune diseases: (1) antigen delivery; (2) idiotypic vaccination; and (3) cytokine modulation. However, the elucidation of mechanisms responsible for the effects reported by these studies needs further work.

7.4. DNA VACCINES AND IMMUNE-MEDIATED PATHOLOGY

In this section we discuss three issues that concern either potential applications or side effects of DNA-based immunization: (1) plasmid-mediated delivery of suppressor cytokines in inflammatory conditions associated with infection; (2) induction of autoimmune responses using plasmid-based administration of self-antigens; and (3) induction or enhancement of anti-DNA antibodies subsequent to inoculation of microbial DNA.

Administration of cytokines via plasmid-based expression vectors is not a very recent issue and was first applied in the context of vaccination against microbes (Xiang and Ertl, 1995a). A recently tested model for plasmid-mediated cytokine delivery is the herpetic stromal keratitis. This is a condition due to postherpetic scarring of cornea, triggered by DTH reaction to local antigen. Previous studies suggested that while antigen-specific Th1 cells are important for the induction of stromal keratitis, local inoculation of the suppressor cytokine IL-10 was followed by significant inhibition of the lesions in a mouse model. The beneficial effect was associated with reduced local IL-2 and IL-6, but interestingly, the mechanisms responsible for the virus clearance were not affected (Tumpey et al., 1994). More recently, the protective effect of IL-10 against stromal keratitis was demonstrated in a similar model by local application of cytokine-expressing plasmid (Daheshia et al., 1997). A subsequent study published by the same group showed that local administration of IL-4-expressing plasmid had a similar suppressor effect on stromal keratitis (Chun et al., 1998). As an interesting finding, only preadministration of plasmid-expressing IL-4, but not IL-10, was followed by Th switch, although each of them inhibited the Th1-mediated DTH reaction to herpes virus. In contrast, IL-10 produced by transduced antigen-presenting cells probably acts by silencing the specific T-cells, a situation that may be reversed by exposure to IL-2 (Chun et al., 1999). This result underscores the multiplicity of immune suppressive pathways that might be therapeutically employed. Another recent report from the same group showed that nasal inoculation of plasmid-expressing TGF-β, while inducing significant protection against subsequently triggered herpes keratitis, was followed by impaired ability of mice to clear the virus (Kuklin et al., 1998). However, the administration of the plasmid after virus infection was not followed by protection against keratitis. Together, these results strengthen the conclusion that plasmid-mediated delivery of cytokines can be an effective way of immune modulation. A recent evaluation in adult and newborn mice gave positive results regarding the safety profile of IL-4- and IFN-γ-expressing plasmids administered in doses resulting in immune modulation (K.J. Ishii et al., 1999).

The strategy of plasmid-mediated delivery of antigens offered the opportunity to study the response of the immune system to self-antigens that are expressed in an ectopic manner. Of course, besides the expression subsequent to in $vivo$ transfection, plasmid inoculation is associated with strong Th1-promoting adjuvant effects that might trigger and/or enhance immune responses. An early paper, discussed in more detail in the next chapter, showed for the first time that inoculation into mice of a plasmid expressing the variable region of k light chain elicited anti-k chain antibodies (Watanabe et al., 1993). However, the k light chain used for immunization originated from a human leukemia library, so that the humoral response might have been directed to human determinants. A more recent report looked at the immunogenicity of CD4 protein as delivered via DNA or recombinant protein (Attanasio et al., 1997). Interestingly, DNA immunization of mice with CD4 was followed by induction of higher titers of antibodies that recognized conformational determinants, which means native CD4. The authors explained this result based on the potential advantage of DNA immunization to promote endogenous synthesis of native protein. Whereas both DNA and recombinant protein delivery were able to break the tolerance to CD4, the Th profiles of the immune responses were significantly different in accordance with other numerous observations. A recent and very interesting report studied the immune response of mice immunized with a plasmid expressing the human thyrotropin receptor (hTSHR). The original aim of the study was to take advantage of DNA-based immunization strategy to raise antibodies against conformational epitopes of hTSHR, otherwise a difficult task to accomplish by inoculation of recombinant protein (Costagliola et al., 1998). Mice immunized with DNA developed hTSHR-specific antibodies that displayed a blocking or activating function on the mouse receptor. In spite of the lack of significant endocrine disturbances, the mice displayed massive lymphocytic infiltration in the thyroid gland. Thus, ectopic expression of the human homologue of TSHR triggered cellular and humoral immune responses to the mouse TSHR. Again, the immunogenic role of human-specific epitopes might be a determinant of the results. Besides theoretical applications of such an approach to generate autoimmune responses, there are very few practical uses. Among these is the induction of antibodies against sex hormones or gamete antigens, with the purpose of immunocontraception (Ramway and Ramshaw, 1997).

Bacterial DNA displays antigenic properties that may contribute to induction or elevation of anti-DNA antibody titers known to have pathogenic effects, for example, in SLE. Recent studies showed that whereas antibodies in SLE patients bind to ss and ds DNA from many prokaryotic and eukaryotic species, anti-DNA antibodies encountered in certain normal individuals display restricted binding to microbial DNA (Wu et al., 1997). A study addressing whether DNA vaccines induce pathogenic anti-DNA antibodies and lupus-like syndrome found that in spite of the modest elevation of anti-DNA antibodies by plasmid vaccines, no glomerulonephritis of autoimmunity was triggered (Mor et al., 1997). Furthermore, no antimuscle cell antibodies or myositis were induced. Even DNA immunization of lupus-prone (NZBxNZF)F1 mice did not lead to alteration of the course of disease (Mor et al., 1997). Our studies showed the lack of anti-ds DNA antibodies in sera of mice immunized as newborns or adults with plasmids. We recently extended this observation to baboons immunized as neonates with a mixture of plasmids expressing hemagglutinin and nucleoprotein of influenza virus (Bot et al., 2000, submitted). However, it is unknown whether the DNA vaccines may induce clinically significant levels of pathogenic anti-DNA antibodies in lupus-prone individuals (Pisetsky, 1997).

Another legitimate concern of DNA vaccines is the triggering of Th1-mediated, organ-specific autoimmune diseases, since bacterial DNA has strong adjuvant activity. Simultaneous exposure to bacterial plasmid and self or self-modified antigens may lead to a break in immune ignorance or tolerance. A single report examined this possibility and found that MBP-specific *T*-cells in the presence of IL-12 became pathogenic when adoptively transferred into EAE-susceptible mice (Segal and Shevach, 1996). However, the authors were able to induce an IL-12-dependent pathogenic phenotype of the MBP-specific *T*-cells only by *in vitro* treatment.

A somewhat disturbing complexity in the mechanisms of immune-mediated pathology triggered by microbial infection, with direct implications on therapeutic strategies, has been recently revealed in a model of encephalomyelitis triggered by mouse infection with the Theiler's murine virus (Tolley et al., 1999). Thus, whereas DNA vaccination of mice—prior to infection—with VP2 and VP3 resulted in suppression of disease, immunization with the VP1 antigen of Theiler's virus resulted in significant aggravation. This important study pinpointed the need to understand the identity of epitopes that are involved in immune-mediated pathology prior to designing antigen-based immune modulating regimens. However, interestingly, this observation may open an avenue for the prevention of microbe-induced immune-mediated pathology using rationally designed vaccines against protective but not pathogenic nonself epitopes.

Prior to the development of new DNA purification methods, contamination of bacterial plasmid with lipopolysaccharide (LPS) used to pose a certain challenge related to the deleterious effects of endotoxin (i.e., fever, neutropenia, Schwartzman phenomenon, or septic shock, due to induction of TNF-α, IL-1, and IL-6). However, recent studies showed that even highly purified bacterial DNA may exhibit some LPS-like effects (Sparwasser et al., 1997a, 1997b). A subsequent study even described CpG motifs able to induce IL-12 and TNF-α in a differential manner (Lipford et al., 1997b). Thus, besides obvious theoretical implications for the mechanisms of innate immunity, this finding would allow for the use of bacterial DNA CpG motifs with IL-12-stimulating activity and devoid of TNF-α-inducing activity that may precipitate septic shock in sensitized individuals.

7.5. CONCLUSIONS AND PERSPECTIVES

The discovery that certain CpG motifs of bacterial DNA stimulate the innate immunity led researchers in the field of DNA-based vaccines toward new areas such as allergies and autoimmunity. A closer look at this aspect of genetic vaccines facilitated two important scientific achievements: first, a deeper understanding on how the immune system comes in contact with the microbes, leading to the detection of infectious non-self; and second, the astonishing finding that CpG-based ODN, when administered together with conventional vaccines, can reproduce the immune effects seen with plasmid-mediated antigen delivery. A few groups showed that CpG ODN may facilitate the CTL priming. The mechanism of CTL stimulation by CpG ODN is not yet understood. The answer to this question might very well be given by a closer look to the mechanisms of cross-priming as well as hsp-assisted processing and presentation. The second question is more practical and regards the eventual superiority of conventional vaccines formulated with CpG ODN compared to genetic vaccines, since in this case, the *in vivo* transfection will not be a limiting factor.

Independent of the answers to these questions, based on the accumulated scientific evidence, it is reasonable to assume that the strong Th1-adjuvant properties of microbial DNA may be of use in preventing or suppressing allergies. However, more work is needed to assess the potential suppressive effect after sensitization. Desensitization might be performed by coinoculation of allergen with CpG ODN, genetic immunization with plasmids expressing allergens, or CpG ODN administration during seasons when environmental exposure to allergens is increased.

An intriguing application for DNA vaccines is the field of autoimmune diseases. The reason behind this is precisely the strong Th1-adjuvant activity of bacterial DNA. Clearly, more work is needed to fully evaluate the potential practical value of such an application, supported only by a few published studies. Generation of Th2 immunity by plasmid-mediated delivery of self-antigens or idiotypes is still poorly understood. Efforts should be focused on characterizing the conditions associated with DNA vaccination that promote autoimmunity versus suppression or tolerance. This would eventually allow safer application of genetic immunization in autoimmune diseases. In spite of the recognized Th1-promoting adjuvant activity, plasmids have been shown to mediate successfully local delivery of immune suppressive cytokines leading to prevention of pathogenic Th1-mediated inflammation. This is still another area that might prove fruitful from a practical point of view.

Finally, an important question is whether genetic vaccines are safe immunogens, devoid of risk of autoimmunity, uncontrollable inflammation, or even septic shock. Recent studies showing an increased TNF-α production by macrophages that recognize bacterial DNA, raised legitimate concerns about possible side effects. However, it is important to realize that scientific information is being continuously generated and used to increase the safety while maintaining the efficiency of DNA vaccines. For example, studies on mechanisms of bacterial DNA recognition by the innate immune system led to characterization of CpG motifs that selectively stimulate IL-12 and not TNF-α. From the perspective of autoimmune diseases, it would be tremendously useful to characterize conditions in which plasmid-based immunization triggers suppressive Th2 responses or even tolerance.

Chapter 8

Genetic Immunization against Tumors

8.1. IMMUNITY AGAINST TUMORS

There is not yet a unified theory that explains the poor immunogenicity of most tumors for essentially two reasons: First, genetic instability of tumoral cells allows the emergence and selection of mutant cells that may evade immunity; second, there is a tremendous heterogeneity in the mechanisms responsible for immune system evasion by tumor cells, including tolerance of tumor antigens that may not be discriminated from self-antigens.

The factors responsible for the poor immunogenicity of tumors can be classified into two general categories: decreased immunogenicity and/or antigenicity of tumor cells, or suppression of the immune cells. Understanding the molecular basis of these mechanisms may allow for the design of effective antitumoral vaccines used for the prevention or therapy of primary lesions and metastases. Conversely, such knowledge may allow definition of the limits of the strategies based on immune manipulation, against various forms of cancer.

Tumor cells may lose the ability to stimulate or to be detected by immune cells subsequent to acquiring phenotypic modifications due to genetic mutations. For example, they may lose the expression of Class I and/or II molecules, or the ability to process and present epitopes through either the endogenous or exogenous pathway (Restifo and Wang, 1996). Furthermore, they may lose the expression of costimulatory or accessory molecules. These defects may lead to qualitatively or quantitatively defective stimulation of T-cells. When tumor-specific immune responses are generated early in the course of disease, the progressive or sudden loss of the ability of tumor cells to present antigens may spare them from immune effectors such as CTL.

Defective stimulation of T-cells due to the lack of costimulation may result in anergy (Harding et al., 1992; Linsley and Ledbetter, 1993). Thus, the emergence of tumor cells endowed with reduced immunogenicity may lead to immune unresponsiveness. There are instances when the tumor-associated antigens are proteins normally expressed in the ontogenic life (i.e., carcino-embrionic antigen [CEA], melanoma associated antigens). In these cases, the antigen-specific lymphocytes might have been deleted during the ontogeny. Thus, specific defects in the T-cell repertoire, created by thymic or peripheral negative selection, may account for low response to tumor-associated antigens. A more recently described mechanism that may be responsible for defective antitumor responses, at least in some cases, is immune deviation (Rocken and Shevach, 1996; Hu et al., 1998). Instead of Th1-regulated immune responses, certain tumors may lead to Th2 responses that are ineffective (Hu et al., 1998). Thus, further priming of tumor-specific Th1 or Tc1 cells may be subsequently impaired. Furthermore, the production of IL-4 and IL-10 by Th2 cells, or TGF-β by Th3 cells or even tumor cells, may exert a bystander suppressor effect on the eventual tumor-specific lymphocytes endowed with the ability to destroy transformed cells.

Therapeutic vaccination against tumors is a particularly difficult task, since one has to circumvent the low responsiveness of tumor-specific lymphocytes as well as the reduced antigenicity of tumor cells. A proper immunotherapeutic strategy should take into account multiple factors such as the type of tumor and the state of the immune system. For example, inducing or enhancing immune responses against poorly immunogenic tumors may imply, first, delivery of tumor-associated antigens in the context of strong costimulation, and second, the upregulation of MHC-peptide complexes in tumor cells. The aim of inducing immune effectors able to destroy tumor cells may not be attained if either one of these strategies is overlooked. Other tumors, in spite of the fact that they are immunogenic, may elicit shifted immune responses that are ineffective against the tumor. In that case, one should take advantage of the immunogenicity of tumor-associated antigens and try to shift the immune response toward an effective strategy (i.e., by cytokine codelivery). Obviously, there are limits to the potential effectiveness of immune therapeutic strategies against cancer, for example, in the case of tumors that lack strong tumor-associated antigens (i.e., sarcomas) and are refractory to immune effector mechanisms. Factors such as the kinetics of tumor growth and genetic instability that regulate the balance between tumor expansion and the immune response may be decisive for the success of immune therapy. From a practical point of view, protocols comprising surgery followed by immune therapy may be followed by increased likelihood of success in suppressing the course of disease or preventing metastases.

Certain characteristics of nucleic-acid-based expression vectors (either plasmid DNA or mRNA) make them appealing as vectors for immune therapy against cancer. First, obviously, is the advantage of low immunogenicity of the vector that may allow subsequent boosts as well as increased life span of transfected APC. Second, microbial DNA is endowed with intrinsic ability to stimulate the production of Th1-promoting cytokines, leading to more effective activation of NK and CTL. Third, such expression vectors may allow delivery of antigens as well as cytokines or costimulatory molecules. However, the rate of *in vivo* transfection may be an important limiting step, particularly when tumor cells or rare APC are targeted. Protocols comprising *ex vivo* transfection of professional APC or tumor cells may circumvent to a certain extent this drawback of naked DNA vaccination, leading to enhanced tumor immunogenicity, although they may not address the aim of increasing the tumor antigenicity.

Various protocols of genetic vaccination have been employed therefore in multiple experimental models of tumors. One category focused on *in vivo* transfection of tumor cells with genes expressing immune-enhancing molecules, with the aim of increasing immunogenicity and antigenicity of the transformed cells. Another consists in genetic vaccination with tumor-associated antigens, with or without costimulatory factors, with the aim of increasing the immune response by *in vivo* transfecting APC. Some groups optimized this strategy by performing *ex vivo* transfection of professional APC. Finally, *ex vivo* transfection of tumor cells with immune enhancer molecules may preclude the requirement of identifying tumor-associated antigens.

8.2. STRATEGIES TO ELICIT OR ENHANCE TUMOR-SPECIFIC IMMUNITY BY NUCLEIC-ACID-BASED DELIVERY OF TUMOR ANTIGENS

Genetic immunization consisting of *in vivo* administration of expression vectors has been shown to induce immunity against tumors in various experimental models (Table 8.1): (1) tumor-associated antigens representing idiotypes; (2) antigens derived from experimental tumors of nonlymphoid origin; (3) antigens of transforming viruses; and (4) surrogate

Table 8.1. DNA-Mediated Antigen Delivery in Tumor Models

Type of antigen		Associated stimuli	References
Tumor-associated antigens	Idiotypes	IL-2	Watanabe et al., 1993
		GM-CSF	Syrengelas et al., 1996
		IL-1 beta	Hakim et al., 1996
		Tetanus toxin	Spellberg et al., 1997
		CpG ODN	Weiner et al., 1997
	CEA	—	Conry et al., 1994
		B7-1/GM-CSF	Conry et al., 1996b
	Melanoma antigens	B7-1/GM-CSF	Bueler and Mulligan, 1996
		IL-12/IFN-α	Tuting et al., 1998
		—	Bronte et al., 2000
	Mutant p53	—	Ciernik et al., 1996a
	erbB2/Neu	—	Concetti et al., 1996
		IL-2	Chen et al., 1998a
	P815A	—	Rosato et al., 1997
	hCG-beta	—	Geissler et al., 1997a
	Combination of antigens	—	de Zoeten et al., 1998
Antigens of oncogenic viruses	SV40 T-Ag	—	Bright et al., 1995
			Schirmbeck et al., 1996
	HPV L1-Ag	—	Donnelly et al., 1996
	HPV E7-Ag	—	Chen et al., 1999
	HTLV-1		Grange et al., 1997
	EBV EBNA-4	IFN-γ	Charo et al., 1999
Surrogate tumor antigens[a]	HLA-B7	—	Nabel et al., 1993
	LacZ	—	Lu et al., 1994
		IL-2/IL-6/IL-7/IL-12	Irvine et al., 1996
	Luciferase	—	Conry et al., 1995c
	HBsAg	—	Bohm et al., 1997
	Ovalbumin	B7-1/B7-2	Corr et al., 1997
	CAT	—	Nomura et al., 1997
	NP of influenza virus	—	Iwasaki and Barber, 1998

[a]Antigens of nontumor origin, such as microbial antigens, expressed on tumor cells.

antigens expressed by genetically manipulated tumors. Certain protocols tested the co-administration of expression vectors that encode cytokines or costimulatory molecules.

8.2.1. Genetic Immunization with Expression Vectors Encoding Tumor Idiotypes

B- and T-cells express membrane-bound antigen B-cell receptors (BCR) and T-cell receptors (TCR). The variable domains of BCR and TCR comprise epitopes (idiotypes) that are recognized by the immune system. Such epitopes encoded by V genes of BCR and TCR are appealing targets for vaccination against tumors because of the high specificity of expression of idiotypes that may allow for fine discrimination between tumor (idiotype$^+$) and nontumor (idiotype$^-$) lymphoid cells. Obviously, this strategy is limited in the treatment of B-cell lymphoma and T-cell leukemia. However, a drawback to using idiotypes as targets is the difficulty of defining and manipulating them in a clinical setting, particularly due to their high specificity for the tumor clone. The design of idiotypic vaccines would require, therefore, the isolation of tumor-associated Fv segments from patients that can be assembled into expression vectors. Effective anti-idiotypic immunization may require coadministration of certain factors such as cytokines.

The first attempt to induce immunity by genetic immunization against an idiotypic determinant took advantage of an IgV segment isolated from human IgM antibodies expressed by chronic lymphocytic leukemia cells (Watanabe et al., 1993). Inoculation in mice of a plasmid expression vector encompassing the Hum vK 325 germline kappa chain gene resulted in induction of anti-idiotype antibodies. Furthermore, coadministration of a plasmid expressing IL-2 led to increased antibody responses to the idiotype as well as detectable DTH responses. One cannot rule out, however, an eventual immunogenic role of xenogenic determinants associated with this human IgV segment. This observation has been confirmed in a similar model, and the potential utilization of cytokines as enhancers for immunity elicited by idiotypic vaccines was extended to GM-CSF (Stevenson et al., 1995).

A new generation of anti-idiotypic vaccines was introduced based on the observation that fusion proteins between single-chain Fv (scFv) fragments isolated from B-cell tumors and cytokines display enhanced ability to induce anti-idiotype antibodies (Syrengelas et al., 1996). Two such cytokines were GM-CSF and IL-1β, and even fragments of them were immunologically active. However, whereas an scFv-GM-CSF fusion construct was effective only when injected as protein, scFv-IL-1β was effective against tumor challenge even when inoculated as plasmid-based vector (Hakim et al., 1996). Thus, these two studies introduced two new aspects: first, that genetic vaccines expressing BCR-derived idiotypes may be protective against tumor challenge in a mouse model of lymphoma, and second, that idiotype–cytokine fusion constructs may improve immunogenicity of idiotype-based genetic vaccines. The principle of using scFv-fusion constructs as means to increase immunogenicity has been recently extended to "strong" antigens, such as the C' fragment of tetanus toxin (Spellerberg et al., 1997). This study showed that immunization of mice with a prototype idiotype–tetanus fusion construct, expressed by plasmid, elicited higher titers of anti-idiotype antibodies that bound tumor cells from which scFv was isolated (Spellerberg et al., 1997). A subsequent study showed that another prototype antigen, keyhole limpet hemocyanin, displayed enhanced immunogenicity when fused to a human scFv and delivered via plasmid into mice (Caspar et al., 1997).

The mechanism of action of anti-idiotypic immunity elicited by antitumor genetic vaccines is mediated by antibodies against BCR. This is suggested by previous preclinical and clinical studies that characterized the therapeutic ability of monoclonal anti-idiotypic antibodies in lymphoma models or patients (Caspar et al., 1997). This conclusion was further strengthened by the fact that relapsing patients treated with anti-idiotypic antibodies displayed mutated tumor-associated BCR that precluded the binding of therapeutic antibody. More recent evidence obtained in a model of murine B-cell lymphoma pinpointed the role of complement-mediated tumor cytotoxicity, triggered by tumor-specific antibodies resulting from idiotypic DNA vaccination (Syrengelas and Levy, 1999). Two characteristics of genetic immunization may offer significant advantages over the strategy of anti-idiotypic antibodies. First, since inoculation of idiotypes elicits polyclonal responses, the emergence of mutated BCR that escape the immune surveillance is less probable (Caspar et al., 1997). Second, immune stimulatory motifs in the bacterial DNA may enhance the activity of effector mechanisms. For example, in a therapeutic model of lymphoma, co-administration of anti-idiotype antibodies with CpG ODN was followed by stimulation of antibody-dependent tumor lysis due to activation of FcR$^+$ cells such as macrophages and NK cells (Wooldridge et al., 1997). In a distinct model, immunization of mice with idiotype together with CpG ODN was followed by protection against challenge with idiotype$^+$ B-lymphoma cells (Weiner et al., 1997).

However, there are still drawbacks to genetic immunization with idiotypes: Reduced *in vivo* transfection rate, despite a continuous production of idiotype, may lead to clearance of the low titer anti-idiotypic antibodies, precluding a therapeutic effect (Stevenson et al., 1995). Furthermore, as in the case of other tumor-associated antigens, the responsiveness of the immune system may be decreased in affected recipients. Of course, this effect is not evident in most of the experimental models mentioned earlier, consisting in immunization of naive animals followed by tumor challenge. The unresponsiveness may be broken by coadministration of immune stimulating factors. Third, most of the vaccine models described earlier employed inoculation of human idiotypes into mice; thus, a possible stimulating effect of xenogenic determinants may have been underestimated in such models. In contrast, whereas the anti-idiotype antibody-based therapy evidently circumvents these drawbacks, it posses significant practical problems due to the natural genetic variation of idiotypes expressed on tumor cells (i.e., selection of idiotype-mutated variants).

8.2.2. Genetic Immunization with Expression Vectors Encoding Other Tumor-Derived Antigens

One of the most investigated tumor-associated antigens in protocols of genetic immunization has been the human carcinoembryonic antigen (CEA). An early report showed humoral and cellular immunity elicited by immunization of mice with a plasmid-expressing human CEA under CMV promoter (Conry et al., 1994). T-cells primed by genetic immunization produced IL-2 and IL-4 rather than IFN-γ subsequent to *in vitro* stimulation with

CEA. Not all the immunized mice displayed significant responses, suggesting that in spite of possible xenogenic determinants, genetic immunization with CEA was suboptimal. Subsequent studies were aimed at optimizing the schedule of immunization and the dose of plasmid. It was shown that mice immunized with the plasmid-expressing human CEA were protected against challenge with a syngeneic line of colon carcinoma cells transduced with human CEA (Conry et al., 1995a). That was associated with induction of cellular and humoral responses against CEA in 100% of immunized mice (Conry et al., 1995b). A further attempt to improve the immunity conferred by CEA-expressing plasmid was carried out by codelivery of B7-1 or GM-CSF (Conry et al., 1996a). Interestingly, codelivery of CEA and B7-1 expressed by the same, but not different, plasmids was followed by increased humoral tumor-specific responses. Inoculation of GM-CSF-expressing plasmid into the skin of mice, 3 days prior to genetic immunization with CEA, was followed by induction of increased humoral and cellular responses (Conry et al., 1996b).

Other antigens tested in models of genetic immunization were the melanoma-associated antigens MAGE-1 and MAGE-3. Either genetic immunization with plasmids expressing MAGE-1 and MAGE-3 or inoculation of antigen-transduced fibroblasts was followed by induction of antigen-specific $CD4^+$ and $CD8^+$ T-cells (Bueler and Mulligan, 1996). Again, coinoculation of plasmids expressing GM-CSF or B7-1 was followed by increased protection against tumor challenge. A recent study was aimed at inducing melanoma-specific immunity through a different strategy, namely, *ex vivo* transfection of human dendritic cells with antigens such as MART-1/Melan-A, pMel-17/gp100, tyrosinase, MAGE-1 or MAGE-3 (Tuting et al., 1998). Such *in vitro* transfected dendritic cells primed human autologous CTL against melanoma antigens. Cotransfection of dendritic cells with plasmids expressing cytokines such as IL-12 or IFN-α was followed by increased priming of virus-specific CTL. DNA immunization of mice with a melanoma-associated antigen, gp100/pmel17, resulted in limited but significant protection against tumor challenge (Nawrath et al., 1999). One potential consequence of immunization against melanoma-associated antigens is a systemic autoimmune reaction against melanocytes that results in vitiligo. Thus, ideally, immune therapeutic strategies in melanoma should be directed against antigens strongly expressed by tumor cells but weakly expressed by normal melanocytes. Interestingly, a very recent report showed that in contrast to the outcome in the case of immunization against TRP-1/gp75, DNA vaccination against the melanoma antigen "tyrosinase-related protein 2" (TRP-2) resulted in protection against tumor challenge devoid of vitiligo as a side effect (Bronte et al., 2000).

Other groups examined the immunogenicity of plasmid-based constructs expressing p185, a mammary tumor associated antigen, encoded by the erbB2/neu gene. Immunization of mice with a plasmid expressing the rat p185 antigen was followed by induction of low levels of antigen-specific IgG that promoted *in vitro* antibody-dependent cellular cytotoxicity of tumor cells (Concetti et al., 1996). Surprisingly, genetic immunization with p185 was not followed by toxicity caused by reactivity of antigen-specific antibodies to host cells expressing low levels of neu. A more recent study showed that mice immunized with plasmids expressing whole-length or fragments of neu were protective against challenge with a neu-expressing tumor (Chen et al., 1998a). Interestingly, whereas coinoculation of an IL-2-expressing plasmid improved the protection ability of the genetic vaccine, it was not associated with an enhancement of the tumor-specific antibody titers. This observation pinpointed an eventual role for cellular immunity in the protection against neu-expressing tumors, besides the already recognized role of antibodies (Concetti et al., 1996). Another study involving coadministration of IL-2 and antigen (ovarian carcinoma-associated antigen folate receptor-α) expressing DNA vectors, showed significant suppressor effect on lung metastases in a tumor regression model (Neglia et al., 1999).

A few recent studies have approached genetic immunization against other tumor-associated antigens. Immunization of mice with a plasmid expressing single epitopes originating from gp120 of HIV-1 and mutated p53 resulted in generation of tumor-specific CTL (Ciernik et al., 1996a). The immunity that afforded protection against tumor challenge was enhanced when the epitopes were fused to an ER targeting signal. Another study showed that genetic immunization with P815A antigen induced CTL and protected mice against lethal challenge with P815 tumor cells (Rosato et al., 1997). More recently, it was shown that DNA vaccination against a paraneoplastic antigen (HuD), associated with small-cell lung cancer in a mouse model of adenocarcinoma, resulted in significant control of tumor size (Ohwada et al., 1999a).

Finally, another report showed that genetic immunization of mice with a plasmid-expressing human chorionic gonadotropin β subunit, an antigen commonly expressed by lung, bladder, and pancreatic tumors, resulted in significant humoral and cellular responses (Geissler et al., 1997b). Although some mice immunized with hCG-expressing plasmid were protected against challenge with hCG-transfected tumor cells, one cannot rule out the role of eventual xenogenic determinants in the immunogenicity of the construct.

8.2.3. Genetic Immunization against Oncogenic Viruses

The onset and evolution of certain tumors are promoted by infection with oncogenic viruses. Usually, these viruses induce transformation by one of the following mechanisms: (1) expression of virus oncogenes directly leading to deregulation of cell cycle; and (2) disruption of the host genome due to insertional mutagenesis, leading to inactivation of suppressor genes and transformation. Examples include certain large DNA viruses that are dependent on host-cell proliferation, and retroviruses that lead to insertion of viral genetic material into chromosomes. A potentially useful strategy to prevent or suppress tumors associated with oncoviruses consists in vaccination against viral antigens. DNA immunization against viruses has been discussed in detail in Chapter 5. Here, we briefly present three examples regarding DNA immunization against oncoviruses.

Papillomaviruses are associated with approximately 90% of human cervical carcinomas. Methods to prevent infection with papillomaviruses may lead to decreased incidence of cervical carcinoma. DNA vaccination has been studied as a method to induce immunity against papillomavirus in a cottontail rabbit papillomavirus model (Donnelly et al., 1996) (Table 8.1). Inoculation of a plasmid expressing the major viral capsid protein L1 resulted in not only antibody response but also protection against papilloma formation subsequent to virus infection. More recently, an interesting study carried out in a tumor regression model showed that mouse DNA vaccination with a fusion construct composed of the HPV-E7 antigen attached to the lysosomal sorting signal of LAMP-1 was effective in controlling liver and lung metastasis by inducing strong CTL and humoral immunity (Chen et al., 1999). In a distinct experimental model comprising another member of the family

Papovaviridae, DNA vaccination of mice with a plasmid expressing the SV40 T-Ag was followed by both induction of specific CTL and rejection of P815/T tumor grafts (Schirmbeck et al., 1996). Other groups demonstrated induction by DNA immunization with plasmids expressing the envelope protein of humoral and cellular immunity against the retrovirus HTLV-1, involved in *T*-cell leukemia and spastic paraparesis (Grange et al., 1997; Agadjanyan et al., 1998). Interestingly, another group took advantage of the *in vivo* transfection technique with naked DNA to study the role of various HTLV-1 genes in the virulence (Zhao et al., 1996). Thus, they defined genes important for infection by inoculating plasmids expressing the whole-length genome of HTLV-1 variants.

If mass vaccination against viruses with oncogenic potential, such as papillomavirus, may contribute to the reduction in the incidence of certain cancers, it is not clear yet whether such a strategy would be successful as a therapeutic vaccination. Since the development of tumors comprises a multistep pathogenesis, the dependence of the malignant cells on expression of virus antigens may decrease and, thus, the sensitivity of tumor cells to virus-specific immune effectors may be lost.

8.2.4. Genetic Immunization in Tumor Models Comprising Surrogate Tumor Antigens

Various tumor models were established that comprise transformed cells engineered to express reporter genes or strong antigens, usually of microbial origin. Such models circumvented the need to previously define tumor-associated antigens in the process of studying various strategies of vaccination against tumors. The drawback of these methods is that, usually, genuine tumor-associated antigens are weak immunogens.

An earlier report approached the feasibility of *in vivo* transfection of human breast cancer xenografts in nude mice with reporter genes using mRNA-liposome-mediated delivery (Lu et al., 1994). This study showed that the efficacy of *in vivo* transfection of capped and polyadenylated mRNA was similar to that of plasmid DNA, when complexed with liposomes. The mRNA may present the advantage of reduced potential side effects due to systemic localization of recombinant DNA. However, the *ex vivo* and *in vivo* stability of mRNA is very low. This might be of particular importance in the case of vaccination with tumor antigens having oncogenic potential, such as HER2/neu, by avoiding a prolonged exposure (Conry et al., 1996a). A subsequent study tested the immunogenicity of an mRNA-based vaccine expressing CEA in mice that were later challenged with CEA-expressing tumor cells (Conry et al., 1995c). Interestingly, most of the mice immunized with mRNA and challenged with tumor, developed CEA-specific antibodies, whereas control mice did not develop a humoral response. However, this study failed to provide information as to whether immunization with mRNA is effective in protecting against tumor challenge.

Another study approached the efficacy of DNA vaccination against metastases in a model of β-galactosidase-transfected tumor cell line of murine origin (Irvine et al., 1996). The results showed that whereas DNA immunization with β-gal has little effect on the already established lung metastases, coadministration of plasmids expressing IL-12, and to a limited extent IL-2, IL-6, and IL-7, was followed by significant reduction in the number of lung metastases. Adoptive transfer experiments suggested that β-gal-specific lymphocytes were responsible for this effect. This is one of the few studies that reported significant therapeutic effects of DNA vaccination in a tumor model.

A pioneering study that represented an early clinical trial regarding DNA immunization studied the feasibility, safety, and therapeutic potential for direct transfer of HLA-B7 gene via liposome-DNA complexes into melanoma tumors of HLA-B7-negative patients (Nabel et al., 1993). All the five patients displayed expression of HLA-B7 in the injected nodules, but most importantly, immune responses to allogeneic HLA-B7 as well as against the autologous tumor. One of the patients displayed regression of the injected tumors as well as the metastases. A more recent study that attempted a similar strategy of vaccination against tumors, consisted of engineering strong antigens (HBsAg) in weakly immunogenic tumors such as P815 (Bohm et al., 1997). Mice immunized with DNA expressing HBsAg and challenged with P815 tumor cells, were inoculated into the tumor with either plasmid or engineered tumor cells expressing HBsAg. Interestingly, such treatment resulted in induction of CTL immunity against P815 cells, as well as tumor rejection. This might have been due to the intermolecular epitope spreading to weakly immunogenic tumor-associated antigens of an immune response triggered by HBsAg. Such a mechanism is consistent with the limited efficacy of *in vivo* transfection of tumor cells (Nomura et al., 1997), making it unlikely that tumor rejection was mediated solely by virus-specific lymphocytes. Somewhat similar observations were made by another study that showed the development of effective immunity against P815 mastocytoma cells after immunization with a plasmid-expressing NP of influenza virus and boost with NP epitope–transfected P815 cells (Iwasaki and Barber, 1998).

DNA immunization against surrogate tumor antigens has been tested in other models as well. For example, DNA vaccination of mice with ovalbumin (OVA)-expressing plasmid, together with B7-1 costimulatory molecule, provided relative protection against challenge with OVA-expressing tumor cells (Corr et al., 1997).

Thus, besides the obvious role of the models comprising surrogate tumor antigens in understanding mechanisms that govern antitumor immunity, an intriguing possibility with practical implications emerged from few recent studies, namely, the use of immunity to strong surrogate tumor antigens in order to break unresponsiveness and to promote effective immunity to otherwise weak tumor antigens.

8.3. INDUCTION OR ENHANCEMENT OF TUMOR-SPECIFIC IMMUNITY BY NUCLEIC-ACID-MEDIATED DELIVERY OF CYTOKINES OR OTHER IMMUNE STIMULATORS

Rather than using tumor-associated antigens to promote antitumor immunity, some groups approached this aim indirectly, by administering cytokines or costimulatory molecules. This approach, aimed at circumventing the need for the characterization of tumor-associated antigens, implied that such determinants exist and the immune system is unable, for various reasons, to mount effective responses against them. Such reasons may include the improper presentation of tumor-derived antigens to lymphocytes, in the absence of costimulation, that leads to anergy rather than activation.

Table 8.2. DNA-Mediated Delivery of Cytokines and Other Immune Enhancers in Tumor Models

Delivery	Examples	Model	References
In vivo	IL-2, IL-6, IFN-γ, TNF-α	Fibrosarcoma/carcinoma	Sun et al., 1995
	IL-12	Various tumors	Rakhmilevich et al., 1996
			Tan et al., 1996
	IL-2, IL-6, GM-CSF	—	Keller et al., 1996
	CpG ODN	Lymphoma	Wooldridge et al., 1997
In vitro	GM-CSF	B16 melanoma	Mahvi et al., 1996
		Sarcoma and melanoma	Mahvi et al., 1997
	IFN-γ	D122 lung carcinoma	Clary et al., 1997
	GM-CSF, IL-6, TNF-α	Burkitt's lymphoma	Mucke et al., 1997
	IL-7	Alveolar carcinoma	Sharma et al., 1997
	IL-2	Various tumors	Stopeck et al., 1998

A few studies showed that direct injection of cytokine-expressing plasmids into tumors may lead to inhibition of tumor growth (Table 8.2). A relatively early study showed the efficacy of IL-6 in reducing the growth of methylcholanthrene-induced fibrosarcoma in a mouse model, as well as that of IL-2 and IFN-γ in reducing the growth of a renal carcinoma (Sun et al., 1995). Although the local expression of these cytokines was documented, data regarding the mechanism of action were lacking. A subsequent study elegantly addressed this point in the case of IL-12 (Rakhmilevich et al., 1996), namely, gene-gun mediated delivery of a vector expressing IL-12 gene to the skin above implanted intradermal tumors resulted in local IL-12 expression and tumor regression, depending on tumor-specific CD8[+] CTL. Another study demonstrated the ability of the same cytokine IL-12, when administered via plasmid to the skin of mice, to significantly delay the onset of a tumor (renal carcinoma) inoculated at a distant site (Tan et al., 1996). This study elegantly revealed that improper priming, rather than lack of immunogenic tumor-associated antigens, may be responsible for the impaired response to certain tumors. Another report showed the feasibility of epidermal delivery, via plasmid-coated particles, of cytokines such as IL-2, IL-6, and GM-CSF in larger animals such as dogs (Keller et al., 1996).

Other reports described a different strategy, namely, *ex vivo* engineering of tumoral or antigen-presenting cells to express cytokines, costimulatory, or MHC molecules that may lead to effective immunity when the cells are reinoculated into organism. That way, one may enhance the effectiveness of breaking the unresponsiveness to tumor antigens, simply because of the colocalization of tumor-derived antigens with immune stimulators. An elegant study showed that *in vitro* transfection of B16 melanoma cells with GM-CSF-expressing plasmid, followed by irradiation and inoculation into mice, was followed by significant protection against challenge with nontransfected B16 tumor cells (Mahvi et al., 1996). In a subsequent study, *in vitro* transfection of murine lung cancer cells with an adeno-associated virus-based plasmid expressing IFN-γ, followed by irradiation and vaccination of mice, resulted in relative protection of the mice against lung metastases subsequent to tumor challenge (Clary et al., 1997). Fairly recently, a phase I/IB clinical trial was begun that comprised *ex vivo* transfection of autologous sarcoma or melanoma cells with GM-CSF-expressing gene, followed by cellular vaccination of the patients (Mahvi et al., 1997). The advantage of using plasmid-based transfection compared, for example, with retrovirus-mediated gene transfer is that no long-term *in vitro* cell culture would be required in order to promote cellular proliferation. An obvious advantage of *ex vivo* versus *in vivo* transfection of tumor cells is that the former may allow engineering of cells originating from nonsolid tumors to produce cytokines. A recent report looked at the effectiveness of a plasmid comprising both the Epstein–Barr virus latent gene EBNA1 and the origin of replication (oriP), in transfecting *ex vivo* human non-Hodgkin's lymphoma cells (Mucke et al., 1997). Such cells, transfected with this prototype plasmid-based expression vector encoding cytokines such as GM-CSF, IL-6, and TNF-α, upon transfer into nude mice, produced sustained levels of cytokines. However, a drawback of this plasmid is that the expression advantage conferred by EBV-derived elements requires cellular proliferation. A recent study showed that various human tumor cell lines can be successfully engineered to express IL-2, another cytokine thought to help in promoting antitumor immunity (Stopeck et al., 1998).

A recent report describes a method to induce enhanced antitumor immunity using variants of the strategies mentioned earlier: *ex vivo* transfection of antigen presenting cells; use of tumor-associated antigens; and use of syngeneic and heterogenic Class I molecules to enhance the immune response. Thus, mouse allogeneic fibroblasts *in vitro* transduced to express a cDNA library from B16 melanoma cells, as well as syngeneic Class I determinants were shown to suppress the growth of already established melanoma tumors upon cellular vaccination (de Zoeten et al., 1998). Multiple mechanisms are likely responsible for the significant therapeutic effect of this cellular vaccine: the presence of allogeneic MHC determinants leading to immunity against nonself antigens that may facilitate intermolecular epitope spreading; colocalization of tumor antigens in the same cells; and the presence of syngeneic MHC determinants on the vaccine cells, leading to direct priming of tumor-specific lymphocytes. An interesting idea approached in other studies is transfection of antigen presenting cells with tumor-derived genetic material, thus precluding the requirement for antigen characterization.

An approach to increase the effectiveness of antitumor vaccines would be to target tumor antigens to professional antigen-presenting cells (pAPC) such as dendritic cells (DC). A report showed that coinoculation of activated DC with tumor cells engineered to express IL-7 and herpes simplex thymidine kinase, led not only to protection against tumor challenge but also to remission of 5-day-old tumors (Sharma et al., 1997).

Thus, various approaches for plasmid-mediated delivery of cytokines, or other molecules with roles in the immune response, were shown to be effective to certain extent either in preventing or treating experimental tumors.

8.4. CONCLUSIONS AND PERSPECTIVES

In spite of the tremendous variety of approaches for DNA-based vaccination or immunotherapy against tumors, most of the published studies reported relative efficacy in preventing tumor formation subsequent to challenge, rather than inducing remission of the already established tumors. A few studies reported the induction of remission and decline in tumor growth or ability to give metastases, circumstances that are more relevant for clinics.

The reason behind this situation is mainly the difficulty in promoting effective tumor-specific immunity in organisms already affected by that specific tumor. Various recombinant DNA methods are being employed to break the unresponsiveness against tumor antigens. Of the more appealing methods based on the emerging literature, theoretical as well as practical considerations include (1) taking advantage of the bystander surrogate antigens (microbial antigens, allogeneic, or xenogenic determinants) that can both trigger strong systemic responses and be delivered to tumor cells; (2) expression of tumor-associated antigens in the context of strong costimulation, in order to break unresponsiveness to tumor; (3) relatively rapid generation of therapeutic anti-idiotypic humanized monoclonal antibodies by genetic vaccination of rodents expressing human Ig.

A significant number of clinical trials consisting of recombinant DNA-mediated immune therapy of tumors was initiated, the rationale being that in spite of the modest preclinical results, the potential benefit–risk ratio in patients with certain tumors was still favorable. Such studies, Phase I/II clinical trials on smaller samples of advanced-stage tumor patients, are particularly aimed at characterizing the safety of procedures based on recombinant DNA. There are ongoing trials involving DNA vaccination with idiotypes in lymphoma and myeloma patients, gene-mediated *in vivo* delivery of cytokines in melanoma and head-and-neck cancers, gene-mediated *in vivo* delivery of MHC molecules in melanoma patients, gene-mediated delivery of idiotype-carrier constructs in lymphoma, gene-mediated delivery in kidney and prostate cancer, and a recently initiated clinical trial comprising melanoma antigen delivery via DNA plus IL-2 administered systemically. Initial rounds of clinical trials initiated by Vical (San Diego, CA) and collaborators are focused on DNA-based delivery into the tumor of immune enhancers such as IL-2 (Leuvectin®). It is expected that another generation of anticancer therapeutics based on tumor antigen-expressing DNA vectors will find its way through clinical trials; such an example is the prostate-specific membrane antigen (PSMA) that recently showed promising results in preclinical trials. A few of the clinical studies have already reported good safety data, allowing the design of more advanced Phase II/III clinical trials that can reliably answer questions regarding efficiency in humans.

Chapter 9

Genetic Vaccination of Neonates

9.1. CHARACTERISTICS OF THE NEONATAL IMMUNE SYSTEM

It is well known that newborns and infants respond poorly to the majority of vaccines. The poor response is related to immaturity of the immune system and/or to high susceptibility of young lymphocytes to tolerogenic signals. The understanding of the effect of neonatal genetic immunization requires a general review of information on the characteristics of the neonatal immune system.

The major function of the immune system is to discriminate foreign antigens from self-antigens leading to induction of humoral and cellular responses against foreign macro-molecules and to unresponsiveness in the case of self-molecules. This property is acquired during the development of the immune system.

Burnet (1959) proposed that the self-reactive clones are eliminated during the development of the immune system. This theory was strongly supported by various findings, such as the induction of a long-lasting tolerance by maternal antiallotype (Dray, 1962) or anti-idiotype (Nisonoff and Bangasser, 1975) antibodies, or by fetal exposure to erythrocytes during fetal life.

Owen (1958) showed that nonidentical calf twins that shared a placenta failed to reject skin grafts during their adult life. Modern studies using congenic and transgenic mice also showed that the exposure during fetal life of lymphocytes to MLS or other cellular antigens led to deletion of T- or B-cell clones bearing receptors specific for self-antigens (Mac-Donald et al., 1988; Kiselow et al., 1988; Hartly et al., 1991). In addition, it was considered that neonatal lymphocytes can be also easily tolerized. Billingham et al. (1956) showed that newborns injected with allogenic hematopoietic cells failed to reject a skin graft during adulthood, indicating induction of tolerance to alloantigens. There are important quantitative and qualitative differences between neonatal and adult immune systems (Bona and Bot, 1997).

In mice, Ridge et al. (1996) showed that the neonatal spleen virtually does not contain T-cells after birth, and their number increases gradually after 4 days. Our analysis of T-cells in TCR-HA transgenic mice showed that only a few cells can be detected in the spleen of 3- to 7-day-old mice. The B-cells are present after birth in peripheral organs but they exhibit an immature phenotype.

Neonatal *T*-cells differ qualitatively in numerous ways from those of adults.

1. Autoreactive cells are present in the peripheral organs of neonates but they are not usually found in adults (Andreu-Sanchez et al., 1991). This is probably related to a delay of establishment of thymic deletion process, which is prolonged in perinatal life (Jones et al., 1990; Ando et al., 1991). Delayed thymic deletion process indicates that neonatal *T*-cells can either undergo maturation or deletion in periphery.

2. Neonatal CD4 *T*-cells lack Qa-2 antigen but express Class I and CD28 molecules interacting with costimulatory molecules borne by APCs (Ramsdel et al., 1991).

3. Neonatal *T*-cells exhibit a strong bias for production of Th2-type lymphokines after stimulation with anti-CD3 antibodies (Adkins et al., 1993). Lack of differentiation to Th1-type cells may be related to the poor expression of CD40-L observed in the case of human neonatal lymphocytes (Durandy et al., 1995). Studies have shown that the secretion of IL-12, which stimulates the Th1-type cells, is dependent of interaction with CD40 on APC, which in turn upregulates the expression of B.7 molecules. Actually, it was shown that neonatal *T*-cells stimulated with anti-CD3 and anti-CD28 monoclonal antibodies, representing a B.7 surrogate, display significantly increased synthesis of INFγ (Sornasse et al., 1996).

4. Both human and murine neonatal cells easily undergo apoptosis after *in vitro* stimulation with polyclonal agents (Aggarwal et al., 1997; Adkins et al., 1996).

5. Delayed expression of TdT, which is detected only in the second week of life (Gregoire et al., 1979; Rothenberg and Trigila, 1983), is mirrored in the limited N-region diversity of TCR from neonatal *T*-cells (Feeney, 1991).

6. The immunization of neonates with T-dependent antigens either induces unresponsiveness or elicits a very poor response. Based on this observation, several studies attempted neonatal regimens of immunization with autoantigens to prevent autoimmune diseases. Thus, it was shown that the injection of SJL mice after birth with myelin basic protein (Sun et al., 1989), or with peptide corresponding to the epitopes recognized by *T*-cells (Clayton et al., 1989), prevents experimental allergic encephalitis. Injection of glutamic acid decarboxylase in NOD neonates was able to delay the occurrence of disease in this strain, genetically prone to develop diabetes a few months after birth (Petersen et al., 1994).

However, in other studies the injection of autoantigens or peptides had a different effect. The treatment of NZB/NZW F1 mice with a peptide derived from an autoantigen induced a Th2 response that was associated with production of pathogenic anti-DNA antibodies (Singh et al., 1996). Similarly, neonatal injection of B6AF1 female mice with a peptide derived from ZP3 ovarian antigen induced an autoimmune oophoritis associated with strong proliferation and Th1–Th2 responses (Garza et al., 1997).

The paradigm of neonatal unresponsiveness was challenged by various observations demonstrating the ability of neonatal *T*-cells to mount an immune response against foreign antigens.

The first evidence was provided by Rubinstein et al. (1982), who showed that the injection of low doses of a myeloma protein bearing a given idiotype in 1- to 21-day-old mice was able to prime CD4 *T*-cells. Cells from animals immunized after birth with A48 protein helped TNP-specific *B*-cells to mount an anti-TNP antibody response in the presence of A48–TNP conjugate. Table 9.1 illustrates these results.

Table 9.1. Demonstration of A48 Id-Specific *T*-Cells
in Mice Treated at Birth with 10 μg of A48 Myeloma Protein

Nude mice infused with	Immunization of nude mice with	Anti-TNP pfc/spleen
Nil	Nil	492
Nil	TNP-Ficoll	90,200
Nil	TNP-A48	0
Nil	TNP-M384	0
Normal *T*-cells	TNP-A48	490
Normal *T*-cells	TNP-M384	212
A48 *T*-cells	TNP-A48	1,674
A48 *T*-cells	TNP-M384	0

Note. *T*-cells were purified on nylon-wool columns from 1-month-old mice immunized at birth with 10 μg A48 monoclonal protein. The anti-TNP response was studied 7 days after infusion of *T*-cells into nude mice injected with TNP-conjugates.

T-cell-mediated responses were also observed following injection of neonates with foreign proteins. Thus, Th1- and virus-specific CTL responses were observed after neonatal injection of tolerogenic doses of lysozyme with adjuvant (Forsthuber et al., 1996) or low dose of CAS, a murine leukemic virus, respectively (Sarzotti et al., 1996). Apparently, the presentation of peptides by dendritic cells plays an important role in induction of *T*-cell-mediated responses in neonates. Ridge et al. (1996) demonstrated effective induction of Y-specific CTL response in newborn females infused with dendritic cells from adult males.

It is noteworthy that cellular immune responses can be induced after the vaccination of newborns or infants with BCG or vaccinia. Thus, we can conclude that neonates in certain conditions are able to mount a cellular immune response. The low responsiveness of neonates can be related to the immaturity of *T*-cells or, alternatively, to the fact that in newborns, the *T*-cells belong to a different lineage, which is replaced during the maturation of the immune system.

Neonatal *B* cells also differ from adult *B* cells in the following ways:

1. Neonatal lymphocytes exhibit an immature phenotype: B220^{lo}, sIgM^{hi}, compared to adult *B*-cells which are B220^{hi}, sIgM^{lo}, and sIgD^{hi} (Osmond, 1986). A small transitional stage of maturation exhibits a particular phenotype: HSA^{br}, B220^{lo}, CD44^{hi}, and sIgD^{-}. This population is most likely to be the target of tolerogenic signals (Carsetti et al., 1995). In addition, at birth, the *B*-cells are devoid of Class II molecules, which are expressed in 43% of the *B*-cells 4 days later (Lam and Stall, 1994).

2. Neonatal *B*-cells have little or no TdT (Rothenberg and Triglia, 1983), which explains infants' more restricted antibody response compared to adults.

3. Neonatal *B*-cells are characterized by a poor proliferative response induced by anti-IgM antibodies, lack of response to TI2 antigens, and weak responses to TD antigens. Lack of stimulation by anti-IgM antibodies may be related to defective signaling pathways of neonatal *B*-cells, in which the signaling through sIgM is not coupled to the inositol–phospholipid cascade (Yellen et al., 1991), as well as to the poor expression of src-tyrosine kinase (Wechsler and Monroe, 1995).

4. Neonatal *B*-cells do not respond to CD38 ligand (Lund et al., 1995).

5. Neonatal *B*-cells cannot be stimulated by certain TI2 antigens such as TNP-Ficoll (Cohen et al., 1976), Type III pneumococcal polysaccharides (Amsbaugh et al., 1972) or phosphorylcholine (Mond et al., 1977). This phenomenon is related to an ontogenic delay of a subset of lymphocytes bearing the Lyb5 marker. The development of this subset is under control of the xid gene (Mosier et al., 1976). The best example is the anti-inulin antibody response that can be elicited only in 28-day-old mice (Bona et al., 1979). Figure 9.1 illustrates the ontogenic delay of anti-inulin response and the expression of idiotypes. While polyclonal activators such lipopolysaccharides can break down the tolerance of B cells, the anti-inulin antibody response cannot be rescued by NWSM, which is also a strong *B*-cell polyclonal activator.

Shain and Cebra (1981) have shown that the delayed acquisition in expression of anti-inulin response is preceded by an increase in frequency of inulin-specific *B*-cells, between the ages of 3 and 5 weeks. The expansion of inulin-specific lymphocytes can be related to the exposure to environmental antigens during the perinatal life.

Neonatal B cells are more sensitive to tolerogenic signals. Thus, a long lasting suppression can be induced by injection after birth of anti-allotype (Dray, 1962) or anti-idiotypic antibodies (Nisonoff and Bangasser, 1975), leading to inability to produce the corresponding allotype or idiotype(s). The unresponsiveness can be broken by *B*-cell mitogens.

A high dosage of antigen administered after birth also causes a long-lasting specific unresponsiveness. The injection of neonates with 1 mg bacterial levan, a β2-6 and β2-1 fructosan, caused inability of adult mice to mount an immune response following challenge with levan (Bona et al., 1979). Figure 9.2 illustrates these results. Several hypotheses were

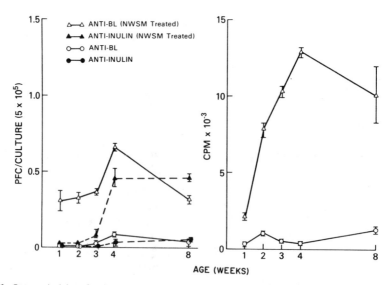

Figure 9.1. Ontogenic delay of anti-inulin antibody response. Balb/c mice were immunized with bacterial levan at age of 1, 2, 3, and 4 weeks and PFC response (left) or proliferative response (right) were measured in presence or absence of NWSM (from Bona et al., *J. Immunol.*, 1979, 123:1484–1490).

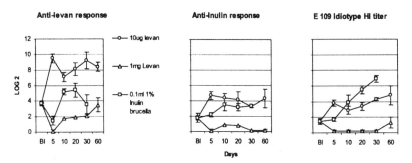

Figure 9.2. High dose tolerance induced by bacterial levan (from Bona et al., *J. Immunol.*, 1979, 123:1484–1490).

advanced to explain the unresponsiveness of neonatal *B*-cells. The most plausible explanation is that neonatal *B*-cells lacking sIgD cannot deliver an activation signal coupled to the inositol–phospholipid signaling pathway (Yellen et al., 1991). This concept is strongly supported by data demonstrating that stripping adult lymphocytes of IgD makes them more sensitive to tolerogenic signals (Kettman et al., 1979). However, there are observations demonstrating that the injection of certain antigens after birth or during the perinatal period can elicit low but significant responses.

Howard and Hale (1976) first demonstrated that adult animals injected as newborns with small doses of polysaccharide antigen can mount an antibody response. Hiernaux et al. (1987) showed that an antibody response against levan can be induced by injection of neonates with anti-idiotype antibodies expressed on antilevan antibodies. Figure 9.3 illustrates the results of these experiments in which the injection of 1-day-old mice with anti-A48 Id antibodies increased significantly the number of antilevan PFC and corresponding A48 idiotype.

Antibody responses were elicited in 1-day-old mice injected with 1-3 dextran (Fernandez and Moller, 1979), with galactan (Bona, 1979), or with TNP-LPS (Bona, 1980). Figure 9.4 illustrates the induction of a long-lasting response of 1-day-old mice immunized with 10 μg arabinogalactan. Specific antibody synthesis was also noted following immunization of 7-day-old mice with phosphorylcholine (Sigal et al., 1997) or with phenylarsenate-protein conjugate (Nutt et al., 1979).

Finally, it was proved that Sabin polio or hepatitis B vaccines are able to induce protective antibodies in infants, while others, such as influenza and polysaccharide vaccines administered to newborns or infants fail to induce protection.

The IgM isotype predominates in the neonatal humoral response. The IgM response is generally encoded by V-genes in genomic configuration. This is associated with two factors: (1) Little or lack of expression of TdT, which contributes to N-region diversity in adult repertoire by addition or deletion of nucleotides in CDR3 (Desiderio et al., 1984; Komori et al., 1996); and (2) delayed mechanism mediating the somatic mutations. However, recently Giorgetti and Press (1998) showed that the cells from neonates injected after birth with NP-CGG or a synthetic polypeptide exhibited somatic mutation, demonstrating that the somatic mutation machinery is activated in neonatal *B*-cells. Neonates can utilize

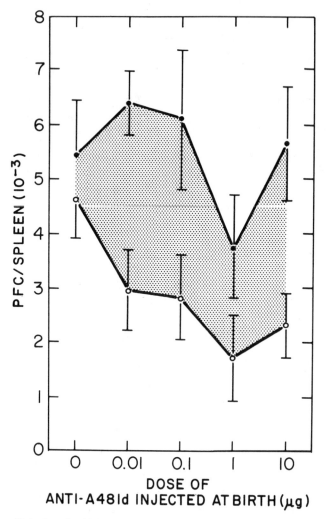

Figure 9.3. Effect of injection after birth of minute amounts of anti-A48 idiotypic antibodies. Hatchered area represents A48Id⁺ PFC (from Bona et al., *J. Immunol.*, 1979, 123:1484–1490).

somatic mutation not only to diversify the germline repertoire but also to produce high affinity antibodies (Giorgetti, 1998, in press).

9.2. EFFECT OF NEONATAL GENETIC IMMUNIZATION

Bot et al., (1996a) first reported that injection of a plasmid-expressing influenza virus nucleoprotein in 1-day-old newborn mice primed NP-specific CTLs that were able to confer protection against challenge with a lethal dose of virus several weeks after birth. In the

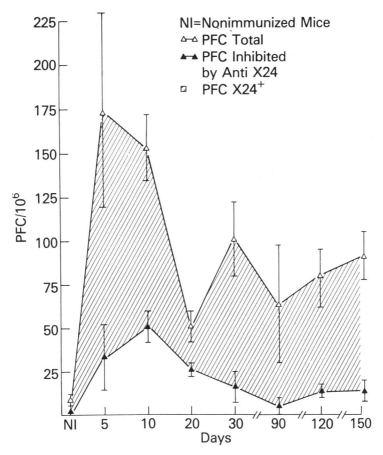

Figure 9.4. Anti-galactan antibody response of 1-day-old mice injected with 10 μg of arabinogalactan. The number of anti-galactan PFC and those expressing X24Id was determined at various ages after immunization.

ensuing years, this observation has been confirmed by several investigators, who demonstrated the ability of naked DNA to elicit humoral and cellular responses when injected into neonates.

9.2.1. Humoral Responses

Monteil et al. (1996) have studied anti-gD-specific antibody response following immunization of 1-day-old piglets with a plasmid expressing the gD gene of pseudorabies virus. An age-dependent increase of antibody titer was observed until the age of challenge (i.e., 70 days after immunization). However, in spite of the fact that the animals produced antibodies, no protection was observed following challenge. The reason for failure of genetic immunization to induce a protective response in this experiment may be related to low expression of gD gene in transfected cells. Wang et al. (1997a) had studied the immune response of mice injected after birth with a plasmid-expressing full-length rabies virus glycoprotein under the control of the SV40 promoter. After boost, these mice developed a higher antibody response compared to those injected with control plasmid. It is noteworthy that the majority of anti-gP antibodies were of IgG2a isotype, suggesting a participation of *T*-cells. Successful responses were also elicited by neonatal immunization of chimpanzees with plasmids encoding hepatitis B surface antigen (Prince et al., 1997) or HIV-1 gag/pol genes (Bagarazzi et al., 1997). In the case of hepatitis B virus, specific antibodies were detected between 15 and 21 weeks after immunization and remained at a constant level until 70 weeks. Challenge of these animals with 100 doses of CID_{50} virus at 33 weeks elicited an anamnestic response. Failure of detection of hepatitis core protein in serum clearly demonstrated that the immunization with plasmid stimulated *B*-cells at birth and produced protective antibodies. In the case of HIV-1 virus, the antibody response was evident as early as 4 weeks following immunization. The magnitude of the response of animals immunized as neonates was comparable to that of immunized adult animals. Studies in our laboratory focused on immune response against influenza virus. The rationale of studying this system was based on epidemiological observations showing that neonates or infants respond poorly or not at all to vaccination with inactivated influenza vaccine. In the case of influenza virus, antihemagglutinin (HA) antibodies prevent the infection by binding to viral HA, thereby inhibiting the binding of virus to the sialoprotein cell receptor. Antineuraminidase antibodies prevent only the spreading of virus and have minor protective properties. While the immunization of adult animals with live or inactivated influenza virus elicited a strong immune response, Antohi et al. (1998) showed that the immunization of neonates with UV-inactivated virus caused a long-lasting anergy. One- to 3-month-old animals injected with virus at birth did not produce anti-HA antibodies after challenge. By contrast, Bot et al. (1997b) showed the occurrence of low amounts of antibodies in mice injected three times (Days 1, 3, and 6 after birth) with a plasmid encoding the HA gene of WSN virus (pHA). However, the mice challenged at the age of 3 months produced an amount of antibodies similar to that of adults primed and challenged with virus. These results demonstrated that neonatal immunization has a strong priming effect on the precursors of anti-HA antibody-forming cells that generated memory cells. Comparison of isotypes of anti-HA antibodies produced by adults and neonates immunized with pHA showed significant differences. While during the secondary response of adults, IgG2a and IgG2b were predominant isotypes, in the animals immunized as neonates, the response was mainly dominated by IgG3 and IgG1. The major question addressed in these studies was to evaluate whether neonatal genetic immunization is able to induce the expansion of memory *B*-cells to the same extent as vaccination of adults and produce a prompt protective antibody response. This question was addressed by measuring the virus lung titer, the loss of weight, and survival of animals challenged with a lethal dose of virus 1 month after the completion of immunization. In these experiments, at Day 3, mice immunized with pHA showed higher virus titers that those immunized with WSN virus. However, by Day 7, they completely cleared the virus compared with mice not primed or those injected with control plasmid. Sixty percent of mice immunized at birth with pHA survived after the challenge with lethal dose. The results of this study are summarized in Table 9.2.

Table 9.2. Correlation between Anti-HA Antibodies
and Protective Responses of Mice Injected as Newborns with pHA

Immunization at birth with	Challenge after 1 mo. with	HI titer	Virus lung titer		Survival
			d3	d7	
Nil	Nil	0	0	0	7/7
Nil	WSN	8.2	5.4	3.7	NS
pC	Nil	0	0	0	7/7
pC	WSN	7.0	4.5	NS	NS
pHA	Nil	5.2	0	0	7/7
pHA	WSN	9.4	4.7	0.8	4/7

Note. Data expressed as $\log_2$ dilution of serum in the case of HI titer and as $\log_{10}$ viral titer in $TCID_{50}$ units. NS = no survivals.

The reduced pulmonary virus titers, increased survival, and weight recovery in a significant proportion of mice immunized as neonates with pHA and challenged with a lethal dose of virus are indicative of a protective humoral and cellular response. Factors that may contribute to efficient priming of *B*-cells by naked DNA include the following: First, sustained presence of low amount of antigen produced by transfected cells suffices to prime the *B*-cells that mature during perinatal life. The low dosage of antigen produced by transfected cells favors the differentiation, avoiding induction of high-dose tolerance. Second, there is the possibility of accelerated replacement of neonatal with adult repertoire. In the case of anti-HA response, Cancro et al. (1979) showed that some clonotypes present in neonates disappeared in adults. Analysis of clonotype specificity pattern of HA-specific clones showed that in animals immunized as neonates with pHA, there is a rapid replacement of restricted clonotypes characteristic for the neonatal repertoire (Antohi et al., 1998).

9.2.2. CTL Responses

While antibodies specific for membrane-associated viral or bacterial proteins are protective by virtue of their ability to prevent the penetration of microbes into cells, favoring phagocytosis, lysis of bacteria, or neutralization of microbial toxins, the CTLs play a major role in recovery from infection caused by either viruses or obligatory intracellular microbes. The expansion of CTL precursors requires the activation of CD4 *T*-cells, which provide growth factors for CD8 *T*-cells. In addition, the NK cells that recognize foreign antigens present on the surface of infected cells may play a role. The role of various populations of lymphocytes was best dissected during the response against influenza virus.

Adoptive transfer experiments showed that influenza-specific CD8 *T*-cell clones can mediate the recovery from influenza virus infection (Taylor and Askonas, 1986; Lukacher et al., 1984; MacKenzie et al., 1989). This concept is supported by other findings.

Bot et al. (1996a) showed that while RAG2$-/-$ and SCID mice are unable to clear the virus from lungs and do not survive after challenge with live virus, JhD$-/-$ mice survived and completely recovered. In addition to CD8 T-cells, the CD4 T-cells also play a role in recovery process. This was shown in β2-microglobulin$-/-$ mice, which were able to recover from a lethal challenge in the absence of CD8 T-cells (Eichelberger et al., 1991).

While the number of NK cells was increased in the lungs of SCID mice infected with influenza virus, the depletion of NK1.1 cells did not affect the overall survival, suggesting that NK cells play a minor role in the recovery process (Bot et al., 1996a).

Because of the inability of inactivated influenza vaccine to induce a CTL immune response, Bot et al. (1996a) evaluated the cellular response induced by the immunization of neonates with a plasmid-encoding influenza nucleoprotein (NPVI). In mice, about 80% of CTL is specific for an allelic Class I peptide (Townsend et al., 1986). Newborn mice immunized with NPVI plasmid developed cytotoxicity comparable to that displayed by adult mice injected with the same dose of plasmid. The cytotoxic activity was related to the expansion of precursors assessed by measuring pCTL frequency, 1 month after immunization of adults or neonates with NPVI plasmid. The data depicted in Table 9.3 show that the pCTL frequency was lower in animals immunized with plasmid than in those immunized with virus, but it increased dramatically after virus boost. This demonstrates the strong priming effect of neonatal genetic immunization on CTL precursors. It is noteworthy that the CTL from animals immunized as neonates with NPVI plasmid and stimulated *in vitro* with virus displayed broad cross-reactivity, being able to lyse cells infected with various Type A influenza strains. Challenge with a lethal dose of influenza virus of animals immunized with NPVI was followed by a drastic reduction of viral titer by Day 7 following infection. Sarzotti et al. (1997) also demonstrated that immunization of neonates with a plasmid-expressing full-length CAS-Br-M genome induced long-lasting, virus-specific, CD8 CTL protective response.

In summary, these findings demonstrate that neonatal genetic immunization primes CTL responses, as in adults. The protectivity conferred by genetic immunization may be related to prolonged stimulation of the immune system that circumvents the requirement of boost and to a better recruitment of virus-specific cells at the site of replication of infectious agent (Bot et al., 1998a).

Table 9.3. Frequency of CTL Precursors after Immunization with NPVI or pHA

| | | 1/CTL frequency | | | |
| | | Newborn | | Adult | |
Immunization with	Boost	WSN	PR8	WSN	PR8
pC	Nil	$>1.0 \times 10^6$		$>1.0 \times 10^6$	
pC	WSN	5.8×10^4		8.7×10^3	
pHA	Nil	$>1.0 \times 10^6$		$>1.0 \times 10^6$	
pHA	WSN	1.7×10^4		4.2×10^3	
Nil	PR8		1.2×10^4		1.2×10^4
NPVI	Nil		1.9×10^5		2.3×10^4
NPVI	PR8		5.0×10^3		2.5×10^3

9.2.3. Cytokine Response

CD4 *T*-cell populations are heterogeneous and composed of phenotypically distinct minute subsets exhibiting different functions: Th1, secreting IL-2 and IFNγ; Th2, secreting IL-4, IL-5; Th3, secreting mainly TGFβ; and an additional subset secreting IL-10.

The activation of these subsets subsequent to immunization creates a network of interactions between various cells involved in the immune responses. Whereas some cytokines provide positive signals, others provide negative signals for the activation and differentiation of antigen-specific lymphocytes as well as for the cells involved in nonspecific immunity, such as NKs, macrophages, neutrophils, eosinophiles, or basophiles. Both Th1 and Th2 cells of adult animals are activated subsequent to immunization with microbial antigens, with the exception of some parasites that activate only a subset (Revillard, 1998).

In contrast, there is a definitive bias of cytokine production in neonates. Neonatal *T*-cells stimulated *in vitro* with anti-CD3, a polyclonal activator (Adkins et al., 1993), or with antigen in the case of transgenic mice (Bot et al., 1997a), produced high levels of IL-4 but little or no IFNγ and IL-2. Similarly, a Th2-biased response was reported by Barrios et al. (1996), who studied the isotypes of antibodies produced subsequent to immunization of neonates with various antigens (measles, canary pox vector, BCG) or peptides derived from tetanus toxoid. The neonatal responses differed from those of adult by an impaired production of antigen-specific IgG2a antibodies and low secretion of IFNγ. These observations predict that while the vaccination stimulates both Th1 and Th2 responses in adults, the response in neonates is polarized toward Th2. Neonatal Th2-skewed response can be circumvented by genetic immunization (Martinez et al., 1997). As in adult mice, administration to neonates of plasmid-encoding measles virus HA, Sendai virus NP, or a fragment of the tetanus toxin gene, induced mixed Th1/Th2 responses as assessed by the isotype of antibodies and by increased IFNγ and decreased IL-5 secretion.

Bot et al. (1997b, 1998c) have studied *in vitro* production of lymphokines by lymphocytes from mice injected after birth with two different plasmids: pHA encoding WSN virus HA, expressing the immunodominant epitopes recognized by CD4 *T*-cells; and NPVI plasmid encoding nucleoprotein, bearing immunodominant epitopes recognized by CD8 *T*-cells. Lymphokine response was studied on negatively selected CD4 *T*-cells in the case of animals immunized with pHA. While the immunization with WSN virus of neonates or adults induced *in vitro* synthesis, upon incubation with the virus, of both IFNγ and IL-4, only low concentrations were detected in cultures of lymphocytes originating from animals immunized with pHA or pC. This clearly showed that the expansion of CD4 *T*-cells by virus immunization is stronger.

However, the pattern of cytokine production was different after boost with WSN virus of animals immunized as adults or neonates with pHA. While the lymphocytes from mice immunized with pHA as neonates displayed a mixed Th1/Th2 response that was augmented after *in vitro* exposure to virus, the lymphocytes from adults displayed a Th1-biased response. This contrasts with lymphocytes from animals primed and boosted with WSN virus, which produced more IL-4 than IFNγ.

CD8 *T*-cells from mice immunized as neonates with NPVI and stimulated *in vitro* with the NP147-155 peptide secreted IFNγ but not IL-4, like *T*-cells from adult animals

Table 9.4. Cytokine Production by Lymphocytes
from Mice Injected with pHA as Adults or Neonates

| Mice immunized with | Boost | Four days of incubation | | | |
| | | IFNγ | | IL-4 | |
		Nil	WSN	Nil	WSN
A. Adults					
Nil		0	0	0	0
WSN		52	214	48	181
WSN	WSN	10	127	218	235
pC		0	11	0	0
pC	WSN	24	158	89	261
pHA		9	60	0	29
pHA	WSN	19	284	54	31
B. Newborn					
Nil		ND	ND	ND	ND
WSN		103	51	132	248
WSN	WSN	9	61	228	594
pC		14	22	0	0
pC	WSN	89	261	198	141
pHA		0	29	38	179
pHA	WSN	19	284	138	257

Note. Concentration of cytokines was determined by ELISA and expressed
as pg/ml.

immunized with virus (Table 9.4). Apparently, the pattern of cytokine production differs in the case of CD4 and CD8 *T*-cells. While CD4 *T*-cells from neonates immunized with DNA or virus secrete both IFNγ and IL-4, the CD8 *T*-cells secrete mainly IFNγ. Together, these observations show that DNA immunization of neonates stimulates the activation of Th1 and Tc1 cells, that produce cytokines involved in antiviral immunity:

1. IFNγ may inhibit virus replication.
2. IL-2 favors the growth of CD8 *T*-cells and Th cells, and provides the signals required for the differentiation of *B*-cells into antibody-forming cells.

Table 9.5 summarizes various reported information on immune response and protection conferred by neonatal genetic immunization.

9.2.4. Augmentation of Protective Defensive Reactions by Coimmunization of Neonates with Plasmids Encoding Antigens Expressing Epitopes Recognized by *B*- and *T*-Cells

Immunization of neonates with pHA encoding influenza HA expressing major epitopes recognized by *B*- and CD4 *T*-cells, while having a definitive priming effect, did

Table 9.5. Immune Response and Protection Conferred
by Neonatal Inoculation of Plasmids Expressing Microbial Antigens

Microbe	Antigen	Species	Immune response	Protection	Reference
Influenza virus	NP	Mouse	CTL	Yes	Bot et al., 1996a
	HA	Mouse	Abs, Th	Yes	Bot et al., 1997b
	NP + HA	Mouse	Abs, CTL, Th	Yes	Bot et al., 1998a
		Nonhuman primate[a]	Abs[a]	ND[a]	Bot et al., 1999
	HA	Mouse	Abs	ND	Pertmer and Robinson, 1999
Plasmodium yoelii	CSP	Mouse	Tolerance[b]	ND	Mor et al., 1996
Pseudorabies virus	gD glycoprotein	Pig	Abs[c]	No	Monteil et al., 1996
Rabies virus	Glycoprotein	Mouse	Abs, Th	Yes	Wang et al., 1997b
Hepatitis B virus	HBsAg	Nonhuman primate	Abs	Yes	Prince et al., 1997
Murine retrovirus	Cas-Br-M antigen	Mouse	CTL	Yes	Sarzotti et al., 1997
HIV	Env, Gag-pol	Nonhuman primate	Abs	ND	Bagarazzi et al., 1997
Measles virus	Hemagglutinin	Mouse	Abs, Th	ND	Martinez et al., 1997
Sendai virus	NP	Mouse	Abs, CTL	ND	Martinez et al., 1997
Clostridium tetanii	C fragment of tetanus toxoid	Mouse	Abs, Th	ND	Martinez et al., 1997
Respiratory syncytial virus	F antigen	Mouse	Abs, CTL	ND	Martinez et al., 1999
Herpes simplex	gB of *Herpes simplex*	Mouse	Abs, Th	Yes	Manickan et al., 1997a
LCMV	NP	Mouse	Abs, CTL	Yes	Hassett et al., 1997, 2000

[a]Follow-up study in progress.
[b]Previous studies showed that in contrast to most of the other studies, single intramuscular inoculation of plasmid-expressing PyCSP in adult mice was followed by Th2 rather than Th1 responses (Mor et al., 1995).
[c]Antibodies were detected only in animals boosted at the age of 42 days.
ND = not done.

confer only a partial protection in a large cohort of mice studied. A similar result was observed after immunization with NPVI plasmid encoding influenza NP, which expresses major epitopes recognized by CD8 *T*-cells.

Since the aim of vaccination is to protect the entire population, Bot et al. (1998a) have studied the protective response elicited by vaccination of neonates with pHA and NPVI plasmids. Coinjection of both plasmids was followed by induction of CTL exhibiting cross-reactivity against various Type A virus strains, expansion of CD4 *T*-cells specific for epitopes shared by virus and drift variants, and production of antibodies specific for the HA encoded by pHA. Data depicted in Table 9.6 show a complete protection paralleled by clearing of virus in animals vaccinated as adults or newborns with a mixture of equal amounts of pHA and NPVI plasmids. Further, in spite of the lack of PR8 HA-specific antibodies, the protection against the PR8 drift variant was almost complete. These ob-

Table 9.6. Effect of Immunization of Newborns with pHA and NPVI Plasmids, on Humoral and Protective Responses against Influenza Virus

Newborns immunized with	HI titer ($\log_2$)	Lung virus titer ($\log_{10}$ of $TCID_{50}$, mean $\pm$ SD)			Survival
		Day 3	Day 7	Day 20	
pC	0	4.2 ± 0.5	NS	NS	0/7
NPVI	0	4.7	NS	NS	0/7
pHA	5.2 ± 0.3	4.0 ± 0.6	1.0	0	4/7
NPVI + pHA	2.2 ± 0.8	3.4 ± 1.2	1.0	0	7/7
UV–WSN	0	ND	ND	ND	0/7

NS = no survivors, ND = not done.

servations suggest that cellular immunity is the most important arm in the protection against influenza virus induced by genetic immunization of adults or neonates, although antibodies play a definitive role.

This information is particularly important, since it demonstrates that the coadministration of a cocktail of plasmids encoding proteins bearing relevant protective epitopes can be successfully used to protect a large population against diseases caused by infectious agents. Prevention of infectious diseases that affect children during the first months of life requires effective vaccines for this population. It clearly appears that in contrast to current vaccines that are unable to confer a protective immunity in children, genetic immunization is able to overcome the unresponsiveness of infants or newborns by priming the immune system efficiently, enabling it to respond promptly to infectious agents.

We have recently pursued a study in baboons (*Papio*) addressing the ability of neonatal vaccination with expression vectors encoding the HA of A/WSN/32 H1N1 virus and the conserved NP of H1N1 subtype to trigger persisting humoral and cellular immunity (Bot et al., 2000, submitted). We showed that intramuscular injection of the plasmid mixture (priming on Day 1 and boosts on Days 14 and 28) triggered virus-specific IgG antibodies of a magnitude and persistence strongly and directly dependent on the vaccine dose. Only at doses of 1 mg/plasmid/inoculation did we note IgG titers in the serum that persisted at substantial levels up to the age of 6 months. This correlated with detectable titers of hemagglutination-inhibiting antibodies. The antibody levels gradually declined until the age of 1½ years. However, a boost using live WSN virus, which abortively infects the respiratory tract of baboons, triggered significantly enhanced levels of antibodies compared to those of baboons inoculated with control negative plasmid as neonates. Most importantly, in the group preimmunized with DNA vaccine and boosted with live virus, we could detect virus-specific antibodies in the respiratory tract. Antigen stimulation of peripheral blood mononuclear cells was associated with increased proliferation and IFN-γ production in the case of baboons preimmunized with DNA vaccine as neonates. These baboons displayed *T*-cell reactivity against syngeneic cells infected with NP-recombinant vaccinia virus, but not with a control vaccinia virus. In conclusion, neonatal DNA vaccination of baboons with influenza antigens (HA and NP) triggered humoral and cellular responses that persisted as immune memory, beyond the infant stage. A combination of systemic neonatal priming with DNA vaccine, followed by boost with live vaccine administered via the respiratory tract later in life, is likely to confer a more optimal immunity at reduced risk for side effects, optimizing protection against influenza virus infection during infancy and childhood.

9.3. EFFECT OF MATERNAL ANTIBODIES ON IMMUNE RESPONSE OF NEONATES AND INFANTS

Maternal IgG, via the placenta, and IgA via the colostrum, can be transferred to newborns. Maternal antibodies exert various effects on host defense reactions and on the development of the immune system of newborns.

9.3.1. Protective Ability of Maternal Antibodies

There is a large body of evidence that maternal antibodies protect newborns and infants against infectious diseases during the postnatal life when their immune systems are immature. From multiple sources of evidence, we have chosen two examples in which the role of IgG antibodies was thoroughly investigated, namely, influenza and HIV viruses.

Influenza viruses are a significant cause of disease in human infants. Protection of infants in the early months of life depends upon transmission of maternal immunity via the placenta and postnatally via colostrum and milk. The role of maternal antibodies in prevention of influenza infection was demonstrated in humans as well as various animal models.

Masurel et al. (1978) showed that newborns born to mothers with high titers of anti-HA antibodies also had significant titers. Puck et al. (1980) confirmed this observation and demonstrated that the protection is time-limited. Maximal half-life of protection was 21 days in the case of infants with high concentrations of antibodies. Murphy et al. (1989) reported that the infection in the presence of low amounts of maternal antibodies was mild. Studies carried out in animals provided additional evidence on protective properties of maternal antibodies.

The ferrets represent a good animal model since intranasal administration of virus proved to be invariably fatal subsequent to severe involvement of upper respiratory tract and influenza pneumonia. Husseini et al. (1984) showed that the challenge of newborn ferrets born to mothers immunized with virulent or attenuated viruses resulted in complete protection. No virus replicated in their lungs, and little or no virus was isolated from their nasal turbinates. A good correlation was noted between the degree of protection and the titer of anti-influenza antibodies. In the case of newborns to mothers immunized 3 weeks prepartum with formalin-inactivated vaccine, the level of protection varied from partial to complete, depending upon the number of doses used to immunize the mother, administered with or without adjuvant. The protection of newborns was transient. They were completely protected at 2 weeks, but susceptibility returned to nasal epithelium at 5 weeks and to lung at 7 weeks (Sweet et al., 1987). Apparently, the protection was conferred by milk IgG rather than by antibodies transferred via the placenta, since 1-day-old ferrets born to nonimmu-nized mothers, and fostered on immune mothers, exhibited a similar level of protection to ferrets born to and suckled by immune mothers.

It is noteworthy that the protection is conferred solely by anti-HA antibodies. This was elegantly demonstrated by experiments in which the prepartum immunization of females was carried out with vaccinia recombinants expressing HA, NA, polymerases (PB1, PB2, or PAC), matrix protein (M1 or M2), and NP or nonstructural NS1 or NS2 proteins. Only recombinants encoding the HA protected newborns against intranasal challenge (Jakeman et al., 1989). Ali et al. (1988) showed that breast-fed guinea pigs from immune mothers were partially protected against influenza virus when compared to guinea pigs born to non-immune mothers.

Similar results were obtained in mice. Nossal (1957) showed that maternal anti-HA antibodies are transferred to progeny by breast-feeding. Reuman et al. (1983) carried out a study aimed at characterizing the defense reaction and the immune response of mice born to immunized mothers. This study concluded that maternal antibodies are life saving, and the lung viral titer of these mice appeared to correlate inversely with the amount of serum antibodies transferred to newborns. Mbawuike et al. (1990) also found that the protection is conferred by breast milk, since it was also achieved by cross-fostering. A majority of maternal antibodies transferred to blood by colostrum or milk are of IgG isotype. This is surprising, since the IgA are found in high concentration in the colostrum. However, this is probably related to a better uptake by the gut of IgG compared to IgM or IgA.

The role of maternal antibodies was also studied in HIV-1 infection in which the virus is vertically transmitted to newborns. Ugen et al. (1997a) found that the antibodies transmit-ted from mother are mainly directed against the C-terminal region of gp41 protein. Rossi et al. (1989), in a study carried out on 33 children born to HIV-infected mothers, and whose clinical outcome was known at the time of analysis, showed that anti-gp120 antibodies might play a role in preventing mother-to-child transmission of HIV-1 virus. The protective ability of maternal antibodies was also revealed in the case of bacteria, such as *N. meningitis* (Lifely et al., 1989), and viral infections caused by gastroenteritis virus (Gough et al., 1983), rotavirus (Sheridan et al., 1992), HSV (Kohl and Loo, 1984), and rabies virus (Xiang and Ertl, 1992).

In conclusion, these data clearly demonstrate that the maternal antibodies exhibit a protective role against various infectious agents.

9.3.2. Regulatory Properties of Maternal Antibodies via Idiotype Interactions

Some observations suggest that maternal antibodies induce an imprint to nascent immune systems. The effect of maternal IgG on the development of B lineage was studied in progenies born to mMt/mMT (Ig$^-$) or mMT/$^+$ (Ig$^+$) females and males. The offspring born to Ig$^+$ females but not to Ig$^-$ females exhibited an increased number of pre-B-cells in bone marrow as well as splenic B-cells, 7 days after birth (Malanchere et al., 1997). The increased number of pre-B-cells cannot be explained by a direct interaction with maternal IgG, since the pre-B-cells lack Ig receptors, but rather may be explained by an effect on cells producing cytokines endowed with growth factor properties.

In contrast, maternal IgG has no effect on the rate of maturation of B-cells from offspring. A study carried out on the same type of crosses as described earlier showed that no differences were observed in the endogenous production of IgM or IgG, nor of Vh repertoire, between the offspring born to Ig$^+$ and Ig$^-$ mothers (Delassus et al., 1997). These observations suggest that while maternal IgG exhibits a positive regulatory role in the early phase of the development of B-lineage, they do not influence the maturation of B-cells.

Maternal antibodies are also able to modulate antigen-specific clones. Winkler et al. (1980) showed that offspring rabbits born to mothers immunized with *M. luteus* produced antibodies sharing the mother's idiotypes, whereas rabbits born to nonimmunized mothers expressed other idiotypes.

Rubinstein et al. (1982, 1984) demonstrated that maternal Igs can expand silent clones via idiotype interactions. This study was carried out on offspring born to mothers injected during the last week of pregnancy with UPC10 or A48 monoclonal proteins. These levan-specific proteins express A48 IdX, which is not expressed on antilevan antibodies elicited following immunization with bacterial levan, indicating that the clones expressing this idiotype are silent. An increased number of levan-specific antibody-forming cells expressing A48 IdX was observed in offspring born to mothers injected with either A48 or UPC10 proteins. The expansion of A48Id$^+$ clones was related to induction by maternal antibodies of A48Id$^+$-specific Th cells. Lemke et al. (1994) also showed that maternal antibodies specific for 2-phenyl-oxazolone influence the antibody response of not only F1 but also F2 offspring born to immunized mothers.

These observations showed that the passive influx of maternal idiotypes in the immune system of a fetus or newborn by placental transfer or milk feeding influences clonal distribution by favoring the expansion of those clones that produce idiotypes similar to the dominant maternal ones. This condition is interesting from both physiological and theoretical points of view. In physiological terms, it is clearly an advantage to have the mother's immunological experience transmitted to the next generation to develop a more vigorous response against pathogens prevailing in the species during a given period. In theoretical terms, this constitutes an example of the inheritance of acquired immunity not only as a passive acquisition of maternal antibodies but also in terms of priming the immune system to a better response against antigens previously encountered by the mother (Bona and Pernis, 1984).

9.3.3. Inhibitory Effect of Maternal Antibodies

In contrast to their positive regulatory effects, the maternal antibodies specific for antigenic determinants expressed on lymphocyte's receptors exhibit a strong suppressive effect. This is well illustrated in three different systems. First, Dray (1962) demonstrated that maternal antibodies specific for father allotype induced a long-lasting suppression of the expression of father allotype in F1 rabbits. Second, several authors showed that maternal anti-idiotypic antibodies specific for idiotypes expressed on the Ig receptor or TCR determinants of B- and T-cells, respectively, are inhibitory. Thus, Weiller et al. (1977) showed that maternal anti-J558 IdX antibodies induced suppression that lasted for 4–5 months. Rothstein and Vastola (1984) induced idiotype suppression by injection during pregnancy of monoclonal antibodies specific for CRI expressed by antiarsonate antibodies. These observations suggest that maternal antibodies can regulate the expression of *B*-cell receptors.

Wang and Shlomchik (1998) showed that maternal IgG mediates neonatal tolerance to rheumatoid factor, an autoantibody specific for IgG. In these experiments, a series of reciprocal genetic crosses of mice expressing different allotypes were used. Mice without maternal IgG, but with the endogenous capacity to express the IgG allotype, did not exhibit the deletion of RF-producing *B*-cells. In contrast, those having maternal IgG, deleted RF-specific autoreactive *B*-cells. McKeever et al. (1997) recently demonstrated that maternal antibodies specific for a clonotype (idiotype) antigenic determinant expressed on TCR, caused also a long-term suppression of *T*-cells bearing the corresponding idiotype.

It is noteworthy that maternal antibodies specific for antigens associated with the cellular membrane do not affect the expression of them. We reported (Braun et al., 1976) that maternal anti-Thy1.2 antibodies did not affect the expression of this *T*-cell antigen in offspring born to mothers producing anti-Thy antibodies.

9.3.4. Inhibitory Effect of Maternal Antibodies on Vaccination of Infants

It is well established that passive administration of specific antibodies induces the suppression of the immune response when the antigen is concomitantly injected for immunization (Uhr and Moller, 1968). Antibodies against a few or one epitope of a macromolecule suffice to induce suppression. This was clearly demonstrated by Cerottini et al. (1969), who injected antibodies specific for Fab or Fc fragments of IgG, followed by the immunization with whole IgG. Both antibodies prevented an anti-IgG response.

The suppression of immune responses by specific antibodies explains the failure of vaccination of infants. The vaccine failures is inversely correlated with the amount of maternal antibodies transferred via the placenta, colostrum, or milk.

Xiang and Ertl (1992) showed that the inhibition of the immune response elicited by rabies virus outlasts the time during which maternal antibodies are present. Siegrist et al. (1998) made similar observations in a study carried out on offspring born to dams immunized with a live recombinant canary pox vector expressing influenza HA, or with attenuated measles vaccine.

The mechanisms mediating immunosuppression by natural or artificial passive immunity are poorly understood. Uhr and Moller (1968) proposed that the suppression is due to immunocomplexes of specific antibodies with antigen or vaccine. This explanation is challenged by more recent data. It is well known that the immunocomplexes display a high affinity for FcR expressed on the surface of professional antigen-presenting cells.

Liu et al. (1996) demonstrated that multimeric complexes composed of antitetanus antibodies and tetanus toxoid internalized via FcR by human blastoid line enhanced the presentation of peptide to *T*-cells 100- to 1000-fold compared with tetanus toxoid alone. This observation is in agreement with the results reported by Zagouhani et al. (1993a), who showed that the FcR mediated internalization of a chimeric IgG expressing an influenza virus, HA-derived peptide, was more efficient than the synthetic peptide alone to activate CD4 *T*-cells.

Data concerning the effect of antibodies on *T*-cell presentation are contradictory (Bot et al., 1996a). Harte and Playfair (1983) proposed that the failure of malaria vaccination in mice born to immunized mothers is related to generation of suppressor cells by maternal IgG. The suppressor T-cells specifically inhibited the development of memory Th cells and persisted until the mice were 8 weeks of age.

Prolonged suppression of antigen-specific proliferation of T-cells by maternal anti-bodies was described upon immunization of offspring with malaria (Harte and Playfair, 1983), rabies and Sendai viruses (Xiang and Ertl, 1992). In contrast, Siegrist et al. (1998) found that the maternal antibodies did not affect the induction of vaccine-specific Th1, Th2, or CTLs. In conclusion, (proper) planning of the vaccination schedules for infants should take into account the inhibitory effects of maternal antibodies.

9.4. EFFECT OF MATERNAL ANTIBODIES ON IMMUNE RESPONSE OF OFFSPRING BORN TO DAMS IMMUNIZED WITH VIRUS OR PLASMID DNA

Although maternal antibodies provide short-time protection to neonates, they may contribute to vaccine failure in infants by inactivating the vaccines or suppressing the B-cells. It is therefore of great interest to determine the immune response of offspring born to virus- or naked DNA-immunized dams.

We have studied the anti-influenza virus immune response in offspring born to dams previously immunized with either WSN virus or with a plasmid bearing the WSN HA (pHA) gene. Offspring of various ages (i.e., 2 weeks, and 1, 3, and 6 months) were immu-nized with UV-inactivated WSN virus, and the HI titer of anti-HA antibodies was mea-sured. The data depicted in Table 9.7 show that 1-month-old mice exhibit higher HI titers

Table 9.7. Effect of Maternal Antibodies on Anti-Influenza Virus Response of Offspring Born to Dams Immunized with Live Virus or Plasmid DNA

Dams immunized with	Age at time of prebleeding and immunization	Prebleeding		7 days after immunization	
		WSN	PR8	WSN	PR8
Saline	2 wks.	0^a	0	1.0 ± 1.2	0
	1 mo.	0	0	3.3 ± 0.6	1.0 ± 1.0
pC	2 wks.	0	0	3.7 ± 1.8	0.5 ± 0.8
	1 mo.	0	0	3.8 ± 0.5	1.8 ± 2.4
pHA	2 wks.	2.4 ± 0.5	0	1.3 ± 0.5	0
	1 mo.	0	0	4.4 ± 1.7	0.2 ± 0.5
	3 mos.	0	0	4.8 ± 1.5	1.2 ± 0.4
	6 mos.	0	0	7.3 ± 0.6	2.7 ± 0.6
WSN virus	2 wks.	5.2 ± 0.9	0	4.3 ± 1.1	0
	1 mo.	3.8 ± 1.2	0	2.2 ± 0.5	0
	3 mos.	0	0	3.5 ± 0.6	1.3 ± 0.9
	6 mos.	0	0	5.8 ± 0.5	3.3 ± 0.5

^{a}HI titer ($\log_2$ dilution); 0 = less than 1/40 dilution of sera.

than 2-week-old mice born to nonimmunized females. This is in agreement with previous data showing that 1 month after birth, mice develop a significant primary immune response following the immunization with inactivated virus. Similar results were observed in 2-week- and 1-month-old mice born to dams injected with control plasmid. In the case of mice born to pHA immunized dams, anti-HA antibodies were detected only in 2-week-old mice. The titer was smaller after boosting than before, and probably represents residual maternal antibodies; 1-, 3-, and 6-month-old mice had no detectable HI titers before boost, but exhibited a gradual and age-dependent increase of HI titers after boost.

In the group of mice born to WSN-virus immunized dams, the HI titers were observed before the boost in 2-week- and 1-month-old mice but not in 3- or 6-month-old mice. After boost, the HI titers of 2-week- and 1-month-old mice were smaller than before boost, suggesting again that they represent residual maternal antibodies. Three-month-old mice had no detectable HI titers before the boost but developed a weaker response than 6-month-old mice after boost. Taken together, these results suggest that the lag time period of unresponsiveness of mice born to dams immunized with plasmid DNA is shorter than of mice born to virus-immunized dams. This probably is related to the lower amount of antibodies produced by animals immunized with DNA vaccines, compared to that of mice immunized with attenuated or inactivated vaccines.

9.5. EFFECT OF MATERNAL ANTIBODIES ON THE IMMUNE RESPONSE OF YOUNG AND ADULT ANIMALS ELICITED BY GENETIC IMMUNIZATION

It clearly appears that the maternal antibodies, besides having a transient protective effect, may have an inhibitory effect on antigen-specific lymphocytes and are responsible for failure of vaccination of infants. Thus, some investigators tried to address an important practical question, namely, whether genetic immunization might redress infants' response to vaccines in the presence of maternal antibodies. Unfortunately, the information concerning this question is quite contradictory.

Manickan et al. (1997a) have studied the immune response of neonates born to dams immunized with HSV: 4- to 6-week-old progeny were then immunized with a plasmid expressing a full-length HSV gB gene. The DNA-vaccinated progeny born to immunized dams exhibited a high concentration of antibodies. It is noteworthy that the virus-vaccinated progeny born to HSV-immunized dams failed to produce antibodies. This result suggests that the antibody response of progeny having detectable amounts of maternal antibodies can be redressed by genetic immunization.

Several studies attempted to determine the effect of maternal antibodies on cellular immune responses. Manickan et al. (1997a) and Siegrist et al. (1998) showed that maternal antibodies do not affect the induction of vaccine-specific Th1 or Th2 cells when the offspring was immunized with plasmid but not conventional vaccine.

Similarly, maternal antibodies specific for antigen vaccine have no effect on generation of CTLs following genetic immunization. Hassett et al. (1997) carried out a comparative study of LCMV-NP-specific cytotoxic activity in progeny born to dams immunized or not with nonlethal dose of LCMV. The progeny were then immunized with pCMV-NP or control plasmids at 6 to 8 weeks of age, and NP-specific CTL activity was measured. This study showed that mice born to and suckled on immune dams exhibiting anti-NP antibodies were able to develop an active cellular immunity following a single injection of pCMV-NP administered 1- and 14-days postpartum. In LCMV infection, while antibodies do not play a vital role, the protection is mediated by CTLs.

Induction of CTLs in progeny born to LCMV-immunized dams with high titers of anti-NP antibodies was paralleled by a reduction of virus concentration in the spleen and an increased survival of mice upon challenge with a lethal dose of LCMV. Lack of inhibition by maternal antibodies of CTL activity of progeny born to LCMV-immunized dams was predictable, since the protein encoded by NP gene expressed in plasmid is processed into endogenous pathway that cannot be affected by anti-NP antibodies. In addition, anti-NP antibodies cannot interfere with the recognition of MHC-peptide complex by T-cells, since it is known that while anti-MHC antibodies can prevent the activation of T-cells by APC, antibodies specific for the nominal peptide associated with MHC molecules have no effect.

In contrast with these data described, other investigators found that genetic immunization of newborns or infants is ineffective in the presence of maternal antibodies.

Monteil et al. (1996) injected 400 µg of plasmid expressing the gene encoding cD glycoprotein into 1-day-old piglets born to sows immunized or not with pseudorabies virus. The animals were boosted on Day 42 and challenged on Day 115. Piglets from immunized sows neither developed antibody response nor were they primed against the virus. Wangy et al. (1998) also reported that mice born to rabies virus-immune dams exhibited an impaired antibody response subsequent to genetic immunization at 6 weeks of age. These results do not agree with those reported by Manickan et al. (1997a), suggesting that the type of virus might differentially affect the outcome of genetic immunization in presence of maternal antibodies.

Additional studies are required in different systems to address this important problem for the vaccination of newborns or infants, namely, whether or not the genetic vaccines circumvent the inhibitory effect of maternal antibodies on neonatal, conventional vaccination.

References

Abastado, J. P., Casrouge, A., and Kourilsky, P. Differential role of conserved and polymorphic residues of the binding groove of Class I molecules in the selection of peptides. *J. Immunol.* (1993), **151**, 3569–3575.

Acsadi, G., Dickson, G., Love, D. R., Jani, A., Walsh, F. S., Gurusinghe, A., Wolff, J. A., and Davies, K. E. Human dystrophin expression in mdx mice after intramuscular injection of DNA constructs. *Nature* (1991a), **352**, 815–818.

Acsadi, G., Jiao, S. S., Jani, A., Duke, D., Williams, P., Chong, W., and Wolff, J. A. Direct gene transfer and expression into rat heart *in vivo*. *New Biol.* (1991b), **3**, 71–78.

Adam, A. *Synthetic adjuvants*. John Wiley & Sons, New York, (1985), pp. 59–85.

Adkins, B., Ghanei, A., and Hamilton, K. Developmental regulation of IL-4, IL-2 and interferon gamma production by murine peripheral T lymphocytes. *J. Immunol.* (1993), **151**, 6117–6126.

Adkins, B., and Du, R.-Q. Newborn mice develop balanced Th1/Th2 primary effector responses *in vivo* but are biased to Th2 secondary responses. *J. Immunol.* (1998), **160**, 4217–4224.

Adkins, B., Chun, K., Hamilton, K., and Nassiri, M. Naive murine neonatal T cells undergo apoptosis in response to primary stimulation. *J. Immunol.* (1996), **157**, 1343–1354.

Agadjanyan, M. G., Trivedi, N. N., Kudchodkar, S., Bennett, M., Levine, W., Lin, A., Boyer, J., Levy, D., Ugen, K. E., Kim, J. J., and Weiner, D. B. An HIV type 2 DNA vaccine induces cross-reactive immune responses against HIV type 2 and SIV. *AIDS Res. Hum. Retrovir.* (1997), **13**, 1561–1572.

Agadjanyan, M. G., Wang, B., Nyland, S. B., Weiner, D. B., and Ugen, K. E. DNA plasmid based vaccination against the oncogenic human T cell leukemia virus type 1. *Curr. Top. Microbiol. Immunol.* (1998), **226**, 175–192.

Aggarwal, S., Gupta, A., Nagata, S., and Gupta, S. Programmed cell death in cord blood lymphocytes. *J. Clin. Immunol.* (1997), **17**, 63–71.

Alberti, E., Acosta, A., Sarmiento, M. E., Hidalgo, C., Vidal, T., Fachado, A., Fonte, L., Izquierdo, L., Infante, J. F., Finlay, C. M., and Sierra, G. Specific cellular and humoral immune response in BALB/c mice immunized with an expression library of *Trypanosoma cruzi*. *Vaccine* (1998), **16**, 608–612.

Ali, H. M., Scott, R., and Thoms, G. L. The susceptibility of breast-fed and cow's milk formula-fed infant guinea pigs to upper tract infection with influenza virus. *Br. J. Exp. Path.* (1988), **69**, 563–575.

Allison, A. G. Mechanisms of tolerance and autoimmunity. *Ann. Rheum. Dis.* (1973), **32**, 283–293.

Ambriovic, A., Adam, M., Monteil, M., Paulin, D., and Eloit, M. Efficacy of replication-defective adenovirus-vectored vaccines: Protection following intramuscular injection is linked to promoter efficiency in muscle representative cells. *Virology* (1997), **238**, 327–335.

Amsbaugh, D. F., Hansen, C. T., Presscot, B., Stashak, P. W., Barthold, D. R., and Baker, P. J. Genetic control of antibody response to type III pneumococcal polysaccharide in mice. *J. Exp. Med.* (1972), **136**, 931–949.

Anderson, E. D., Mourich, D. V., Fahrenkrug, S. C., LaPatra, S., Shepherd, G., and Leong, J. A. Genetic immunization of rainbow trout (*Oncorhynchus mykiss*) against infectious hematopoietic necrosis virus. *Mol. Mar. Biol. Biotechnol.* (1996a), **5**, 114–122.

Anderson, E. D., Mourich, D. V., and Leong, J. A. Gene expression in rainbow trout (*Oncorhynchus mykiss*) following intramuscular injection of DNA. *Mol. Mar. Biol. Biotechnol.* (1996b), **5**, 105–113.

Anderson, R., Gao, X. M., Papakonstantinopoulou, A., Fairweather, N., Roberts, M., and Dougan, G. Immunization of mice with DNA encoding fragment C of tetanus toxin. *Vaccine* (1997), **15**, 827–829.

Anderson, R., Gao, X. M., Papakonstantinopoulou, A., Roberts, M., and Dougan, G. Immune response in mice following immunization with DNA encoding fragment C of tetanus toxin. *Infect. Immunol.* (1996), **64**, 3168–3173.

Ando, T., Yoshikai, Y., Matsuzaki, G., Takimoto, H., and Nomoto, K. The stage of negative selection in tolerance induction in neonatal mice. *Immunology* (1991), **74**, 638–646.

Andre, S., Seed, B., Eberle, J., Schraut, W., Bultmann, A., and Haas, J. Increased immune response elicited by DNA vaccination with a synthetic gp120 sequence with optimized codon usage. *J. Virol.* (1998), **72**, 1497–1503.

Andreu-Sanchez, J. L., Moreno de Alboran, I. M., Marcos, M. A., Sanchez-Movilla, A., Martinez, A. C., and Kromer, G. Interleukin-2 abrogates the T cells expressing a forbidden TCR repertoire and induces autoimmune disease in neonatally thymectomized mice. *J. Exp. Med.* (1991), **173**, 1323–1330.

Angus, C. W., Klivington, D., Wyman, J., and Kovacs, J. A. Nucleic acid vaccination against *Toxoplasma gondii* in mice. *J. Eukaryot. Microbiol.* (1996), **43**, 117S.

Anitescu, M., Chace, J. H., Tuetken, R., Yi, A. K., Berg, D. J., Krieg, A. M., and Cowdery, J. S. Bacterial DNA induces secretion of Interleukine-12. *J. Interferon-Cytokine Res.* (1997), **17**, 781–788.

Antohi, S., Bot, A., Manfield, L., and Bona, C. The reactivity pattern of hemagglutinin-specific clonotypes from mice immunized as neonates or adults with naked DNA. *Int. Immunol.* (1998), **10**, 663–668.

Arichi, T., Saito, T., Major, M. E., Belyakov, I. M., Shirai, M., Engelhard, V. H., Feinstone, S. M., and Berzofsky, J. A. Prophylactic DNA vaccine for hepatitis C virus (HCV) infection results in HCV-specific cytotoxic T lymphocyte induction and protection from HCV-recombinant vaccinia infection in an HLA-A2.1 transgenic mouse model. *Proc. Natl. Acad. Sci. USA* (2000), **97**, 297–302.

Armaleo, D., Ye, G. N., Klein, T. M., Shark, K. B., Sanford, J. C., and Johnston, S. A. Biolistic nuclear transformation of *Saccharomyces cerevisiae* and other fungi. *Curr. Genet.* (1990), **17**, 97–103.

Asakura, Y., Hamajima, K., Fukushima, J., Mohri, H., Okubo, T., and Okuda, K. Induction of HIV-1 Nef-specific cytotoxic T lymphocytes by Nef-expressing DNA vaccine. *Am. J. Hematol.* (1996), **53**, 116–117.

Asakura, Y., Hinkula, J., Leandersson, A. C., Fukushima, J., Okuda, K., and Wahren, B. Induction of HIV-1 specific mucosal immune responses by DNA vaccination. *Scand. J. Immunol.* (1997), **46**, 326–330.

Atanasiu, P. Production des tumeurs chez le hamster par inocculation d'acide desoxyribonucleique extrait de cultures de tissus infectee par le virus du polyoma. *C.R. Acad Sci.* (1962), **254**, 4228–4230.

Atassi, M. Z. Antigenic structure of myoglobin: The complete immunochemical anatomy of a protein. *Immunochemistry* (1975), **12**, 423–438.

Attanasio, R., Pehler, K., and Scinicariello, F. DNA-based immunization induces anti-CD4 antibodies directed primarily to native epitopes. *FEMS Immunol. Med. Microbiol.* (1997), **17**, 207–215.

Avery, O. T., MacLeod, C. M., and MacCarty, M. Studies on the chemical nature of the substance inducing transformation of pneumococcal types. *J. Exp. Med.* (1944), **79**, 137–158.

Babbit, B. P., Allen, P. M., Matsueda, G., Haber, G., and Unanue, E. Binding of immunogenic peptides to Ia histocompatibility molecules. *Nature* (1985), **317**, 359–366.

Bagarazzi, M. L., Boyer, J. D., Javadian, M. A., Chattergoon, M., Dang, K., Kim, G., Shah, J., Wang, B., and Weiner, D. B. Safety and immunogenicity of intramuscular and intravaginal delivery of HIV-1 DNA constructs to infant chimpanzees. *J. Med. Primatol.* (1997), **26**, 27–33.

Ballas, Z. K., Rasmussen, W. I., and Krieg, A. M. Induction of NK activity in murine and human cells by CpG motifs in ODN and bacterial DNA. *J. Immunol.* (1996), **157**, 1840–1845.

Ban, E. M., van Ginkel, F. W., Simecka, J. W., Kiyono, H., Robinson, H. L., and McGhee, J. R. Mucosal immunization with DNA encoding influenza hemagglutinin. *Vaccine* (1997), **15**, 811–813.

Barnett, S. W., Rajasekar, S., Legg, H., Doe, B., Fuller, D. H., Haynes, J. R., Walker, C. M., and Steimer, K. S. Vaccination with HIV-1 gp120 DNA induces immune responses that are boosted by a recombinant gp120 protein subunit. *Vaccine* (1997), **15**, 869–873.

Barr, M., Glenny, A. T., and Randall, K. J. Diphtheria immunization in young babies. *Lancet* (1950), **1**, 6–10.

Barrios, C., Brawand, P., Berney, M., Brandt, C., Lambert, P.-H., and Siegrist, C.-A. Neonatal and early life immune response to various form of vaccines qualitatively differ from adult. *Eur. J. Immunol.* (1996), **26**, 1489–1496.

Barry, M. A., Lai, W. C., and Johnston, S. A. Protection against mycoplasma infection using expression-library immunization. *Nature* (1995), **377**, 632–635.

Barthel, F., Remy, J. S., Loeffler, J. P., and Behr, J. P. Gene transfer optimization with lipospermine-coated DNA. *DNA Cell Biol.* (1993), **12**, 553–560.

Benimetskaya, L., Loike, J. D., Khaled, Z., Loike, G., Silverstein, S. C., el Khoury, J., Cai, T. G., and Stein, C. A. Mac-1 is an oligonucleotide-binding protein. *Nat. Med.* (1997), **3**, 414–420.

Bennett, R. M., Gabor, G. T., and Merritt, M. J. DNA binding to human leukocytes. *J. Clin. Invest.* (1985), **78**, 2182–2189.

Bennett, R. M., Kotzin, B. L., and Merritt, M. J. DNA receptor dysfunction in systemic lupus erythematosus and kindered disorders. *J. Exp. Med.* (1987), **166**, 850–863.

Bensch, K., Gordon, G., and Miller, L. Electronmicroscopical and cytochemical studies on DNA-containing particles phagocytized by mammalian cells. *Trans. N.Y. Acad. Sci.* (1966), **28**, 712–725.

Berns, K. I., and Giraud, C. Adenovirus and adeno-associated virus as vectors for gene therapy. *Ann. N.Y. Acad. Sci.* (1995), **772**, 95–104.

Billingham, R., Brent, L., and Medawar, P. Quantitative studies on tissue transplantation immunity: III. Actively acquired tolerance. *Proc. Roy. Soc. Lond.* (1956), **239**, 44–45.

Bird, A. P. CpG islands as gene markers in the vertebrate nucleus. *Trends Genet.* (1987), **3**, 342–346.

Boccaccio, G. L., Mor, F., and Steinman, L. Non-coding plasmid DNA induces IFN-gamma *in vivo* and suppresses autoimmune encephalomyelitis. *Int. Immunol.* (1999), **11**, 289–296.

Bohm, W., Kuhrober, A., Paier, T., Mertens, T., Reimann, J., and Schirmback, R. DNA vector constructs that prime hepatitis B surface antigen-specific cytotoxic T lymphocyte and antibody responses in mice after intramuscular injection. *J. Immunol. Meth.* (1996), **193**, 29–40.

Bohm, W., Schirmbeck, R., and Reimann, J. Targeting an anti-viral CD8+ T cell response to a growing tumor facilitates its rejection. *Cancer Immunol. Immunother.* (1997), **44**, 230–238.

Bona, C. Modulation of immune responses by Nocardia immunostimulants. *Prog. Allerg.* (1979), **26**, 97–102.

Bona, C. Sequential activation of V genes during postnatal life. *Am. J. Repr. Immunol.* (1980), **1**, 35–39.

Bona, C., and Bot, A. Neonatal immunoresponsiveness. *The Immunologist* (1997), **5**, 5–9.

Bona, C., and Cazenave, P.-A. Release from maternally-induced allotypic suppression in rabbit by Nocardia water-soluble mitogen. *J. Exp. Med.* (1997), **146**, 881–886.

Bona, C., and Pernis, B. Idiotypic networks. In *Fundamental Immunology* (W. E. Paul, ed.), Raven Press, New York, 1984, pp. 577–592.

Bona, C., Anteunis, A., Robineaux, R., and Astesano, A. Transfer of antigenic molecules from macrophages to lymphocytes. *Immunology* (1972), **23**, 799–816.

Bona, C., Liberman, R., Chien, C. C., Mond, J. J., House, S., Green, I., and Paul, W. E. Immune response to levan: I. Kinetics and ontogeny of anti-levan and anti-inulin response and expression of cross-reactive idiotype. *J. Immunol.* (1978), **120**, 1436–1432.

Bona, C., Liberman, R., House, S., Green, I., and Paul, W. E. Immune response to levan: II. T-independence of suppression of cross-reactive idiotypes by anti-idiotype antibodies. *J. Immunol.* (1979), **122**, 1614–1619.

Bona, C. A., Casares, S., and Brumeanu, T.-D. Towards development of T-cell vaccines. *Immunol. Today* (1998), **19**, 126–133.

Bonato, V. L., Lima, V. M., Tascon, R. E., Lowrie, D. B., and Silva, C. L. Identification and characterization of protective T cells in hsp65 DNA-vaccinated and *Mycobacterium tuberculosis*-infected mice. *Infect. Immunol.* (1998), **66**, 169–175.

Bot, A., Antohi, S., and Bona, C. Immune response of neonates elicited by somatic transgene vaccination with naked DNA. *Frontiers in Biosciences* (1997), **2**, 173–188.

Bot, A., Antohi, S., Bot, S., Garcia-Sastre, A., and Bona, C. Induction of humoral and cellular immunity against influenza virus by immunization of newborn mice with a plasmid bearing a hemagglutinin gene. *Int. Immunol.* (1997), **9**, 1641–1650.

Bot, A., Bot, S., and Bona, C. Enhanced protection against influenza virus of mice immunized as newborns with a mixture of plasmids expressing hemagglutinin and nucleoprotein. *Vaccine* (1998a), **16**, 1675–1682.

Bot, A., Bot, S., and Bona, C. A. Protective role of gamma interferon during the recall response to influenza virus. *J. Virol.* (1998b), **72**, 6637–6645.

Bot, A., Bot, S., Garcia-Sastre, A., and Bona, C. DNA immunization of newborn mice with a plasmid-expressing nucleoprotein of influenza virus. *Viral Immunol.* (1996a), **9**, 207–210.

Bot, A., Bot, S., Garcia-Sastre, A., and Bona, C. Protective cellular immunity against influenza virus induced by plasmid inoculation of newborn mice. *Develop. Immunol.* (1998c), **5**, 197–210.

Bot, A., Rechlin, A., Isobe, H., Bot, S., Schulman, J., Yokoyama, W. M., and Bona, C. Cellular mechanisms involved in protection and recovery from influenza virus infection in immunodeficient mice. *J. Virol.* (1996b), **70**, 5668–5672.

Bot, A., Shearer, M., Bot, S., Woods, C., Limmer, J., Kennedy, R., and Casares, S. Induction of antibody response by DNA immunization of newborn baboons against influenza virus. *Viral Immunol.* (1999), **12**, 91–96.

Bot, A., Stan, A.-C., Inaba, K., Steinman, R., and Bona, C. Dendritic cells at a DNA vaccination site express an encoded nucleoprotein and prime CD8 cytolytic lymphocytes upon adoptive transfer. *Int. Immunol.* (2000), **12**, 825–832.

Bourne, N., Stanberry, L. R., Bernstein, D. I., and Lew, D. DNA immunization against experimental genital herpes simplex virus infection. *J. Infect. Dis.* (1996), **173**, 800–807.

Boyer, J. D., Chattergoon, M. A., Ugen, K. E., Shah, A., Bennett, M., Cohen, A., Nyland, S., Lacy, K. E., Bagarazzi, M. L., Higgins, T. J., Baine, Y., Ciccarelli, R., Ginsberg, R. S., MacGregor, R. R., and Weiner, D. B. Enhancement of cellular immune response in HIV-1 seropositive individuals: A DNA-based trial. *Clin. Immunol.* (1999), **90**, 100–107.

Boyer, J. D., Ugen, K. E., Chattergoon, M., Wang, B., Shah, A., Agadjanyan, M., Bagarazzi, M. L., Javadian, A., Carrano, R., Coney, L., Williams, W. V., and Weiner, D. B. DNA vaccination as anti-human immunodeficiency virus immunotherapy in infected chimpanzees. *J. Infect. Dis.* (1997a), **176**, 1501–1509.

Boyer, J. D., Ugen, K. E., Wang, B., Agadjanyan, M., Gilbert, L., Bagarazzi, M. L., Chattergoon, M., Frost, P., Javadian, A., Williams, W. V., Refaeli, Y., Ciccarelli, R. B., McCallus, D., Coney, L., and Weiner, D. B. Protection of chimpanzees from high-dose heterologous HIV-1 challenge by DNA vaccination. *Nat. Med.* (1997b), **3**, 526–532.

Boyer, J. D., Wang, B., Ugen, K. E., Agadjanyan, M., Javadian, A., Frost, P., Dang, K., Carrano, R. A., Ciccarelli, R., Coney, L., Williams W. V., and Weiner, D. B. *In vivo* protective anti-HIV immune responses in non-human primates through DNA immunization. *J. Med. Primatol.* (1996), **25**, 242–250.

Boyle, C. M., Morin, M., Webster, R. G., and Robinson, H. L. Role of different lymphoid tissues in the initiation and maintenance of DNA-raised antibody responses to the influenza virus H1 glycoprotein. *J. Virol.* (1996), **70**, 9074–9078.

Braciale, T. L., and Braciale, V. L. Antigen presentation: Structural theme and functional variations. *Immunol. Today* (1992), **12**, 124–129.

Braun, C., Mahouy, G., Bona, C., Goujec-Zalc, C., Tuffrey, M., Crewe, P., and Barnes, R. Failure to suppress theta antigenic expression in progeny derived from pre-immunized maternal recipients. *J. Immunogenetics* (1976), **3**, 307–314.

Bretscher, P., and Cohn, M. A theory of self–nonself discrimination. *Science* (1970), **169**, 1042–1049.

Bright, R. K., Shearer, M. H., and Kennedy, R. C. Nucleic acid vaccination against virally induced tumors. *Ann. N.Y. Acad. Sci.* (1995), **772**, 241–251.

Bronte, V., Appoloni, E., Ronca, R., Zamboni, P., Overwijk, W. W., Surman, L., Restifo, N. P., and Zanovello, P. Genetic vaccination with self tyrosinase-related protein 2 caused melanoma eradication but not vitiligo. *Cancer Res.* (2000), **15**, 253–258.

Brown, F. A synthetic peptide vaccine for foot and mouth disease. In *Recombinant and Synthetic Vaccines* (G. V. Talwar, K. V. S. Rao, and V. S. Chauan, eds.). Narosa, New Delhi, 1994, pp. 21–29.

Brumeanu, T.-D., Bot, A., Bona, C. A., Dehazya, P., Wolf, I., and Zaghouani, H. Engineering of doubly antigenized immunoglobulins expressing T and B viral epitopes. *Immunotechnology* (1996), **2**, 85–95.

Bueler, H., and Mulligan, R. C. Induction of antigen-specific tumor immunity by genetic and cellular vaccines against MAGE: Enhanced tumor protection by coexpression of granulocyte-macrophage colony-stimulating factor and B7-1. *Mol. Med.* (1996), **2**, 545–555.

Burkholder, J. K., Decker, J., and Yang, N. S. Rapid transgene expression in lymphocyte and macrophage primary cultures after particle bombardment-mediated gene transfer. *J. Immunol. Meth.* (1993), **165**, 149–156.

Burnet, M. The clonal selection theory of acquired immunity. Vanderbilt University Press, Nashville, TN, 1959.

Burstyn, D. G., Baraff, L. J., Peppler, M. S., Leake, R. D., St. Geme, J., and Manclark, C. R. Serological response to filamentous hemagglutinin and lymphocytosis-promoting toxin of *Bordetella pertussis*. *Infect. Immunol.* (1983), **41**, 1150–1156.

Cai, Z., Brunmark, A., Jackson, M. R., Loh, D., Peterson, P. A., and Sprent, J. Transfected Drosophila cells as a probe for defining the minimal requirements for stimulation of unprimed CD8 T cells. *Proc. Natl. Acad. Sci. USA* (1996), **93**, 1436–1439.

Calarota, S., Bratt, G., Nordlund, S., Hinkula, J., Leandersson, A. C., and Sandstrom, E. Cellular cytotoxic response induced by DNA vaccination in HIV-1 infected patients. *Lancet* (1998), **351**, 1320–1325.

Calarota, S. A., Leandersson, A. C., Bratt, G., Hinkula, J., Klinman, D. M., Weinhold, K. G., Sandstrom, E., and Wahren, B. Immune responses in asymptomatic HIV-1-infected patients and HIV-DNA immunization followed by highly active antiretroviral treatment. *J. Immunol.* (1999), **163**, 2330–2338.

Cancro, M. P., Wilie, D. E., Gerhard, W., and Klinman, N. R. Pattern acquisition of antibody repertoire: Diversity of hemagglutinin specific B cell repertoire in neonatal BALB/c mice. *Proc. Natl. Acad. Sci. USA* (1979), **76**, 6577–6581.

Carbone, F. R., and Bevan, M. J. Class I-restricted processing and presentation of exogenous cell-associated antigen *in vivo. J. Exp. Med.* (1990), **171**, 377–387.

Cardoso, A. I., Blixenkrone-Moller, M., Fayolle, J., Liu, M., Buckland, R., and Wild, T. F. Immunization with plasmid DNA encoding for the measles virus hemagglutinin and nucleoprotein leads to humoral and cell-mediated immunity. *Virology* (1996), **225**, 293–299.

Carsetti, R., Kohler, G., and Lammers, M. C. Transitional B cells are target of negative selection in B cell compartment. *J. Exp. Med.* (1995), **181**, 2129–2140.

Casares, S., Brumeanu, T.-D., Bot, A., and Bona, C. Protective immunity elicited by vaccination with DNA encoding for a B cell and T cell epitope of the A/PR/8/34 influenza virus. *Viral Immunol.* (1997a), **10**, 129–136.

Casares, S., Inaba, K., Brumeanu, T.-D., Steinman, R. M., and Bona, C. Antigen presentation by dendritic cells after immunization with DNA encoding a major histocompatibility complex class II-restricted viral epitope. *J. Exp. Med.* (1997b), **186**, 1481–1486.

Casares, S., Bona, C. A., and Brumeanu, T. D. Engineering and characterization of a murine MHC class II-immunoglobulin chimera expressing an immunodominant CD4 T viral epitope. *Prot. Eng.* (1997), **10**, 1295–1301.

Caspar, C. B., Levy, S., and Levy, R. Idiotype vaccines for non-Hodgkin's lymphoma induce polyclonal immune responses that cover mutated tumor idiotypes: Comparison of different vaccine formulations. *Blood* (1997), **90**, 3699–3706.

Casten, L. A., and Pierce, S. K. Receptor-mediated B cell antigen processing. *J. Immunol.* (1988), **140**, 404–410.

Cerottini, J.-Ch., McCooaney, P. J., and Dixon, F. Specificity of immunosuppression caused by passive administration of antibody. *J. Immunol.* (1969), **103**, 268–275.

Chace, J. H., Hooker, N. A., Mildenstein, K. L., Krieg, A. M., and Cowdery, J. S. Bacterial DNA-induced NK-cell IFN-gamma production is dependent on macrophage secretion of IL-12. *Clin. Immunol. Immunopathol.* (1997), **84**, 185–193.

Chaplin, P. J., De Rose, R., Boyle, J. S., McWaters, P., Kelly, J., Tennent, J. M., Lew, A. M., and Scheerlinck, J. P. Targeting improves the efficacy of DNA vaccine against *Corynebacterium pseudotuberculosis* in sheep. *Infect. Immunol.* (1999), **67**, 6434–6438.

Charo, J., Ciupitu, A. M., Le Chevalier De Preville, A., Trivedi, P., Klein, G., Hinkula, G., and Kiessling, R. A long-term memory obtained by genetic immunization results in full protection from a mammary adenocarcinoma expressing an EBV gene. *J. Immunol.* (1999), **163**, 5913–5919.

Chattergoon, M. A., Robinson, T. M., Boyer, J. D., and Weiner, D. B. Specific immune induction following DNA-based immunization through *in vivo* transfection and activation of macrophages/antigen-presenting cells. *J. Immunol.* (1998), **160**, 5705–5718.

Chen, C. H., Ji, H., Suh, K. W., Choti, M. A., Pardoll, D. M., and Wu, T. C. Gene gun-mediated DNA vaccination induces antitumor immunity against human papillomavirus type 16 E7-expressing murine tumor metastases in the liver and lungs. *Gene Ther.* (1999), **6**, 1972–1981.

Chen, C. H., Wang, T. L., Hung, C. F., Yang, Y., Pardoll, D. M., and Wu, K. Enhancement of DNA vaccine potency by linkage of antigen gene to an HSP70 gene. *Cancer Research* (2000), **60**, 1035–1042.

Chen, S. C., Fynan, E. F., Robinson, H. L., Lu, S., Greenberg, H. B., Santoro, J. C., and Herrmann, J. E. Protective immunity induced by rotavirus DNA vaccines. *Vaccine* (1997), **15**, 899–902.

Chen, S. C., Jones, D. H., Fynan, E. F., Farrar, G. H., Clegg, J. C., Greenberg, H. B., and Herrmann, J. E. Protective immunity induced by oral immunization with a rotavirus DNA vaccine encapsulated in microparticles. *J. Virol.* (1998), **72**, 5757–5761.

Chen, Y., Hu, D., Eling, D. J., Robbins, J., and Kipps, T. J. DNA vaccines encoding full-length or truncated Neu induce protective immunity against Neu-expressing mammary tumors. *Cancer Research* (1998a), **58**, 1965–1971.

Chen, Y., Webster, R. G., and Woodland, D. L. Induction of CD8[+] T cell responses to dominant and subdominant epitopes and protective immunity to Sendai virus infection by DNA vaccination. *J. Immunol.* (1998b), **160**, 2425–2432.

Chen, Z. R., Wang, Y. H., Alter, H. J., and Shih, J.W.-K. Genetic immunization of mice with plasmids containing hepatitis C virus core protein-encoding DNA. *Vaccine Research* (1995), **4**, 135–144.

Cheng, L., Ziegelhoffer, P. R., and Yang, N. S. *In vivo* promoter activity and transgene expression in mammalian somatic tissues evaluated by using particle bombardment. *Proc. Natl. Acad. Sci. USA* (1993), **90**, 4455–4459.

Chesnut, R. W., Colon, S. M., and H. Grey. Requirements for the processing of antigens by antigen-presenting B cells. *J. Immunol.* (1982), **129**, 2382–2388.

Choi, A. H., Knowlton, D. R., McNeal, M. M., and Ward, R. L. Particle bombardment-mediated DNA vaccination with rotavirus VP6 induces high levels of serum rotavirus IgG but fails to protect mice against challenge. *Virology* (1997), **232**, 129–138.

Chow, Y. H., Chiang, B. L., Lee, Y. L., Chi, W. K., Lin, W. C., Chen, Y. T., and Tao, M. H. Development of Th1 and Th2 populations and the nature of immune responses to hepatitis B virus DNA vaccines can be modulated by codelivery of various cytokine genes. *J. Immunol.* (1998), **160**, 1320–1329.

Chow, Y. W., Huang, W. L., Chi, W. K., Chu, Y. D., and Tao, M. H. Improvement of hepatitis B virus DNA vaccines by plasmids coexpressing hepatitis B surface antigen and interleukin-2. *J. Virol.* (1997), **71**, 169–178.

Chu, R. S., Targoni, O. S., Krieg, A. M., Lehman, P. V., and Harding, C. V. CpG oligonucleotides act as adjuvants that switch on Th1 immunity. *J. Exp. Med.* (1997), **186**, 1623–1631.

Chun, S., Daheshia, M., Kuklin, N. Y., and Rouse, B. T. Modulation of viral immunoinflammatory responses with cytokine DNA administered by different routes. *J. Virol.* (1998), **72**, 5545–5551.

Chun, S., Daheshia, M., Lee, S., Eo, S. K., and Rouse, B. T. Distribution fate and mechanism of immune modulation following mucosal delivery of plasmid DNA encoding IL-10. *J. Immunol.* (1999), **163**, 2393–2402.

Ciernik, I. F., Berzofsky, J. A., and Carbone, D. P. Induction of cytotoxic T lymphocytes and antitumor immunity with DNA vaccines expressing single T cell epitopes. *J. Immunol.* (1996a), **156**, 2369–2375.

Ciernik, I. F., Krayenbuhl, B. H., and Carbone, D. P. Puncture-mediated gene transfer to skin. *Hum. Gene Ther.* (1996b), **7**, 893–899.

Clarke, B. E., Newton, S. E., Caroll, A. R., and Brown, F. Improved immunogenicity of a peptide epitope after fusion to hepatitis B core protein. *Nature* (1987), **320**, 381–384.

Clarke, N. J., Hissey, P., Buchan, K., and Harris, S. pPV: A novel IRES-containing vector to facilitate plasmid immunization and antibody response characterization. *Immunotechnology* (1997), **3**, 145–153.

Clary, B. M., Coveney, E. C., Blazer, D. G., III, Philip, R., Morse, M., Gilboa, E., and Lyerly, H. K. Active immunization with tumor cells transduced by a novel AAV plasmid-based gene delivery system. *J. Immunother.* (1997), **20**, 26–37.

Clayton, J. P., Gammon, G. M., Ando, D. G., Kono, D. H., Hood, L., and Sercarz, E. Peptide-specific prevention of allergic experimental encephalomyelitis. *J. Exp. Med.* (1989), **169**, 1681–1689.

Cohen, P. L., Scher, I., and Mosier, D. E. *In vitro* studies of the genetically determined unresponsiveness to thymus-independent antigens in CBA/N mice. *J. Immunol.* (1976), **116**, 300–311.

Concetti, A., Amici, A., Petrelli, C., Tibaldi, A., Provinciali, M., and Venanzi, F. M. Autoantibody to p185erbB2/neu oncoprotein by vaccination with xenogenic DNA. *Cancer Immunol. Immunother.* (1996), **43**, 307–315.

Condon, C., Watkins, S. C., Celluzi, C. M., Thompson, K., and Falo, L. D. DNA-based immunization by *in vivo* transfection of dendritic cells. *Nat. Med.* (1996), **2**, 1122–1127.

Cone, R. E., and Johnson, A. G. Regulation of the immune system by synthetic polynucleotides. III. Action on antigen-reactive cells of thymic origin. *J. Exp. Med.* (1971), **133**, 665–676.

Coon, B., An, L. L., Whitton, J. L., and von Herrath, M. G. DNA immunization to prevent autoimmune diabetes. *J. Clin. Invest.* (1999), **104**, 189–194.

Conry, R. M., LoBuglio, A. F., and Curiel, D. T. Polynucleotide-mediated immunization therapy of cancer. *Semin. Oncol.* (1996a), **23**, 135–147.

Conry, R. M., LoBuglio, A. F., Kantor, J., Schlom, J., Loechel, F., Moore, S. E., Sumerel, L. A., Barlow, D. L., Abrams, S., and Curiel, D. T. Immune response to a carcinoembryonic antigen polynucleotide vaccine. *Cancer Research* (1994), **54**, 1164–1168.

Conry, R. M., LoBuglio, A. F., Loechel, F., Moore, S. E., Sumerel, L. A., Barlow, D. L., and Curiel, D. T. A carcinoembryonic antigen polynucleotide vaccine has *in vivo* antitumor activity. *Gene Ther.* (1995a), **2**, 59–65.

Conry, R. M., LoBuglio, A. F., Loechel, F., Moore, S. E., Sumerel, L. A., Barlow, D. L., Pike, J., and Curiel, D. T. A carcinoembryonic antigen polynucleotide vaccine for human clinical use. *Cancer Gene Ther.* (1995b), **2**, 33–38.

Conry, R. M., Widera, G., LoBuglio, A. F., Fuller, J. T., Moore, S. E., Turner, J., Yang, N. S., and Curiel, D. T. Selected strategies to augment polynucleotide immunization. *Gene Ther.* (1996b), **3**, 67–74.

Corr, M., Lee, D. J., Carson, D. A., and Tighe, H. Gene vaccination with naked plasmid DNA: Mechanism of CTL priming. *J. Exp. Med.* (1996), **184**, 1555–1560.

Corr, M., Tighe, H., Lee, D., Dudler, J., Trieu, M., Brinson, D. C., and Carson, D. A. Costimulation provided by DNA immunization enhances antitumor immunity. *J. Immunol.* (1997), **159**, 4999–5004.

Costagliola, S., Rodien, P., Many, M.-C., Ludgate, M., and Vassart, G. Genetic immunization against the human thyrotropin receptor causes thyroiditis and allows production of monoclonal antibodies recognizing the native receptor. *J. Immunol.* (1998), **160**, 1458–1465.

Cowdery, J. S., Chace, J. H., Yi, A.-K., and Krieg, A. M. Bacterial DNA induces NK cells to produce IFNγ *in vivo* and increases the toxicity of lipopolysaccharides. *J. Immunol.* (1996), **156**, 4570–4575.

Cox, G. J., Zamb, T. J., and Babiuk, L. A. Bovine herpesvirus 1: Immune responses in mice and cattle injected with plasmid DNA. *J. Virol.* (1993), **67**, 5664–5667.

Cuisiner, A. M., Mallet, V., Meyer, A., Caldora, C., and Aubert, A. DNA vaccination using expression vectors carrying FIV structural genes induces immune response against feline immunodeficiency virus. *Vaccine* (1997), **15**, 1085–1094.

Daheshia, M., Kuklin, N., Kanangat, S., Manickan, F., and Rouse, B. T. Suppression of ongoing ocular inflammatory disease by topical administration of plasmid DNA encoding IL-10. *J. Immunol.* (1997), **159**, 1945–1952.

Danko, I., Fritz, J. D., Jiao, S., Hogan, K., Latendresse, J. S., and Wolff, J. A. Pharmacological enhancement of *in vivo* foreign gene expression in muscle. *Gene Ther.* (1994), **1**, 114–121.

Darji, A., Guzman, C. A., Gerstel, B., Wachholz, P., Timmis, K. N., Wehland, J., Chakraborty, T., and Weiss, S. Oral somatic transgene vaccination using attenuated *S. typhimurium*. *Cell* (1997), **91**, 765–775.

Davis, H. L., Brazolot Millan, C. L., Mancini, M., McCluskie, M. J., Hadchouel, M., Comanita, L., Tiollais, P., Whalen, R. G., and Michel, M. L. DNA-based immunization against hepatitis B surface antigen (HBsAg) in normal and HBsAg-transgenic mice. *Vaccine* (1997), **15**, 849–852.

Davis, H. L., McCluskie, M. J., Gerin, J. L., and Purcell, R. H. DNA vaccine for hepatitis B: Evidence for immunogenicity in chimpanzees and comparison with other vaccines. *Proc. Natl. Acad. Sci. USA* (1996), **93** (14), 7213–7218.

Davis, H. L., Michel, M. L., Mancini, M., Schleef, M., and Whalen, R. G. Direct gene transfer in skeletal muscle: Plasmid DNA-based immunization against the hepatitis B virus surface antigen. *Vaccine* (1994), **12**, 1503–1509.

Davis, H. L., Michel, M. L., and Whalen, R. G. DNA-based immunization induces continuous secretion of hepatitis B surface antigen and high levels of circulating antibody. *Hum. Mol. Genet.* (1993a), **2**, 1847–1851.

Davis, H. L., Schirmbeck, R., Reimann, J., and Whalen, R. G. DNA-mediated immunization in mice induces a potent MHC Class I-restricted cytotoxic T lymphocyte response to the hepatitis B envelope protein. *Hum. Gene Ther.* (1995), **6**, 1447–1456.

Davis, H. L., Weeranta, R., Waldschmidt, T. J., Tygrett, L., Schorr, J., and Krieg, A. M. CpG DNA is a potent enhancer of specific immunity in mice immunized with recombinant hepatitis B surface antigen. *J. Immunol.* (1998), **160**, 870–876.

Davis, H. L., Whalen, R. G., and Demeneix, B. A. Direct gene transfer into skeletal muscle *in vivo*: Factors affecting efficiency of transfer and stability of expression. *Hum. Gene Ther.* (1993b), **4**, 151–159.

Deck, R. R., DeWitt, C. M., Donnelly, J. J., Liu, M. A., and Ulmer, J. B. Characterization of humoral immune responses induced by an influenza hemagglutinin DNA vaccine. *Vaccine* (1997), **15**, 71–78.

Degano, P., Schneider, J., Hannan, C. M., Gilbert, S. C., and Hill, A. V. Gene gun intradermal DNA immunization with modified vaccinia virus *Ankara*: Enhanced CD8+ T cell immunogenicity and protective efficacy in the influenza and malaria models. *Vaccine* (1999), **18**, 623–632.

Dela Cruz, C. S., Chamberlain, J. W., MacDonald, K. S., and Barber, B. H. Xenogeneic and allogeneic anti-MHC immune responses induced by plasmid DNA immunization. *Vaccine* (1999), **17**, 2479–2492.

Delassus, S., Darche, S., Kourilsky, P., and Cumano, A. Maternal immunoglobulins have no effect on the rate of maturation of the B cell compartment of offspring. *Eur. J. Immunol.* (1997), **27**, 1737–1742.

Demeneix, B. A., Abdel-Taweb, H., Benoist, C., Seugnet, I., and Behr, J. P. Temporal and spatial expression of lipospermine-compacted genes transferred into chick embryos *in vivo*. *Biotechniques* (1994), **16**, 496–501.

Demeneix, B. A., Fredriksson, G., Lezual'ch, F., Daugeras-Bernard, N., Behr, J. P., and Loeffler, J. P. Gene transfer into intact vertebrate embryos. *Int. J. Dev. Biol.* (1991), **35**, 481–484.

Denis, O., Tanghe, A., Palfliet, K., Jurion, F., van den Berg, T. P., Vanonckelen, A., Ooms, J., Saman, E., Ulmer,

J. B., Content, J., and Huygen, K. Vaccination with plasmid DNA encoding mycobacterial antigen 85A stimulates a CD4$^+$ and CD8$^+$ T-cell epitopic repertoire broader than that stimulated by *Mycobacterium tuberculosis* H37Rv infection. *Infect. Immunol.* (1998), **66**, 1527–1533.

Desiderio, S. V., Yancopoulos, G. D., Paskind, M., Thomas, E., Boss, M. A., Landau, N., Alt, F. W., and Baltimore, D. Insertion of N-regions into heavy-chain genes is correlated with expression of TdT in B cells. *Nature* (1984), **311**, 752–755.

de Zoeten, E. F., Carr-Brendel, V., and Cohen, E. P. Resistance to melanoma in mice immunized with semiallogeneic fibroblasts transfected with DNA from mouse melanoma cells. *J. Immunol.* (1998), **160**, 2915–2922.

Dhawan, J., Rando, T. A., Elson, S. L., Bujard, H., and Blau, H. M. Tetracycline-regulated gene expression following direct gene transfer into mouse skeletal muscle. *Somat. Cell. Mol. Genet.* (1995), **21**, 233–240.

Dietrich, G., Bubert, A., Gentschev, I., Sokolovic, Z., Simm, A., Catic, A., Kaufmann, S. H., Hess, J., Szalay, A. A., and Goebel, W. Delivery of antigen-encoding plasmid DNA into the cytosol of macrophage by attenuated suicide *Listeria monocytogenes*. *Nat. Biotechnol.* (1998), **16**, 181–185.

Ding, L., and Shevach, E. M. Activation of CD4$^+$ T cells by delivery of the B7 costimulatory signal on bystander antigen-presenting cells. *Eur. J. Immunol.* (1994), **24**, 859–866.

Doe, B., Selby, M., Barnett, S., Baezinger, J., and Walker, C. M. Induction of cytotoxic T lymphocytes by intramuscular immunization with plasmid DNA is facilitated by bone marrow–derived cells. *Proc. Natl. Acad. Sci. USA* (1996), **93**, 8578–8583.

d'Oliveira, C., Feenstra, A., Vos, H., Osterhaus, A. D., Shiels, B. R., Cornelissen, A. W., and Jongejan, F. Induction of protective immunity to *Theileria annulata* using two major merozoite surface antigens presented by different delivery systems. *Vaccine* (1997), **15**, 1796–1804.

Donnelly, J. J., Friedman, A., Martinez, D., Montgomery, D. L., Shiver, J. W., Motzel, S. L., Ulmer, J. B., and Liu, M. A. Preclinical efficacy of a prototype DNA vaccine: Enhanced protection against antigenic drift in influenza virus. *Nat. Med.* (1995), **1**, 583–587.

Donnelly, J. J., Friedman, A., Ulmer, J. B., and Liu, M. A. Further protection against antigenic drift of influenza virus in a ferret model by DNA vaccination. *Vaccine* (1997), **15**, 865–868.

Donnelly, J. J., Martinez, D., Jansen, K. U., Ellis, R. W., Montgomery, D. L., and Liu, M. A. Protection against papillomavirus with a polynucleotide vaccine. *J. Infect. Dis.* (1996), **173**, 314–320.

Doolan, D. L., Hedstrom, R. C., Wang, R., Sedegah, M., Scheller, L. F., Hobart, P., Norman, J. A., and Hoffman, S. L. DNA vaccines for malaria: The past, the present and the future. *Indian J. Med. Res.* (1997a), **106**, 109–119.

Doolan, D. L., and Hoffman, S. L. Pre-erythrocytic-stage immune effector mechanisms in *Plasmodium* spp. infections. *Philos. Trans. R. Soc. Lond. B. Biol. Sci.* (1997b), **352**, 1361–1367.

Doolan, D. L., Sedegah, M., Hedstrom, R. C., Hobart, P., Charoenvit, Y., and Hoffman, S. L. Circumventing genetic restriction of protection against malaria with multigene DNA immunization: CD8$^+$ cell-, interferon gamma-, and nitric oxide-dependent immunity. *J. Exp. Med.* (1996), **183**, 1739–1746.

Dougan, G., Hormaeche, C. E., and Maskel, D. J. Live oral *Salmonella* vaccines: Potential use of attenuated strains as carriers of heterologous antigen to immune system. *Parasite Immunology* (1987), **9**, 151–163.

Dowty, M. E., Williams, P., Zhang, G., Hagstrom, J. E., and Wolf, J. A. Plasmid DNA entry in postmitotic nuclei of primary rate myotubes. *Proc. Natl. Acad. Sci. USA* (1995), **92**, 4572–4576.

Dray, S. Effect of maternal isoantibodies on the quantitative expression of two allelic genes controlling gamma-globulin allotypic specificities. *Nature (London)* (1962), **195**, 677–680.

Dubensky, T. W., Campbell, B. A., and Villareal, L. P. Direct transfection of viral and plasmid DNA into the liver or spleen of mice. *Proc. Natl. Acad. Sci. USA* (1984), **81**, 7529–7533.

Dupre, L., Poulain-Godefroy, O., Ban, E., Ivanoff, N., Mekranfar, M., Schacht, A. M., Capron, A., and Riveau, G. Intradermal immunization of rats with plasmid DNA encoding *Schistosoma mansoni* 28 kDa glutathione S-transferase. *Parasite Immunology* (1997), **19**, 505–513.

Dupuy, C., Buzoni-Gatel, D., Touze, A., Bout, D., and Coursaget, P. Nasal immunization of mice with human papillomavirus type (HPV-16) virus-like particles or with the HPV-16 L1 gene elicits specific cytotoxic T lymphocytes in vaginal draining lymph nodes. *J. Virol.* (1999), **73**, 9063–9071.

Durandy, A., De Saint Basile, G., Lisovska-Grospierre, B., Gauchat, J.-F., Foreville, M., Kroczek, R. A., Bonnefois, J.-Y., and Fischer, A. Undetectable CD40 ligand expression on T cells and B low responses to CD40 binding agonists in human newborns. *J. Immunol.* (1995), **154**, 1560–1568.

Eastman, S. J., Lukason, M. J., Tousignant, J. D., Murray, H., Lane, M. D., St. George, J. A., Akita, G. Y., Cherry, M., Cheng, S. H., and Scheule, R. K. A concentrated and stable aerosol formulation of cationic lipid: DNA complexes giving high level gene expression in mouse lung. *Hum. Gene Ther.* (1997a), **8**, 765–773.

Eastman, S. J., Tousignant, J. D., Lukason, M. J., Murray, H., Siegel, C. S., Constantino, P., Harris, D. J., Cheng, S. H., and Scheule, R. K. Optimization of formulations and conditions for the aerosol delivery of functional cationic lipid DNA complexes. *Hum. Gene Ther.* (1997), **8**, 313–322.

Eichelberger, M., Allan, W., Zijlstra, M., Jaenisch, R., and Doherty, P. C. Clearance of influenza virus infection in mice lacking Class I MHC-restricted CD8$^+$ cells. *J. Exp. Med.* (1991), **174**, 875–880.

Eisenbraun, M. D., Fuller, D. H., and Haynes, J. R. Examination of parameters affecting the elicitation of humoral immune responses by particle bombardment-mediated genetic immunization. *DNA Cell Biology* (1993), **12**, 791–797.

Enami, M., and Palese, P. High efficiency formation of influenza virus transfectants. *J. Virol.* (1991), **65**, 2711–2713.

Erb, K. J., Kirman, J., Woodfield, L., Wilson, T., Collins, D. M., Watson, J. D., and LeGros, G. Identification of potential CD8 T-cell epitopes of the 19 kDa and AhpC proteins from *Mycobacterium tuberculosis*: No evidence for CD8 T-cell priming against the identified peptides after DNA-vaccination of mice. *Vaccine* (1998), **16**, 692–697.

Erbacher, P., Roche, A. C., Monsigny, M., and Midoux, P. The reduction of the positive charges of polylysine by partial glyconoylation increases the transfection efficiency of polylysine/DNA complexes. *Biochim. Biophys. Acta* (1997), **1324**, 27–36.

Etchart, N., Buckland, R., Liu, M. A., and Kaiserlian, D. Class I-restricted CTL induction by mucosal immunization with naked DNA encoding measles virus hemagglutinin. *J. Gen. Virol.* (1997), **78**, 1577–1580.

Evans, D. J., McKeating, J., Meredith, J. M., and Almond, J. W. An engineered poliovirus elicits broadly reactive HIV-1 neutralizing antibodies. *Nature* (1989), **339**, 385–388.

Feeney, A. J. Junctional sequences of fetal T cell receptor beta chains have few N regions. *J. Exp. Med.* (1991), **174**, 115–123.

Felgner, J. H., Kumar, R., Sridhar, C. N., Wheeler, C. J., Tsai, Y. J., Border, R., Ramsey, P., Martin, M., and Felgner, P. L. Enhanced gene delivery and mechanism studies with a novel series of cationic lipid formulations. *J. Biol. Chem.* (1994), **269**, 2550–2561.

Felgner, P. L., and Ringold, G. M. Cationic liposome-mediated transfection. *Nature* (1989), **337**, 387–388.

Feltquate, D. M., Heaney, S., Webster, R. G., and Robinson, H. L. Different T helper cell types and antibody isotypes generated by saline and gene gun DNA immunization. *J. Immunol.* (1997), **158**, 2278–2284.

Fernandez, C., and Moller, G. Immunological unresponsiveness to native dextran B512 in young mice is due to lack of Ig-receptor expression. *J. Exp. Med.* (1978), **147**, 645–655.

Fischer, G. S., Kent, C., Joseph, L. Green, D. R., and Scott, D. W. Anti IgM-mediated growth arrest and apoptosis of murine B lymphomas is prevented by the stabilization of c-myc. *J. Exp. Med.* (1994), **179**, 221–230.

Fooks, A. R., Jeevarajah, D., Warnes, A., Wilkinson, G. W., and Clegg, J. C. Immunization of mice with plasmid DNA expressing the measles virus nucleoprotein gene. *Viral Immunol.* (1996), **9**, 65–71.

Forns, X., Emerson, S. U., Tobin, G. J., Mushahwar, I. K., Purcell, R. H., Bukh, J. DNA immunization of mice and macaques with plasmids encoding hepatitis C virus envelope E2 protein expressed intracellularly and on the cell surface. *Vaccine* (1999), **17**, 1992–2002.

Forsthuber, H. C., Yip, H. C., and Lehman, P. V. Induction of Th1 and Th2 immunity in neonatal mice. *Science* (1996), **271**, 1728–1731.

Freedman, H. H., Nakano, M., and Braun, W. Antibody formation in endotoxin-tolerant mice. *Proc. Soc. Exp. Biol. Med.* (1966), **121**, 1228–1230.

Friend, D. S., Papahadjopoulos, D., and Debs, R. J. Endocytosis and intracellular processing accompanying transfection mediated by cationic liposomes. *Biochim. Biophys. Acta* (1996), **1278**, 41–50.

Fritz, J. D., Herweijer, H., Zhang, G., and Wolff, J. A. Gene transfer into mammalian cells using histone-condensed plasmid DNA. *Hum. Gene Ther.* (1996), **7**, 1395–1404.

Frolov, I., Hoffman, T. A., Pragai, B. M., Dryga, S. A., Huang, H. V., Schlesinger, S., and Rice, C. M. Alphavirus-based expression vectors: Strategies and applications. *Proc. Natl. Acad. Sci. USA* (1996), **93**, 11371–11377.

Fu, T. M., Friedman, A., Ulmer, J. B., Liu, M. A., and Donnelly, J. J. Protective cellular immunity: Cytotoxic T-lymphocyte responses against dominant and recessive epitopes of influenza virus nucleoprotein induced by DNA immunization. *J. Virol.* (1997a), **71**, 2715–2721.

Fu, T. M., Ulmer, J. B., Caulfield, M. J., Deck, R. R., Friedman, A., Wang, S., Liu, X., Donnelly, J. J., and Liu, M. A. Priming of cytotoxic T lymphocytes by DNA vaccines: Requirement for professional antigen presenting cells and evidence for antigen transfer from myocytes. *Mol. Med.* (1997b), **3**, 362–371.

Fuller, D. H., Corb, M. M., Barnett, S., Steimer, K., and Haynes, J. R. Enhancement of immunodeficiency virus-specific immune responses in DNA-immunized rhesus macaques. *Vaccine* (1997a), **15**, 924–926.

Fuller, D. H., and Haynes, J. R. A qualitative progression in HIV type 1 glycoprotein 120-specific cytotoxic cellular and humoral immune responses in mice receiving a DNA-based glycoprotein 120 vaccine. *AIDS Res. Hum. Retrovir.* (1994), **10**, 1433–1441.

Fuller, D. H., Murphey-Corb, M., Clements, J., Barnett, S., and Haynes, J. R. Induction of immunodeficiency virus-specific immune responses in rhesus monkeys following gene-gun-mediated DNA vaccination. *J. Med. Primatol.* (1996), **25**, 236–241.

Fuller, D. H., Simpson, L., Cole, K. S., Clements, J. E., Panicali, D. L., Montelaro, R. C., Murphey-Corb, M., and Haynes, J. R. Gene gun-based nucleic acid immunization alone or in combination with recombinant vaccinia vectors suppresses virus burden in rhesus macaques challenged with a heterologous SIV. *Immunol. Cell. Biol.* (1997b), **75**, 389–396.

Furth, P. A., Shamay, A., Wall, R. J., and Hennighausen, L. Gene transfer into somatic tissues by jet injection. *Anal. Biochem.* (1992), **205**, 365–368.

Fynan, E. F., Robinson, H. L., and Webster, R. G. Use of DNA encoding influenza hemagglutinin as an avian influenza vaccine. *DNA Cell. Biol.* (1993a), **12**, 785–789.

Fynan, E. F., Webster, R. G., Fuller, D. H., Haynes, J. R., Santoro, J. C., and Robinson, H. L. DNA vaccines: Protective immunizations by parenteral, mucosal and gene-gun inoculations. *Proc. Natl. Acad. Sci. USA* (1993b), **90**, 11478–11482.

Gardner, M. J., Doolan, D. L., Hedstrom, R. C., Wang, R., Sedegah, M., Gramzinski, R. A., Aguiar, J. C., Wang, H., Margalith, M., Hobart, P., and Hoffman, S. L. DNA vaccines against malaria: Immunogenicity and protection in a rodent model. *J. Pharm. Sci.* (1996), **85**, 1294–1300.

Garza, K. M., Griggs, N. D., and Tung, K. S. K. Neonatal injection of ovarian peptides induces autoimmune ovarian disease in female mice: Requirement of endogenous neonatal ovaries. *Immunity* (1997), **6**, 89–96.

Geissler, M., Gesien, A., Tokushige, K., and Wands, J. R. Enhancement of cellular and humoral immune responses to hepatitis C virus core protein using DNA-based vaccines augmented with cytokine-expressing plasmids. *J. Immunol.* (1997a), **158**, 1231–1237.

Geissler, M., Tokushige, K., Chante, C. C., Zurawski, V. R., Jr., and Wands, J. R. Cellular and humoral immune response to hepatitis B virus structural proteins in mice after DNA-based immunization. *Gastroenterology* (1997b), **112**, 1307–1320.

Geissler, M., Wands, G., Gesien, A., de la Monte, S., Bellet, D., and Wands, J. R. Genetic immunization with the free human chorionic gonadotropin beta subunit elicits cytotoxic T lymphocyte responses and protects against tumor formation in mice. *Lab. Invest.* (1997c), **76**, 859–871.

Gerdts, V., Jons, A., Macoschey, B., Visser, N., and Mettenleiter, T. C. Protection of pigs against Aujeszky's disease by DNA vaccination. *J. Gen. Virol.* (1997), **78**, 2139–2146.

Gerloni, M., Ballou, W. R., Billetta, R., and Zanetti, M. Immunity to *Plasmodium falsiparum* malaria sporozoites by somatic transgene immunization. *Nat. Biotech.* (1997), **15**, 876–881.

Ghiasi, H., Cai, S., Slanina, S., Nesburn, A. B., and Wechsler, S. L. Vaccination of mice with herpes simplex virus type 1 glycoprotein D DNA produces low levels of protection against lethal HSV-1 challenge. *Antiviral Research* (1995), **28**, 147–157.

Gibb, L., and Kay, E. R. M. Incorporation of DNA by cells of the Ehrlich–Lettre ascites carcinoma. *J. Cell. Biol.* (1968), **38**, 452–454.

Gilbert, M. J., Riddle, S. R., Plachter, B., and Greenberg, P. D. Cytomegalovirus selectively blocks antigen processing and presentation of its immediate early gene product. *Nature* (1996), **383**, 720–722.

Gilkeson, G. S., Grudiewr, J. P., Karouns, D. G., and Pisetsky, D. S. Induction of anti-ds DNA antibodies in normal mice by immunization with bacterial DNA. *J. Immunol.* (1998), **142**, 1482–1486.

Gilkeson, G. S., Pritchard, A.-L., and Pisetsky, D. S. Specificity of anti-DNA antibodies induced in normal mice by immunization with bacterial DNA. *Clin. Immunol. Immunopathol.* (1991), **59**, 288–300.

Giorgetti, C., and Press, J. L. A peptide sequence mimics the epitope on the multideterminant antigen (Tyr, Glu)-Ala-Lys that induces the dominant H10/V kappal$^+$ primary antibody response. *J. Immunol.* (1994), **152**, 136–145.

Giorgetti, C. A., and Press, J. L. Somatic mutation in the neonatal mouse. *J. Immunol.* (1998), **161**, 6093–6104.

Goebels, N., Michaelis, D., Wekerle, H., and Hohlfeld, R. Human myoblasts as antigen-presenting cells. *J. Immunol.* (1992), **149**, 661–667.

Goldstein, J. S., Chen, T., Brunswik, M., Mostowsky, H., and Kozlowski, S. Purified MHC class I and peptide complexes activate naive CD8 T cells independently of the CD28/B7 and LFA-I/ICAM-I costimulatory molecules. *J. Immunol.* (1998), **160**, 3180–3187.

Gough, P. M., Frank, C. J., Moore, D. G., Sagona, M. A., and Johnson, C. J. Lactogenic immunity to transmissible gastroenteritis virus induced by a subunit immunogen. *Vaccine* (1983), **1**, 37–41.

Gonzales Armas, J. C., Morello, C. S., Cranmer, L. D., and Spector, D. H. DNA immunization confers protection against murine cytomegalovirus infection. *J. Virol.* (1996), **70**, 7921–7928.

Graham, F. L., and Prevec, L. Adenovirus-based expression vector and recombinant vaccines. In *Vaccines: New Approaches to Immunological Problems* (R. W. Elis, ed.). Butterworth-Heineman, Boston, (1992), pp. 231–250.

Gramzinski, R. A., Maris, D. C., Doolan, D., Charoenvit, Y., Obaldia, N., Rossan, R., Sedegah, M., Wang, R., Hobart, P., Margalith, M., and Hoffman, S. Malaria DNA vaccines in Aotus monkeys. *Vaccine* (1997), **15**, 913–915.

Grange, M. P., Armand, M. A., Audoly, G., Thollot, D., and Desgranges, C. Induction of neutralizing antibodies against HTLV-1 envelope proteins after combined genetic and protein immunization in mice. *DNA Cell. Biol.* (1997), **16**, 1439–1448.

Gregoire, K. E., Goldschneider, I., Barton, R. W., and Bollum, F. J. Ontogeny of terminal deoxynucleotidyl transferase-positive cells in lymphopoietic tissues of rat and mice. *J. Immunol.* (1979), **123**, 1347–1353.

Gregoriadis, G., Saffie, R., and Hart, S. L. High yield incorporation of plasmid DNA within liposomes: Effect on DNA integrity and transfection efficiency. *J. Drug Target* (1996), **3**, 469–475.

Gregoriadis, G., Saffie, R., and de Souza, J. B. Liposome-mediated DNA vaccination. *FEBS Lett.* (1997), **402**, 107–110.

Grifantini, R., Finco, O., Bartolini, E., Draghi, M., del Giudice, G., Kocen, C., Thomas, A., Abrigani, S., and Grandi, G. Multi-plasmid DNA vaccination avoids antigenic competition and enhances immunogenicity of a poorly immunogenic plasmid. *Eur. J. Immunol.* (1998), **28**, 1225–1232.

Grosjean, I., Caux, C., Bella, C., Berger, I., Wild, F., Banchereau, J., and Kaiserlian, D. Measles virus infects human dendritic cells and blocks their allostimulatory properties for CD4+ T cells. *J. Exp. Med.* (1997), **186**, 801–812.

Gurunathan, S., Sacks, D. L., Brown, D. R., Reiner, S. L., Charest, H., Glaichenhaus, N., and Seder, R. A. Vaccination with DNA encoding the immunodominant LACK parasite antigen confers protective immunity to mice infected with *Leishmania major*. *J. Exp. Med.* (1997), **186**, 1137–1147.

Hahn, C. S., Hahn, Y. S., Braciale, T. J., and Rice, C. M. Infectious *Sindbis* virus transient expression vector for studying antigen processing and presentation. *Proc. Natl. Acad. Sci. USA* (1992), **89**, 2679–2683.

Hakim, I., Levy, S., and Levy, R. A nine-amino acid peptide from IL-1 beta augments antitumor immune responses induced by protein and DNA vaccines. *J. Immunol.* (1996), **157**, 5503–5511.

Hamaoka, T., and Katz, D. H. Mechanism of adjuvant activity of poly A:U on antibody responses to hapten-carrier conjugates. *Cell. Immunol.* (1973), **7**, 246–260.

Hanke, T., Schneider, J., Gilbert, S. C., Hill, A. V., and McMichael, A. DNA multi-CTL epitope vaccines for HIV and *Plasmodium falciparum*: Immunogenicity in mice. *Vaccine* (1998), **16**, 426–435.

Harding, C. V., Collins, D. S., Slot, J. W., Geuze, H. J., and Unanue, E. R. Liposome-encapsulated antigens are processed in lysosomes, recycled, and presented to T cells. *Cell* (1991), **64**, 393–401.

Harding, F. A., McArthur, J. G., Gross, J. A., Raulet, D. H., and Allison, J. P. CD28-mediated signalling co-stimulates murine T cells and prevents induction of anergy in T-cell clones. *Nature* (1992), **356**, 607–609.

Hariharan, M. J., Driver, D. A., Townsend, K., Brumm, D., Polo, J. M., Belli, B. A., Catton, D. J., Hsu, D., Mittelstaedt, D., McCormack, J. E., Karavodin, L., Dubensky, T. W., Jr., Chang, S. M., and Banks, T. A. DNA immunization against herpes simplex virus: Enhanced efficacy using a Sindbis virus based vector. *J. Virol.* (1998), **72**, 950–958.

Harpin, S., Talbot, B., Mbikay, M., and Elazhary, Y. Immune response to vaccination with DNA encoding the bovine viral diarrhea virus major glycoprotein gp53 (E2). *FEMS Microbiol. Lett.* (1997), **146**, 229–234.

Harte, P. G., and Playfair, J. H. L. Failure of malaria vaccination in mice born to immune mothers. II. Induction of specific suppressor cells by maternal IgG. *Clin. Exp. Immunol.* (1983), **51**, 157–164.

Hartl, A., Kiesslich, J., Weiss, R., Bernhaupt, A., Mostbock, S., Scheiblhofer, M., Ebner, C., Ferreira, F., and Thalhamer, J. Immune responses after immunization with plasmid DNA encoding Bet v 1, the major allergen of birch pollen. *J. Allerg. Clin. Immunol.* (1999), **103**, 107–113.

Hartly, S. B., Croslic, R., Brink, R., Kantor, A. B., Basten, A., and Goodnow, C. C. Elimination from peripheral lymphoid tissues of self-reactive lymphocytes recognizing membrane-bound antigens. *Nature* (1991), **353**, 765–769.

Hassett, D. E., Zhang, J., Slifka, M., and Whitton, J. L. Immune responses following neonatal DNA vaccination are long-lived, abundant, and qualitatively similar to those induced by conventional immunization. *J. Virol.* (2000), **74**, 2620–2627.

Hassett, D. E., Zhang, J., and Whitton, J. L. Neonatal DNA immunization with a plasmid encoding an internal viral protein is effective in the presence of maternal antibodies and protects against subsequent viral challenge. *J. Virol.* (1997), **71**, 7881–7888.

He, J., Hoffman, S. L., and Hayes, C. G. DNA inoculation with a plasmid vector carrying the hepatitis E virus structural protein gene induces immune response in mice. *Vaccine* (1997), **15**, 357–362.

Hedstrom, R. C., Doolan, D. L., Wang, R., Gardner, M. J., Kumar, A., Sedegah, M., Gramzinski, R. A., Sacci, J. B., Jr., Charoenvit, Y., Weiss, W. R., Margalith, M., Norman, J. A., Hobart, P., and Hoffman, S. L. The development of a multivalent DNA vaccine for malaria. *Springer Semin. Immunopathol.* (1997), **19**, 147–159.

Hengge, U. R., Walker, P. S., and Vogel, J. C. Expression of naked DNA in human, pig, and mouse skin. *J. Clin. Invest.* (1966), **97**, 2911–2916.

Herrmann, J. E., Chen, S. C., Fynan, E. F., Santoro, J. C., Greenberg, H. B., and Robinson, H. L. DNA vaccines against rotavirus infections. *Arch. Virol. Suppl.* (1996b), **12**, 207–215.

Herrmann, J. E., Chen, S. C., Fynan, E. F., Santoro, J. C., Greenberg, H. B., Wang, S., and Robinson, H. L. Protection against rotavirus infections by DNA vaccination. *J. Infect. Dis.* (1996a), **174**(Suppl. 1), S93–S97.

Hershberg, R. M., Framason, P. E., Cho, D. H., Lee, L. Y., Kovats, S., Beltz, J., Blum, J. S., and Nepom, G. T. Intestinal epithelial cells use two distinct pathways for class II antigen processing. *J. Clin. Invest.* (1997), **100**, 204–215.

Hickman, M. A., Malone, R. W., Lehmann-Bruinsma, K., Sih, T. R., Knoell, D., Szoka, F. C., Walzem, R., Carlson, D. M., and Powell, J. S. Gene expression following direct injection of DNA into liver. *Hum. Gene Ther.* (1994), **5**, 1477–1483.

Hiernaux, J., Bona, C., and Baker, P. Neonatal treatment with low doses of anti-idiotypic antibodies lead to the expression of a silent clone. *J. Exp. Med.* (1981), **153**, 1004–1008.

Hinkula, J., Lundholm, P., and Warren, B. Nucleic acid vaccination with HIV regulatory genes: A combination of HIV-1 genes in separate plasmids induces strong immune responses. *Vaccine* (1997a), **15**, 874–878.

Hinkula, J., Svanholm, C., Schwartz, S., Lundholm, P., Brytting, M., Engstrom, G., Benthin, R., Glaser, H., Sutter, G., Kohleisen, B., Erfle, V., Okuda, K., Wigzell, H., and Wahren, B. Recognition of prominent viral epitopes induced by immunization with human immunodeficiency virus type I regulatory genes. *J. Virol.* (1997b), **71**, 5528–5539.

Hoerr, I., Obs, R., Rammensee, H. G., and Jung, G. *In vivo* application of RNA leads to induction of specific cytotoxic lymphocytes and antibodies. *Eur. J. Immunol.* (2000), **30**, 1–7.

Hoffman, S. L., Doolan, D. L., Sedegah, M., Aguiar, J. C., Wang, R., Malik, A., Gramzinski, R. A., Weiss, W. R., Hobart, P., Norman, J. A., Margalith, M., and Hedstrom, R. C. Strategy for development of a pre-erythryocytic *Plasmodium falciparum* DNA vaccine for human use. *Vaccine* (1997a), **15**, 842–845.

Hoffman, S. L., Doolan, D. L., Sedegah, M., Wang, R., Scheller, L. F., Kumar, A., Weiss, W. R., Le, T. P., Klinman, D. M., Hobart, P., Norman, J. A., and Hedstrom, R. C. Toward clinical trials of DNA vaccines against malaria. *Immunol. Cell. Biol.* (1997b), **75**, 376–381.

Hoffman, S. L., Sedegah, M., and Hedstrom, R. C. Protection against malaria by immunization with a *Plasmodium yoelii* circumsporozoite protein nucleic acid vaccine. *Vaccine* (1994), **12**, 1529–1533.

Hohlfeld, R., and Engel, A. G. Induction of HLA-DR expression on human myoblasts with interferon-gamma. *Am. J. Pathol.* (1990), **136**, 503–508.

Hohlfeld, R., and Engel, A. G. The immunobiology of muscle. *Immunology Today* (1994), **15**, 269–274.

Hong, K., Zheng, W., Baker, A., and Papahadjopoulos, D. Stabilization of cationic liposome-plasmid DNA complexes by polyamines and poly(ethylene glycol)-phospholipid conjugates for efficient *in vivo* gene delivery. *FEBS Lett.* (1997), **400**, 233–237.

Howard, J. G., and Hale, C. Lack of neonatal susceptibility to induction of tolerance to polysaccharide antigens. *Eur. J. Immunol.* (1976), **6**, 486–493.

Hsu, C. H., Chua, K. Y., Tao, M. H., Huang, S. K., and Hsieh, K. H. Inhibition of specific IgE response *in vivo* by allergen–gene transfer. *Int. Immunol.* (1996a), **8**, 1405–1411.

Hsu, C. H., Chua, K. Y., Tao, M. H., Lai, Y. L., Wu, H. D., Huang, S. K., and Hsieh, K. H. Immunoprophylaxis of allergen-induced immunoglobulin E synthesis and airway hyperresponsiveness *in vivo* by genetic immunization. *Nat. Med.* (1996b), **2**, 540–544.

Hu, H.-M., Urba, W. J., and Fox, B. A. Gene-modified tumor vaccine with therapeutic potential shifts tumor-specific T cell response from a Type 2 to a Type 1 cytokine profile. *J. Immunol.* (1998), **161**, 3033–3041.

Husseini, R. H., Sweet, C., Overton, H., and Smith, H. Role of maternal immunity in the protection of newborn ferrets against infection with a virulent influenza virus. *Immunology* (1984), **52**, 389–394.

Huygen, K., Content, J., Denis, O., Montgomery, D. L., Yawman, A. M., Deck, R. R., DeWitt, C. M., Orme, I. M., Baldwin, S., D'Souza, C., Drowart, A., Lozes, E., Vandenbussche, P., Van Vooren, J. P., Liu, M. A., and Ulmer, J. B. Immunogenicity and protective efficacy of a tuberculosis DNA vaccine. *Nat. Med.* (1996), **2**, 893–898.

Ichino, M., Mor, G., Conover, J., Weiss, W. R., Takeno, M., Ishii, K. J., and Klinman, D. M. Factors associated with the development of neonatal tolerance after the administration of a plasmid DNA vaccine. *J. Immunol.* (1999), **162**, 3814–3818.

Inchauspe, G., Vivitsky, L., Major, M. E., Jung, G., Spengler, U., Maisonnas, M., and Trepo, C. Plasmid DNA expressing a secreted or a non-secreted form of hepatitis C virus nucleocapsid: Comparative studies of antibody and T-helper responses following genetic immunization. *DNA Cell. Biol.* (1997), **16**, 185–195.

Indraccolo, S., Feroli, F., Minuzzo, S., Mion, M., Rosato, A., Zamarchi, R., Titti, F., Verani, P., Amadori, A., and Chieco-Bianchi, L. DNA immunization of mice against SIVmac239 Gag and Env using Rev-independent expression plasmids. *AIDS Res. Hum. Retrovir.* (1998), **14**, 83–90.

Irvine, K. R., Rao, J. B., Rosenberg, S. A., and Restifo, N. P. Cytokine enhancement of DNA immunization leads to effective treatment of established pulmonary metastases. *J. Immunol.* (1996), **156**, 238–245.

Ishii, K. J., Weiss, W. R., and Klinman, D. M. Prevention of neonatal tolerance by a plasmid encoding granulocyte-macrophage colony stimulating factor. *Vaccine* (1999), **18**, 703–710.

Ishii, K. J., Weiss, W. R., Ichino, M., Verthelyi, D., and Klinman, D. M. Activity and safety of DNA plasmids encoding IL-4 and IFN-gamma. *Gene Ther.* (1999), **6**, 237–244.

Ishii, N., Fukushima, J., Kaneko, T., Okada, E., Tani, K., Tanaka, S. I., Hamajima, K., Xin, K. Q., Kawamoto, S., Koff, W., Nishioka, K., Yasuda, T., and Okuda, K. Cationic liposomes are a strong adjuvant for a DNA vaccine of human immunodeficiency virus type I. *AIDS Res. Hum. Retrovir.* (1997a), **13**, 1421–1428.

Ishii, N., Sugita, Y., Nakajima, H., Bukawa, H., Asakura, Y., and Okuda, K. Genetic control of immune responses to HIV-1 env DNA vaccine. *Microbiol. Immunol.* (1997b), **41**, 421–425.

Isobe, H., Moran, T., Li, S., Young, A., Nathenson, S., Palese, P., and Bona, C. Presentation by Major Histocompatibility Complex Class I molecules of nucleoprotein peptide expressed in two different genes of an influenza transfectant. *J. Exp. Med.* (1995), **181**, 293–313.

Ito, Y. Heat-resistance of tumorigenic nucleic acids of Shope papilloma. *Virology* (1961), **12**, 596–601.

Iwasaki, A., and Barber, B. H. Induction by DNA immunization of a protective antitumor cytotoxic T lymphocyte response against a minimal-epitope-expressing tumor. *Cancer Immunol. Immunother.* (1998), **45**, 273–279.

Iwasaki, A., Stiernholm, B. J., Chan, A. K., Berinstein, N. L., and Barber, B. H. Enhanced CTL responses mediated by plasmid DNA immunogens encoding costimulatory molecules and cytokines. *J. Immunol.* (1997a), **158**, 4591–4601.

Iwasaki, A., Torres, C. A. T., Ohashi, P. S., Robinson, H. L., and Barber, B. H. The dominant role of bone marrow-derived cells in CTL induction following plasmid DNA immunization at different sites. *J. Immunol.* (1997b), **159**, 11–14.

Jain, V., and Mekalanos, J. J. Use of lambda phage S and R gene products in an inducible lysis system for *Vibrio cholerae* and *Salmonella enterica serovar typhimurinum*-based DNA vaccine delivery systems. *Infect. Immunol.* (2000), **68**, 986–989.

Jakeman, K.J., Smith, H., and Sweet, C. Mechanism of immunity to influenza. *J. Gen. Virol.* (1989), **70**, 1523–1531.

Jelonek, M. T., Maskrey, J. L., Steimer, K. S., Potts, B. J., Higgins, K. W., and Keller, M. A. Maternal monoclonal antibody to the V3 loop alters specificity of the response to a human immunodeficiency virus vaccine. *J. Infect. Dis.* (1996), **174**, 886–889.

Jennings, P. A., Bills, M. M., Irving, D. O., and Mattick, J. S. Fimbriae of *Bacteroides nodosum*: Protein engineering of the structural subunit for production of an exogenous peptide. *Protein Engineering* (1989), **2**, 365–369.

Jiang, C., Magee, D. M., and Cox, R. A. Coadministration of interleukin 12 expression vector with antigen expressing cDNA enhances induction of protective immunity against *Coccidioides immitis*. *Infect. Immunol.* (1999), **67**, 5848–5853.

Jiao, S., Cheng, L., Wolff, J. A., and Yang, N. S. Particle bombardment-mediated gene transfer and expression in rat brain tissues. *Biotechnology* (1993), **11**, 497–502.

Jiao, S., Williams, P., Berg, R. K., Hodgeman, B. A., Liu, L., Repetto, G., and Wolff, J. A. Direct gene transfer into nonhuman primate myofibers *in vivo. Hum. Gene Ther.* (1992), **3**, 21–33.

Johanning, F. W., Conry, R. M., LoBuglio, A. F., Wright, M., Sumerel, L. A., Pike, M. J., and Curiel, D. T. A Sindbis virus mRNA polynucleotide vector achieves prolonged and high level heterologous gene expression *in vivo. Nucleic Acids Res.* (1995), **23**, 1495–1501.

Johnston, S. A. Biolistic transformation: Microbes to mice. *Nature* (1990), **346**, 776–777.

Johnston, S. A., and Tang, D. C. The use of microparticle injection to introduce genes into animal cells *in vitro* and *in vivo. Genet. Eng. (NY)* (1993), **15**, 225–236.

Jones, D. H., Corris, S., McDonald, S., Clegg, J. C., and Farrar, G. H. Poly(DL-lactide-co-glycolide) encapsulated plasmid DNA elicits systemic and mucosal antibody responses to encoded protein after oral administration. *Vaccine* (1997), **15**, 814–817.

Jones, L. A., Chin, L. T., Merriam, G. R., Nelson, L. M., and Kruisbeck, A. M. Failure of clonal deletion in neonatally thymectomized mice: Tolerance is preserved through clonal anergy. *J. Exp. Med.* (1990), **172**, 1277–1285.

Justewicz, D. M., and Webster, R. G. Long term-maintenance of B cell immunity to influenza virus hemagglutinin in mice following DNA based immunization. *Virology* (1996), **224**, 10–17.

Kaiserlian, D., Vidal, K., and Revillard, J. P. Murine enterocytes can present soluble antigen to specific Class II restricted CD4 T cells. *Eur. J. Immunol.* (1989), **19**, 1513–1516.

Kaneko, H., Bednarek, I., Wierzbicki, A., Kiszka, I., Dmochowski, M., Wasik, T. J., Kaneko, Y., and Kozbor, D. Oral DNA vaccination promotes mucosal and systemic immune responses to HIV envelope glycoprotein. *Virology* (2000), **267**, 8–16.

Kasper, L. H., Khan, I. A., Ely, K. H., Buelow, R., and Boothroyd, J. C. Antigen-specific (p30) mouse CD8 T cells are cytotoxic against Toxoplasma gondii-infected peritoneal macrophages. *J. Immunol.* (1992), **148**, 1493–1498.

Kawabata, S., Terao, Y., Fujiwara, T., Nakagawa, I., and Hamada, S. Targeted salivary gland immunization with plasmid DNA elicits specific salivary immunoglobulin A and G antibodies and serum immunoglobulin G in mice. *Infect. Immunol.* (1999), **67**, 5863–5868.

Kawamura, T., and Furue, M. Comparative analysis of B7.1 and B7.2 expression in Langerhans cells: Differential regulation by T helper Type I and T helper Type II cytokines. *Eur. J. Immunol.* (1995), **25**, 1913–1917.

Kay, E. R. M. Incorporation of deoxyribonucleic acid by mammalian cells *in vitro. Nature* (1961), **191**, 387–391.

Kazanji, M., Bomford, R., Bessereau, J. L., Schulz, T., and de The, G. Expression and immunogenicity in rats of recombinant adenovirus 5 DNA plasmids and vaccinia virus containing the HTLV-1 env gene. *Int. J. Cancer* (1997), **71**, 300–307.

Keller, E. T., Burkholder, J. K., Shi, F., Pugh, T. D., McCabe, D., Malter, J. S., MacEwen, E. G., Yang, N. S., and Ershler, W. B. *In vivo* particle-mediated cytokine gene transfer into canine oral mucosa and epidermis. *Cancer Gene Ther.* (1996), **3**, 186–191.

Kettman, J. R., Cambier, J. C., Uhr, J. W., Lipler, F., and Viteta, E. S. The role of receptor IgM and IgD in determining triggering and induction of tolerance in murine B cells. *Immunol. Rev.* (1979), **43**, 69–95.

Kim, J. J., Ayyavoo, V., Bagarazzi, M. L., Chattergoon, M., Boyer, J. D., Wang, B., and Weiner, D. B. Development of a multicomponent candidate vaccine for HIV-1. *Vaccine* (1997a), **15**, 879–883.

Kim, J. J., Ayyavoo, V., Bagarazzi, M. L., Chattergoon, M. A., Dang, K., Wang, B., Boyer, J. D., and Weiner, D. B. *In vivo* engineering of a cellular immune response by coadministration of IL-12 expression vector with a DNA immunogen. *J. Immunol.* (1997b), **158**, 816–826.

Kim, J. J., Bagarazzi, M. L., Trivedi, N., Hu, Y., Kazahaia, K., Wilson, D. M., Ciccarelli, R., Chattergoon, M. A., Dang, K., Mahaligam, S., Chalian, A. A., Agadjanyan, M. B., Boyer, J. D., Wang, B., and Wener, D. B. Engineering of *in vivo* immune response to DNA immunization via codelivery of costimulatory molecule genes. *Nat. Biotechnol.* (1997a), **15**, 641–646.

Kim, J. J., Nottingham, L. K., Tsai, A., Lee, D. J., Maguire, H. C., Oh, J., Dentchev, T., Manson, K. H., Wyand, M. S., Wyand, M. S., Agadjanyan, M. G., Ugen, K. E., and Weiner, D. B. Antigen-specific humoral and cellular immune responses can be modulated in rhesus macaques through the use of IFN-gamma, IL-12, or IL-18 gene adjuvants. *J. Med. Primatol.* (1999a), **28**, 214–223.

Kim, J. J., Trivedi, N. N., Nottingham, L. K., Morrison, L., Tsai, A., Hu, Y., Mahalingam, S., Dang, K., Ahn, L., Doyle, N. K., Wilson, D. M., Chattergoon, M. A., Chalian, A. A., Boyer, J. D., Agadjanyan, M. G., and Weiner, D. B. Modulation of amplitude and direction of *in vivo* immune responses by co-administration of cytokine gene expression cassettes with DNA immunogens. *Eur. J. Immunol.* (1998), **28**, 1089–1103.

Kim, J. J., Tsai, A., Nottingham, L. K., Morrison, L., Cunning, D. M., Oh, J., Lee, D. J., Dang, K., Dentchev, T., Chalian, A. A., Agadjanyan, M. G., and Weiner, D. B. Intracellular adhesion molecule-1 modulates beta-chemokines and directly costimulates T cells *in vivo. J. Clin. Invest.* (1999b), **103**, 869–877.

Kimura, Y., Sonehara, K., Kuramoto, E., Makiano, T., Yamamoto, S., Yamamoto, T., Kataoka, T., and Tokunaga, T. Binding of oligoguanylate to scavenger receptors is required for oligonucleotides to augment NK cell activity and induce IFN. *J. Biochem.* (1994), **1116**, 991–994.

Kiselow, P., Blutham, H., Staerz, U. D., Steinmez, M., and von Boehmer, H. Tolerance in T cells receptor transgenic mice involves delation of $CD4^+$ $CD8^+$ thymocytes. *Nature* (1988), **333**, 742–746.

Klavinskis, L. S., Gao, L., Barnfield, C., Lehner, T., and Parker, S. Mucosal immunization with DNA-liposome complex. *Vaccine* (1997), **15**, 818–820.

Kline, J. N., Waldschmidt, T. J., Businga, T. R., Lemish, J. E., Weinstock, J. V., Thorne, P. S., and Krieg, A. M. Modulation of airway inflammation by CpG oligodeoxynucleotides in a murine model of asthma. *J. Immunol.* (1998), **160**, 2555–2559.

Klinman, D., Yi, A.-K., Beausage, S. L., Conover, J., and Krieg, A. M. CpG motifs in bacterial DNA rapidly induce lymphocytes to secrete IL-6, IL-12 and IFN-gamma. *Proc. Natl. Acad. Sci. USA* (1996), **93**, 2879–2883.

Klinman, D. M., Barnhart, K. M., and Conover, J. CpG motifs as immune adjuvants. *Vaccine* (1999a), **17**, 19–25.

Klinman, D. M., Verthelyi, D., Takeshita, F., and Ishii, K. J. Immune recognition of foreign DNA: A cure for bioterrorism? *Immunity* (1999b), **11**, 123–129.

Klinman, D. M., Yamshikov, G., and Ishgatsubo, Y. Contribution of CpG motifs to the immunogenicity of DNA vaccines. *J. Immunol.* (1997), **158**, 3635–3659.

Knight, S. C., Iqball, S., Roberts, M. S., Macatonia, S., and Bedford, P. A. Transfer of antigen between dendritic cells in the stimulation of primary T Cell proliferation. *Eur. J. Immunol.* (1998), **28**, 1636–1644.

Kochel, T., Wu, S. J., Raviprakash, K., Hobart, P., Hoffman, S., Porter, K., and Hayes, C. Inoculation of plasmids expressing the dengue-2 envelop gene elicit neutralizing antibodies in mice. *Vaccine* (1997), **15**, 547–552.

Kodihalli, S., Haynes, J. R., Robinson, H. L., and Webster, R. G. Cross-protection among lethal H5N2 influenza viruses induced by DNA vaccine to the hemagglutinin. *J. Virol.* (1997), **71**, 3391–3396.

Kohl, S., and Loo, L. S. The relative role of transplacental milk immune transfer in protection against neonatal herpes simplex virus in mice. *J. Infect. Dis.* (1984), **149**, 38–42.

Komori, T., Pricop, L., Hatakeyama, A., Bona, C., and Alt, F. W. Repertoire of antigen receptors in TdT congenitally defective mice. *Int. Rev. Immunol.* (1996), **13**, 257–382.

Kozono, H., White, J., Clements, J., Marrack, P., and Kapller, J. Production of soluble MHC Class II proteins with covalently bound single peptide. *Nature* (1994), **369**, 151–154.

Krasemann, S., Groschup, M., Hunsmann, G., and Bodemer, W. Induction of antibodies against human prion proteins (PrP) by DNA-mediated immunization of PrP0/0 mice. *J. Immunol. Meth.* (1996), **199**, 109–118.

Krieg, A. M. Lymphocyte activation by CpG dinucleotide motifs in prokaryotic DNA. *Trends Microbiol.* (1996), **4**, 73–76.

Krieg, A. M., Matson, S., Cheng, K., Fischer, E., Koretzky, G. A., and Koland, J. G. Identification of an oligonucleotide sequence motif that specifically inhibits phosphorylation by proteinkinases. *Antisense–Nucleic Acid–Drug Dev.* (1997), **7**, 115–123.

Krieg, A. M., Yi, A.-K., Waldschmidt, T. J., Bishop, G., Teasdale, R., Koretzky, G. A., and Klinman, D. S. CpG motifs in bacterial DNA trigger direct B-cell activation. *Nature* (1995), **374**, 546–548.

Kriesel, J. D., Spruance, S. L., Daynes, R. A., and Araneo, B. A. Nucleic acid vaccine-encoding gD2 protects mice from herpes simplex virus Type 2 disease. *J. Infect. Dis.* (1996), **173**, 536–541.

Kuhrober, A., Wild, J., Pudollek, H. P., Chisari, F. V., and Reimann, J. DNA vaccination with plasmids encoding the intracellular (HBcAg) or secreted (HBeAg) form of the core protein of hepatitis B virus primes T cell responses to two overlapping Kb and Kd restricted epitopes. *Int. Immunol.* (1997), **9**, 1203–1212.

Kuklin, N., Daheshia, M., Karem, K., Manickan, E., and Rouse, B. T. Induction of mucosal immunity against herpes simplex virus by plasmid DNA immunization. *J. Virol.* (1997), **71**, 3138–3145.

Kuklin, N. A., Daheshia, M., Chun, S., and Rouse, B. T. Immunomodulation by mucosal gene transfer using TGF-beta DNA. *J. Clin. Invest.* (1998), **102**, 438–444.

Kurar, E., and Splitter, G. A. Nucleic acid vaccination of *Brucella abortus* ribosomal L7/L12 gene elicits immune response. *Vaccine* (1997), **15**, 1851–1857.

Kwiatkowski, D., and Marsh, K. Development of a malaria vaccine. *Lancet* (1997), **350**, 1696–1701.

Lai, W. C., Bennett, M., Johnston, S. A., Barry, M. A., and Pakes, S. P. Protection against *Mycoplasma pulmonis* infection by genetic vaccination. *DNA Cell. Biol.* (1995), **14**, 643–651.

Lai, W. C., Pakes, S. P., Ren, K., Lu, Y. S., and Bennett, M. Therapeutic effect of DNA immunization of genetically susceptible mice infected with virulent *Mycoplasma pulmonis*. *J. Immunol.* (1997), **158**, 2513–2516.

Lam, K. P., and Stall, A. M. MHC Class II expression distinguish two distinct B cell developmental pathways during ontogeny. *J. Exp. Med.* (1994), **180**, 507–516.

Lamb, J. R., and Feldman, M. Essential requirement for major histocompatibility complex recognition in T cell tolerance induction. *Nature (London)* (1984), **308**, 72–74.

Lagging, L. M., Meyer, K., Hoft, D., Houghton, M., Belshe, R. B., and Ray, R. Immune responses to plasmid DNA encoding the hepatitis C virus core protein. *J. Virol.* (1995), **69**, 5859–5863.

Larsen, D. L., Dybdahl-Sissoko, N., McGregor, M. W., Drape, R., Neumann, V., Swain, W. F., Lunn, D. P., and Olsen, C. W. Coadministration of DNA encoding interleukin-6 and hemagglutinin confers protection from influenza virus challenge in mice. *J. Virol.* (1998), **72**, 1704–1708.

Le, T. P., Coonan, K. M., Hedstrom, R. C., Charoenvit, Y., Sedegah, M., Epstein, S., Kumar, S., Wang, R., Doolan, D. L., Maguire, J. D., Parker, S. E., Hobart, P., Norman, J., and Hoffman, S. L. Safety, tolerability and humoral immune responses after intramuscular administration of a malaria DNA vaccine to the adult volunteers. *Vaccine* (2000), **18**, 1893–1901.

Le Borgne, S., Mancini, M., Le Grand, R., Schleef, M., Dormont, D., Tiollais, P., Riviere, Y., and Michel, M. L. *In vivo* induction of specific cytotoxic T lymphocytes in mice and rhesus macaques immunized with DNA vector encoding an HIV epitope fused with hepatitis B surface antigen. *Virology* (1998), **240**, 304–315.

Leclerc, C., Deriaud, E., Rojas, M., and Whalen, R. G. The preferential induction of a Th1 immune response by DNA-based immunization is mediated by the immunostimulatory effect of plasmid DNA. *Cell. Immunol.* (1997), **179**, 97–106.

Leclerc, C., Lo-Man, R., Charbit, A., Martineau, P., Clement, J. M., and Hofung, M. Immunogenicity of viral B- and T-cell epitopes expressed in recombinant bacterial proteins. *Inter. Rev. Immunol.* (1994), **11**, 103–178.

Lee, D. J., Tighe, H., Corr, M., Roman, M., Carson, D. A., Spiegelberg, H. L., and Raz, E. Inhibition of IgE antibody formation by plasmid DNA immunization is mediated by both CD4$^+$ and CD8$^+$ T cells. *Int. Arch. Allerg. Immunol.* (1997), **113**, 227–230.

Lee, Y. L., Tao, M. H., Chow, Y. H., and Chiang, B. L. Construction of vectors expressing bioactive heterodimeric and single-chain murine interleukin-12 for gene therapy. *Hum. Gene Ther.* (1998), **9**, 457–465.

Leitner, W. W., Seguin, M. C., Ballou, W. R., Seitz, J. P., Schultz, A. M., Sheehy, M. J., and Lyon, J. A. Immune responses induced by intramuscular or gene gun injection of protective deoxyribonucleic acid vaccines that express the circumsporozoite protein from *Plasmodium berghei* malaria parasites. *J. Immunol.* (1997), **159**, 6112–6119.

Leitner, W. W., Ying, H., Driver, D. A., Dubensky, T. W, and Restifo, N. P. Enhancement of tumor specific immune response with plasmid DNA replicon vectors. *Cancer Research* (2000), **60**, 51–55.

Lekutis, C., Shiver, J. W., Liu, M. A., and Letvin, N. L. HIV-1 env DNA vaccine administered to rhesus monkeys elicits MHC Class II-restricted CD4$^+$ T helper cells that secrete IFN-gamma and TNF-alpha. *J. Immunol.* (1997), **158**, 4471–4477.

Lemke, H., Lange, H., and Berek, C. Maternal immunization modulates the primary immune response to 2-phenyl-oxazolone in BALB/c mice. *Eur. J. Immunol.* (1994), **24**, 3025–3030.

Le Potier, M. F., Monteil, M., Houdayer, C., and Eloit, M. Study of the delivery of the gD gene of pseudorabies virus to one-day-old piglets by adenovirus or plasmid DNA as ways to by-pass the inhibition of immune response by colostral antibodies. *Vet. Microbiol.* (1997), **55**, 75–80.

Lerner, R. A., Meinke, W., and Goldstein, D. A. Membrane associated DNA in the lymphocyte nucleus. *Proc. Natl. Acad. Sci. USA* (1971), **68**, 1212–1216.

Lewis, J., Lin, K.-Y., Kothavale, A., Flanagan, M., Matteucci, M. D., DePrince, R. B., Mook, R. A., Jr., Hendren, R. W., and Wagner, R. W. A serum-resistant cytofectin for cellular delivery of antisense oligodeoxy-nucleotides and plasmid DNA. *Proc. Natl. Acad. Sci. USA* (1996), **93**, 3176–3181.

Lewis, P. J., Van Drunen, Little-Van Den Hurk, and Babiuk, L. A. Altering the cellular location of an antigen expressed by DNA based vaccine modulates the immune response. *J. Virol.* (1999), **73**, 10214–10223.

Li, S., Polonis, V., Isobe, H., Zaghouani, H., Guinea, R., Moran, T., Bona, C., and Palese, P. Chimeric influenza virus induces neutralizing antibodies and cytotoxic T cells against human immunodeficiency virus Type 1. *J. Virol.* (1993), **67**, 6659–6666.

Lifley, M. R., Esdaile, J., and Moreno, C. Passive transfer of meningococcal group polysaccharide antibodies to the offspring of pregnant rabbits and their protective role against infection with *Escherichia coli*. *Vaccine* (1989), **7**, 17–21.

Lin, Y. L., Chen, L. K., Liao, C. L., Yeh, C. T., Ma, S. H., Chen, J. L., Huang, Y. L., Chen, S. S., and Chiang, H. Y. DNA immunization with Japanese encephalitis virus nonstructural protein NS1 elicits protective immunity in mice. *J. Virol.* (1998), **72**, 191–200.

Linsley, P. S., and Ledbetter, J. A. The role of the CD28 receptor during T cell responses to antigen. *Annu. Rev. Immunol.* (1993), **11**, 191–212.

Lipford, G. B., Bauer, M., Blank, C., Reiter, R., Wagner, H., and Heeg, K. CpG-containing synthetic oligonucleotides promote B and cytotoxic T cell responses to protein antigens. *Eur. J. Immunol.* (1997a), **27**, 3240–3244.

Lipford, G. B., Sparwasser, T., Bauer, M., Zimmermann, S., Koch, E. S., Heeg, K., and Wagner, H. Immunostimulatory DNA: Sequence-dependent production of potentially harmful or useful cytokines. *Eur. J. Immunol.* (1997b), **27**, 3420–3426.

Liu, M. A., Yasutomi, Y., Davies, M. E., Perry, H. C., Freed, D. C., Letvin, N. L., and Shiver, J. W. Vaccination of mice and non-human primates using HIV-gene-containing DNA. *Antibiot. Chemother.* (1996), **48**, 100–104.

Liu, Y., Mounkes, L. C., Liggitt, H. D., Brown, C. S., Solodin, Y., Heath, T. D., and Debs, R. J. Factors influencing the efficiency of cationic liposome-mediated intravenous gene delivery. *Nat. Biotechnol.* (1997), **15**, 167–173.

Livingston, J. B., Lu, S., Robinson, H. L., and Anderson, D. J. The induction of mucosal immunity in the female genital tract using gene-gun technology: Part 1. Antigen expression. *Ann. N.Y. Acad. Sci.* (1995), **772**, 265–267

Lobell, A., Weissert, R., Eltayeb, S., Svanholm, C., Olsson, T., and Wigzell, H. Presence of CpG DNA and the local cytokine milieu determine the efficacy of suppressive DNA vaccination in experimental autoimmune encephalomyelitis. *J. Immunol.* (1999), **163**, 4754–4762.

Lobell, A., Weissert, R., Storch, M. K., Svanholm, C., de Graaf, K. L., Lassmann, H., Andersson, R., Olsson, T., and Wigzell, H. Vaccination with DNA encoding an immunodominant myelin basic protein peptide targeted to Fc of immunoglobulin G suppresses experimental autoimmune encephalomyelitis. *J. Exp. Med.* (1998), **187**, 1543–1548.

Loke, S. L., Stein, C. A., Zhang, X. H., Nakanishi, M., Subasinghe, C., Cohen, J. S., and Neckers, L. M. Characterization of oligonucleotide transport into living cells. *Proc. Natl. Acad. Sci. USA* (1989), **86**, 3474–3478.

Lopes, L. M., and Chain, B. M. Liposomes-mediated delivery stimulates a class I-restricted cytotoxic T Cell response to soluble antigen. *Eur. J. Immunol.* (1992), **22**, 287–290.

Lowrie, D. B., Silva, C. L., Colston, M. J., Ragno, S., and Tascon, R. E. Protection against tuberculosis by a plasmid DNA vaccine. *Vaccine* (1997a), **15**, 834–838.

Lowrie, D. B., Silva, C. L., and Tascon, R. E. DNA vaccines against tuberculosis. *Immunol. Cell. Biol.* (1997b), **75**, 591–594.

Lowrie, D. B., Tascon, R. E., Bonato, V. L., Lima, V. M., Faccioli, L. H., Stavropol, E., Colston, M. J., Hewinson, R. G., Moelling, K., and Silva, C. L. Therapy of tuberculosis in mice by DNA vaccination. *Nature* (1999), **400**, 269–271.

Lowrie, D. B., Tascon, R. E., Colston, M. J., and Silva, C. L. Towards a DNA vaccine against tuberculosis. *Vaccine* (1994), **12**, 1537–1540.

Lozes, E., Huygen, K., Content, J., Denis, O., Montgomery, D. L., Yawman, A. M., Vanderbussche, P., Van Vooren, J. P., Drowart, A., Ulmer, J. B., and Liu, M. A. Immunogenicity and efficacy of a tuberculosis DNA vaccine encoding the components of the secreted antigen 85 complex. *Vaccine* (1997), **15**, 830–833.

Lu, D., Benjamin, R., Kim, M., Conry, R. M., and Curiel, D. T. Optimization of methods to achieve mRNA-mediated transfection of tumor cells *in vitro* and *in vivo* employing cationic liposome vectors. *Cancer Gene Ther.* (1995), **1**, 245–252.

Lu, S., Arthos, J., Montefiori, D. C., Yasutomi, Y., Manson, K., Mustafa, F., Johnson, E., Santoro, J. C., Wissink, J., Mullins, J. I., Haynes, J. R., Letvin, N. L., Wyand, M., and Robinson, H. L. Simian immunodeficiency virus DNA vaccine trial in macaques. *J. Virol.* (1996), **70**, 3978–3991.

Lu, S., Manson, K., Wyand, M., and Robinson, H. L., SIV DNA vaccine trial in macaques: Post-challenge necropsy in vaccine and control groups. *Vaccine* (1997), **15**, 920–923.

Lu, S., Santoro, J. C., Fuller, D. H., Haynes, J. R., and Robinson, H. L. Use of DNAs expressing HIV-1 env and noninfectious HIV-1 particles to raise antibody responses in mice. *Virology* (1995), **209**, 147–154.

Lu, Y., Xin, K. Q., Hamajima, K., Tsuji, T., Aoki, I., Yang, J., Sasaki, S., Fukushima, J., Yoshimura, T., Toda, S., Okada, E., and Okada, K. Macrophage inflammatory protein-1alpha (MIP-1alpha) expression plasmid enhances DNA vaccine-induced immune response against HIV-1. *Clin. Exp. Immunol.* (1999), **115**, 335–341.

Lukacher, A., Braciale, V. L., and Braciale, T. J. *In vivo* effector function of influenza virus-specific clones is highly specific. *J. Exp. Med.* (1984), **160**, 814–826.

Luke, C. J., Carner, K., Liang, X., and Barbour, A. G. An OspA-based DNA vaccine protects mice against infection with *Borrelia burgdorferi*. *J. Infect. Dis.* (1997), **175**, 91–97.

Lund, F. E., Solvason, N. W., Cooke, M. P., Heath, A. W., Grimaldi, J. C., Parkhouse, R. M. E., Goodnow, G. C., and Howard, M. Signaling through murine CD38 is impaired in antigen receptor-unresponsive B cells. *Eur. J. Immunol.* (1995), **25**, 1338–1345.

Lundholm, P., Asakura, Y., Hinkula, J., Lucht, E., and Wahren, B. Induction of mucosal IgA by a novel jet delivery technique for HIV-1 DNA. *Vaccine* (1999), **17**, 2036–2042.

Mabbott, N. A., Farquhar, C. F., Brown, K. L., and Bruce, M. E. Involvement of the immune system in TSE pathogenesis. *Immunology Today* (1998), **19**, 201–203.

MacDonald, H. R., Pedrazzini, T., Schneider, R., Louis, J. A., Zinkernagel, R. M., and Hengartner, H. Intrathymic elimination of MSLa reactive (Vβ6) cells during neonatal tolerance induction to Mlsa-encoded antigens. *J. Exp. Med.* (1988), **167**, 2005–2014.

MacFarlane, D. E., Manzel, L., and Krieg, A. M. Unmethylated CpG-containing oligonucleotides inhibit apoptosis in WEHI 231 B lymphocytes induced by several agents. *Immunology* (1997), **91**, 586–593.

MacGregor, R. R., Boyer, J. D., Ugen, K. E., Lacy, K. E., Bagarazzi, M. L., Chattergoon, M. A., Baine, Y., Higgins, T. J., Ciccarelli, R. B., Coney, L. R., Ginsberg, R. S., and Weiner, D. B. First human trial of a DNA-based vaccine for treatment of HIV-1 infection: Safety and host response. *J. Infect. Dis.* (1998), **178**, 92–100.

MacKenzie, C. D., Taylor, P. M., and Askonas, B. A. Rapid recovery of lung histology correlates with clearance of influenza-specific cells. *Immunology* (1989), **67**, 375–381.

Macklin, M. D., McCabe, D., McGregor, M. W., Neumann, V., Meyer, T., Callan, R., Hinshaw, V. S., and Swain, W. F. Immunization of pigs with a particle-mediated DNA vaccine to influenza A virus protects against challenge with homologous virus. *J. Virol.* (1998), **72**, 1491–1496.

Maecker, H. T., Umetsu, D. T., Dekruyff, R. H., and Levy, S. DNA vaccination with cytokine fusion constructs biases the immune response to ovalbumin. *Vaccine* (1997), **15**, 1687–1696.

Mahvi, D. M., Burkholder, J. K., Turner, J., Culp, J., Malter, J. S., Sondel, P. M., and Yang, N. S. Particle-mediated gene transfer of granulocyte-macrophage colony-stimulating factor cDNA to tumor cells: Implications for a clinically relevant tumor vaccine. *Hum. Gene Ther.* (1996), **7**, 1535–1543.

Mahvi, D. M., Sondel, P. M., Yang, N. S., Albertini, M. R., Schiller, J. H., Hank, J., Heiner, J., Gan, J., Swain, W., and Logrono, R. Phase I/II study of immunization with autologous tumor cells transfected with the GM-CSF gene by particle-mediated transfer in patients with melanoma or sarcoma. *Hum. Gene Ther.* (1997), **8**, 875–891.

Major, M. E., Vitviski, L., Mink, M. A., Schleef, M., Whalen, R. G., Trepo, C., and Inchauspe, G. DNA-based immunization with chimeric vectors for the induction of immune responses against the hepatitis C virus nucleocapsid. *J. Virol.* (1995), **69**, 5798–5805.

Malanchere, E., Huetz, F., and Couthino, A. Maternal IgG stimulates B lineage cell development in the progeny. *Eur. J. Immunol.* (1997), **27**, 788–793.

Mallick-Wood, C. A., Lewis, J. M., Richie, L. I., Owen, M. J., Tigelar, R. E., and Hayday, A. C. Conservation of T cell receptor conformation in epidermal cells with disrupted primary Vγ gene usage. *Science* (1998), **279**, 1729–1732.

Malone, R. W., Felgner, P. L., and Verma, I. M. Cationic liposome-mediated RNA transfection. *Proc. Natl. Acad. Sci. USA* (1989), **86**, 6077–6081.

Mancini, M., Davis, H. L., Tiollais, P., and Michel, M. L. DNA based immunization against the envelope proteins of the hepatitis B virus. *J. Biotechnol.* (1996a), **44**, 47–57.

Mancini, M., Hadchouel, M., Davis, H. L., Whalen, R. G., Tiollais, P., and Michel, M. L. DNA-mediated immunization in a transgenic mouse model of the hepatitis B surface antigen chronic carrier state. *Proc. Natl. Acad. Sci. USA* (1996b), **93**, 12496–12501.

Manickan, E., Kanangat, S., Rouse, R. J., Yu, Z., and Rouse, B. T. Enhancement of immune response to naked DNA vaccine by immunization with transfected dendritic cells. *J. Leukoc. Biol.* (1997a), **61**, 125–132.

Manickan, E., Rouse, R. J., Yu, Z., Wire, W. S., and Rouse, B. T. Genetic immunization against herpes simplex virus. *J. Immunol.* (1995), **155**, 259–265.

Manickan, E., Yu, Z., and Rouse, B. T. DNA immunization of neonates induces immunity despite the presence of maternal antibody. *J. Clin. Invest.* (1997a), **100**, 2371–2375.

Manning, W. C., Paliard, X., Zhou, S., Pat Bland, M., Lee, A. Y., Hong, K., Walker, C. M., Escobedo, J. A., and

Dwarki, V. Genetic immunization with adeno-associated virus vectors expressing herpes simplex virus type 2 glycoproteins B and D. *J. Virol.* (1997), **71**, 7960–7962.

Manthorpe, M., Cornefert-Jensen, F., Hartikka, J., Felgner, J., Rundell, A., Margalith, M., and Dwarki, V. J. Gene therapy by intramuscular injection of plasmid DNA: Studies on firefly luciferase gene expression in mice. *Hum. Gene Ther.* (1993), **4**, 419–425.

Martinez, X., Brandt, C., Saddallah, F., Tougne, C., Barrios, C., Wild, F., Dougan, G., Lambert, P. H., and Siegrist, C. A. DNA immunization circumvents deficient induction of T helper type 1 and cytotoxic T lymphocyte responses in neonates and during early life. *Proc. Natl. Acad. Sci. USA* (1997), **94**, 8726–8731.

Martinez, X., Li, X., Kovarik, J., Klein, M., Lambert, P. H., and Siegrist, C. A. Combining DNA and protein vaccines for early life immunization against respiratory syncytial virus in mice. *Eur. J. Immunol.* (1999), **29**, 3390–3400.

Martins, L. P., Lau, L. L., Asano, M. S., and Ahmed, R. DNA vaccination against persistent viral infection. *J. Virol.* (1995), **69**, 2574–2582.

Masurel, N. J., DeBruijne, J. I., Beunigh, H. A., and Schouten, H. J. A. Hemagglutination-inhibition antibodies against influenza A and B in maternal and neonatal sera. *J. Hyg.* (1978), **80**, 13–19.

Matsue, H., Bergstresser, P. R., and Takashima, A. Keratinocyte-derived IL-7 serves as growth factor for dendritic epidermal T cells in mice. *J. Immunol.* (1993), **151**, 6012–6018.

Matsumoto, Y., Kim, G., and Tanuma, N. Characterization of T cell receptor associated with the development of P2 peptide-induced autoimmune neuritis. *J. Neuroimmunol.* (2000), **102**, 67–72.

Mayer, L. Antigen presentation in the intestine: New rules and regulation. *Am. J. Physiol.* (1998), **274**, G7–G9.

Mbawuike, I. N., Six, H. R., Cate, T. R., and Ciuch, R. B. Vaccination with inactivated influenza A virus during pregnancy protect neonatal mice against lethal challenge by influenza A viruses representing three subtypes. *J. Virol.* (1990), **64**, 1370–1374.

McClements, W. L., Armstrong, M. E., Keys, R. D., and Liu, M. A. Immunization with DNA vaccines encoding glycoprotein D or glycoprotein B, alone or in combination, induces protective immunity in animal models of herpes simplex virus-2 disease. *Proc. Natl. Acad. Sci. USA* (1996), **93**, 11414–11420.

McClements, W. L., Armstrong, M. E., Keys, R. D., and Liu, M. A. The prophylactic effect of immunization with DNA encoding herpes simplex virus glycoproteins on HSV-induced disease in guinea pigs. *Vaccine* (1997), **15**, 857–860.

McCoy, K. L., Noone, M., Inman, J. K., and Stutzman, R. Exogenous antigens internalized through transferrin receptors activate CD4 T cells. *J. Immunol.* (1993), **150**, 1691–1704.

McDaniel, L. S., Loechel, F., Benedict, C., Greenway, T., Briles, D. E., Conry, R. M., and Curiel, D. T. Immunization with a plasmid expressing pneumococcal surface protein A (PspA) can elicit protection against fatal infection with *Streptococcus pneumoniae*. *Gene Ther.* (1997), **4**, 375–377.

McKeever, U., Khandekar, S., Jesson, M., Newcomb, J., Gregory, P., Naylor, J., Haskins, K., and Jones, B. Maternal immunization with a soluble TCR-Ig chimeric protein. *J. Immunol.* (1997), **159**, 5936–5945.

Mendoza, R. B., Cantwell, M. J., and Kipps, T. J. Immunostimulatory effects of a plasmid expressing CD40 ligand (CD154) on gene immunization. *J. Immunol.* (1997), **159**, 5777–5781.

Messina, J. P., Gilkeson, G. S., and Pisetsky, D. S. Stimulation of *in vitro* murine lymphocyte proliferation by bacterial DNA. *J. Immunol.* (1991), **147**, 1759–1764.

Michel, M. L., Davis, H. L., Schleef, M., Mancini, M., Tiollais, P., and Whalen, R. G. DNA-mediated immunization to the hepatitis B surface antigen in mice: Aspects of the humoral response mimic hepatitis B viral infection in humans. *Proc. Natl. Acad. Sci. USA* (1995), **92**, 5307–5311.

Mitrofanova, E. E., Bakhvalova, V. N., Dobrikova, E., Pap, V. A., and Morozova, O. V. Genetic immunization against tick-borne encephalitis virus. *Mol. Biol. (Mosk)* (1997), **31**, 403–406.

Mitsuda, S., Nakagawa, T., Nakazano, H., and Ikai, A. Receptor-linked antigen delivery system. *Biochem. Biophys. Res. Comm.* (1995), **216**, 399–405.

Mond, J. J., Liberman, R., Inman, J. K., Mosier, D. J., and Paul, W. E. Inability of mice with a defect in B-lymphocyte maturation to respond to phosphocholine on immunogenic carriers. *J. Exp. Med.* (1977), **146**, 1138–1142.

Monteil, M., Le Potier, M. F., Guillotin, J., Cariolet, R., Houdayer, C., and Eloit, M. Genetic immunization of seronegative one day old piglets against pseudorabies induces neutralizing antibodies but not protection and is ineffective in piglets from immune dams. *Vet. Res.* (1996), **27**, 443–452.

Montgomery, D. L., Shiver, J. W., Leander, K. R., Perry, H. C., Friedman, A., Martinez, D., Ulmer, J. B., Donnelly, J. J., and Liu, M. A. Heterologous and homologous protection against influenza A by DNA vaccination: Optimization of DNA vectors. *DNA Cell. Biol.* (1993), **12**, 777–783.

Mor, G., Klinman, D. M., Shapiro, S., Hagiwara, E., Sedegah, M., Norman, J. A., Hoffman, S. L., and Steinberg, A. D. Complexity of the cytokine and antibody response elicited by immunizing mice with *Plasmodium yoelii* circumsporozoite protein plasmid DNA. *J. Immunol.* (1995), **155**, 2039–2046.

Mor, G., Singla, M., Steinberg, A. D., Hoffman, S. L., Okuda, K., and Klinman, D. M. Do DNA vaccines induce autoimmune disease? *Hum. Gene Ther.* (1997), **8**, 293–300.

Mor, G., Yamshchikov, G., Sedegah, M., Takeno, M., Wang, R., Houghten, R. A., Hoffman, S., and Klinman, D. M. Induction of neonatal tolerance by plasmid DNA vaccination of mice. *J. Clin. Invest.* (1996), **98**, 2700–2705.

Mosier, D. E., Scher, I., and Paul, W. E. Spleen cells from mice with X-linked defect that precludes immune responses to several thymus independent antigens can respond to TNP-lipopolysaccharide. *J. Immunol.* (1976a), **117**, 1336–1345.

Mosier, D., Scher, I., and Paul, W. E. *In vitro* response of CBA/N mice: Spleen cells with an X-linked defect that precludes immune response to several thymus independent antigens. *J. Immunol.* (1976b), **117**, 788–796.

Moss, B. Vaccinia virus vectors. In *Vaccines: New Approaches to Immunological Problems* (R. W. Elis, ed.). Butterworth-Heineman, Boston, (1992), pp. 345–357.

Mucke, S., Polack, A., Pawlita, M., Zehnpfennig, D., Massoudi, N., Bohlen, H., Doerfler, W., Bornkamm, G., Diehl, V., and Wolf, J. Suitability of Epstein–Barr virus-based episomal vectors for expression of cytokine genes in human lymphoma cells. *Gene Ther.* (1997), **4**, 82–92.

Murakami, M., Tsubata, T., Shinkura, R., Nisitani, S., Okamoto, M., Yoshioka, M., Usui, T., Miyawaki, S., and Honjo, T. Oral administration of LPS activates B-a cells in the peritoneal cavity and lamina propria of the gut and induces autoimmune symptoms in an autoantibody transgenic mouse. *J. Exp. Med.* (1994), **180**, 111–119.

Murphy, T. P., Henderson, F. W., Clyde, W. A., Collier, A. M., and Denny, F. W. Pneumonia: An eleven year study in pediatric practice. *Am. J. Epidemiol.* (1981), **113**, 12–21.

Nabel, E. G., Gordon, D., Yang, Z. Y., Xu, L., San, H., Plautz, G. E., Wu, B. Y., Gao, X., Huang, L., and Nabel, G. J. Gene transfer *in vivo* with DNA-liposome complexes: Lack of autoimmunity and gonadal localization. *Hum. Gene Ther.* (1992a), **3**, 649–656.

Nabel, G. J., Nabel, E. G., Yang, Z. Y., Fox, B. A., Plautz, G. E., Gao, X., Huang, L., Shu, S., Gordon, D., and Chang, A. E. Direct gene transfer with DNA-liposome complexes in melanoma: Expression, biologic activity, and lack of toxicity in humans. *Proc. Natl. Acad. Sci. USA* (1993), **90**, 11307–11311.

Nabel, E. G., Plautz, G., and Nabel, G. J. Transduction of a foreign histocompatibility gene into the arterial wall induces vasculitis. *Proc. Natl. Acad. Sci. USA* (1992b), **89**, 5157–5161.

Nakano, M., and Braun, W. Fluctuation tests with antibody-forming spleen cell populations. *Science* (1966), **151**, 338–340.

Nakano, M., and Braun, W. Cell-released non-specific stimulators of antibody forming spleen cell populations. *J. Immunol.* (1967), **99**, 570–575.

Nawrath, M., Pavlovic, J., Dummet, R., Schultz, J., Strack, B., Heinrich, J., and Moelling, K. Reduced melanoma tumor formation in mice immunized with plasmid expressing the melanoma specific antigen gp100/pmel17. *Leukemia* (1999), **13**(Suppl. 1), S48–S51.

Neglia, F., Orengo, A. M., Cilli, M., Meazza, R., Tomassetti, A., Canevari, S., Colombo, M. P., and Ferrini, S. DNA vaccination against the ovarian carcinoma-associated antigen folate receptor alpha (FRalpha) induces cytotoxic T lymphocytes and antibody responses in mice. *Cancer Gene Ther.* (1999), **6**, 349–357.

Newton, S. M. C., Jacob, C., and Stocker, B. A. D. Immune response to cholera toxin epitope inserted in *Salmonella flagellin. Science* (1989), **247**, 70–72.

Niidome, T., Ohmori, N., Ichinose, A., Wada, A., Mihara, H., Hirayama, T., and Aoyagi, H. Binding of cationic alpha-helical peptides to plasmid DNA and their gene transfer abilities into cells. *J. Biol. Chem.* (1997), **272**, 15307–15312.

Nisonoff, A., and Bangasser, S. A. Immunological suppression of idiotypic specificities. *Transpl. Rev.* (1975), **27**, 100–134.

Nomura, T., Takahura, Y., and Hashida, M. Cancer gene therapy by direct intratumoral injection: Gene expression and intratumoral pharmacokinetics of plasmid DNA. *Gan To Kagaku Ryoho* (1997), **24**, 483–488.

Norman, J. A., Hobart, P., Manthorpe, M., Felgner, P., and Wheeler, C. Development of improved vectors for DNA-based immunization and other gene therapy applications. *Vaccine* (1997), **15**, 801–803.

Noguchi, Y., Noguchi, T., Sato, T., Yokoo, Y., Itho, S., Yoshida, M., Yoshiki, T., Akiyoshi, K., Sunamoto, J., Nakayama, E., and Shiku, H. Priming for *in vitro* and *in vivo* anti-human T lymphotropic virus type I cellular immunity by virus-related protein reconstituted into liposome. *J. Immunol.* (1991), **146**, 3599–3603.

Nossal, G. J. V. The immunological response of foetal mice to influenza virus. *Austral. J. Exp. Biol. Med. Sci.* (1957), **35**, 49–61.

Nutt, N. B., Wiesel, A. N., and Nisonoff, A. Neonatal expression of cross-reactive idiotype associated with anti-phenylarsonate antibodies in strain A mice. *Eur. J. Immunol.* (1979), **9**, 864–868.

Nyika, A., Mahan, S. M., Burridge, M. J., McGuire, T. C., Rurangirwa, F., and Barbet, A. F. A DNA vaccine protects mice against the rickettsial agent *Cowdria ruminantium. Parasite Immunol.* (1998), **20**, 111–119.

O'Callaghan, D., Charbit, A., Martineau, P., Leclerc, C., van der Werf, S., Nauciel, C., and Hofnung, M. Immunogenicity of foreign peptide epitopes expressed in bacterial envelope proteins. *Res. Microbiol* (1990), **141**, 963–969.

Ohashi, P. S., Oehen, S., Buerki, K., Pircher, H., Ohashi, C. T., Odermatt, B., Malissen, B., Zinkernagel, R. M., and Hengartner, H. Ablation of tolerance and induction of diabetes by virus infection in viral antigen transgenic mice. *Cell* (1991), **65**, 305–317.

Ohwada, A., Nagaoka, I., Takahashi, F., Tominaga, S., and Fukuchi, Y. DNA vaccination against HuD antigen elicits antitumor activity against small-cell lung cancer murine model. *Am. J. Respir. Cell. Mol. Biol.* (1999a), **21**, 37–43.

Ohwada, A., Sekyia, M., Hanaki, H., Arai, K. K., Nagaoka, Y., Hori, S., Tomin, J., Hiramatsu, K., and Fukuchi, Y. DNA vaccination by mecA sequence evokes an antibacterial immune response against methicillin-resistant *Staphylococcus aureus. J. Antimicrob. Chemother.* (1999b), **44**, 767–774.

Okada, E., Sasaki, S., Ishii, N., Aoki, I., Yasuda, T., Nishioka, K., Fukushima, J., Miyazaki, J., Wahren, B., and Okuda, K. Intranasal immunization of a DNA vaccine with IL-12 and granulocyte macrophage colony stimulating factor (GM-CSF)-expressing plasmids in liposomes induces strong mucosal and cell mediated immune responses against HIV-1 antigens. *J. Immunol.* (1997), **159**, 3638–3647.

Okuda, K., Xin, K. O., Tsuji, T., Bukawa, H., Tanaka, S., Koff, W. C., Tani, K., Okuda, K., Honma, K., Kawamoto, S., Hamajima, K., and Fukushima, J. DNA vaccination followed by macromolecular multicomponent peptide vaccination against HIV-1 induces strong antigen-specific immunity. *Vaccine* (1997), **15**, 1049–1056.

Oldstone, M. B., Nerenberg, M., Southern, P., Price, J., and Lewicki, H. Virus infection triggers insulin-dependent diabetes mellitus in a transgenic model. *Cell* (1991), **65**, 319–331.

Ono, T., Fujino, Y., Tsuchiya, T., and Tsuda, M. Plasmid DNAs directly injected into mouse brain with lipofectin can be incorporated and expressed by brain cells. *Neurosci. Lett.* (1990), **117**, 259–263.

Osmond, D. G. Population dynamics of bone marrow B lymphocytes. *Immunol. Rev.* (1986), **93**, 103–124.

Owen, R. D. Immunological tolerance. *Fed. Proc.* (1958), **16**, 581–591.

Pachuk, C. J., Arnold, R., Herold, K., Ciccarelli, R. B., and Higgins, T. J. Humoral and cellular immune responses to herpes simplex virus-2 glycoprotein D generated by facilitated DNA immunization of mice. *Curr. Top. Microbiol. Immunol.* (1998), **226**, 79–89.

Pande, H., Campo, K., Tanamachi, B., Forman, S. J., and Zaia, J. A. Direct DNA immunization of mice with plasmid DNA encoding the tegument protein pp65 (ppUL83) of human cytomegalovirus induces high levels of circulating antibody to the encoded protein. *Scand. J. Infect. Dis. Suppl.* (1995), **99**, 117–120.

Pearson, A. M., Rich, A., and Krieger, M. Polynucleotide binding to macrophage scavenger receptors depends on the formation of base-quartet-stabilized four-stranded helices. *J. Biol. Chem.* (1993), **268**, 3546–3554.

Peet, N. M., McKeating, J. A., Ramos, B., Klonisch, T., De Souza, J. B., Delves, P. J., and Lund, T. Comparison of nucleic acid and protein immunization for induction of antibodies specific for HIV-1 gp120. *Clin. Exp. Immunol.* (1997), **109**, 226–232.

Perkins, F. T., Yetts, R., and Gaisford, W. Response of infants given a third dose of poliomyelitis vaccine ten to twelve months after primary immunization. *Br. Med. J.* (1959), **1**, 680–682.

Pertmer, T. M., Eisenbraun, M. D., McCabe, D., Prayaga, S. K., Fuller, D. H., and Haynes, J. R. Gene gun based nucleic acid immunization: Elicitation of humoral and cytotoxic T lymphocyte responses following epidermal delivery of nanogram quantities of DNA. *Vaccine* (1995), **13**, 1427–1430.

Pertmer, T. M., Roberts, T. R., and Haynes, J. R. Influenza virus nucleoprotein-specific immunoglobulin G subclass and cytokine responses elicited by DNA vaccination are dependent on the route of vector DNA delivery. *J. Virol.* (1996), **70**, 6119–6125.

Pertmer, T. M., and Robinson, H. L. Studies on antibody responses following neonatal immunization with influenza hemagglutinin DNA or protein. *Virology* (1999), **257**, 406–414.

Peters, P. J., Neefijes, J. J., Oorschot, V., Ploegh, H. L., and Genze, H. J. Segregation of MHC Class II molecules in the Golgi complex for transport to lysosomal compartment. *Nature* (1991), **349**, 669–675.

Petersen, J. S., Karlsen, A. E., Markholst, H., Worsaae, A., Dyrberg, T., and Michelsen, B. Neonatal tolerization with glutamic acid decarboxylase but not bovine serum albumin delays the onset of diabetes in NOD mice. *Diabetes* (1994), **43**, 1478–1484.

Piedrafita, D., Xu, D., Hunter, D., Harrison, R. A., and Liew, F. Y. Protective immune responses induced by vaccination with an expression genomic library of *Leishmania major*. *J. Immunol.* (1999), **163**, 1467–1472.

Philip, R., Liggitt, D., Philip, M., Dazin, P., and Debs, R. *In vivo* gene delivery: Efficient transfection of T lymphocytes in adult mice. *J. Biol. Chem.* (1993), **268**, 16087–16090.

Phillpotts, R. J., Venugopal, K., and Brooks, T. Immunization with DNA polynucleotides protects mice against lethal challenge with St. Louis encephalitis virus. *Arch. Virol.* (1996), **141**, 743–749.

Pisetsky, D. S. Immune activation by bacterial DNA: A new genetic code. *Immunity* (1996), **5**, 303–310.

Pisetsky, D. S. Specificity and immunochemical properties of antibodies to bacterial DNA. *Methods* (1997), **11**, 55–61.

Porgador, A., Irwine, K. R., Iwasaki, A., Barber, B. H., Restifo, N. P., and Germain, R. N. Predominant role for directly transfected dendritic cells in antigen presentation to CD8 T cells after gene gun immunization. *J. Exp. Med.* (1998), **188**, 1075–1082.

Prayaga, S. K., Ford, M. J., and Haynes, J. R. Manipulation of HIV-1 gp120-specific immune responses elicited via gene gun based DNA immunization. *Vaccine* (1997), **15**, 1349–1352.

Press, J. L. Neonatal immunity and somatic mutation. *Int. Rev. Immunol.* (2000), **19**, 256–287.

Prigozy, T., Dalrymple, K., Kedes, L., and Shuler, C. Direct DNA injection into mouse tongue muscle for analysis of promoter function *in vivo*. *Somat. Cell. Mol. Genet.* (1993), **19**, 111–122.

Prince, A. M., Whalen, R. G., and Brotman, B. Successful nucleic acid based immunization of newborn chimpanzees against hepatitis B virus. *Vaccine* (1997), **15**, 916–919.

Puck, J. M., Glezen, W. P., Frank, A. L., and Six, H. R. Protection of infants from infection with influenza A virus by transplacentally-acquired antibody. *J. Infect. Dis.* (1980), **142**, 844–849.

Qiu, P., Ziegelhoffer, P., Sun, J., and Yang, N. S. Gene gun delivery of mRNA *in situ* results in efficient transgene expression and genetic immunization. *Gene Ther.* (1996), **3**, 262–268.

Quill, H., and Schwartz, R. H. Stimulation of normal inducer T cell clones with antigen presented by purified Ia molecules in planar lipid membranes: Specific induction of a long lived state of proliferative nonresponsiveness. *J. Immunol.* (1987), **138**, 3704–3712.

Radu, D. L., Antohi, S., Bot, A., Weksler, M. E., and Bona, C. Plasmid expressing the influenza HA gene protects old mice from lethal challenge with influenza virus. *Viral Immunol.* (1999), **12**, 217–226.

Ragno, S., Colston, M. J., Lowrie, D. B., Winrow, V. R., Blake, D. R., and Tascon, R. Protection of rats from adjuvant arthritis by immunization with naked DNA encoding for mycobacterial heat shock protein 65. *Arthritis Rheum.* (1997), **40**, 277–283.

Rakhmilevich, A. L., Turner, J., Ford, M. J., McCabe, D., Sun, W. H., Sondel, P. M., Grota, K., and Yang, N. S. Gene-gun mediated skin transfection with interleukin 12 gene results in regression of established primary and metastatic murine tumors. *Proc. Natl. Acad. Sci. USA* (1996), **93**, 6291–6296.

Ramsdel, F., Jenkins, M., Dinh, Q., and Fowlkes, B. J. The majority of CD4+ CD8⁻ thymocytes are functionally immature. *J. Immunol.* (1991), **147**, 1779–1785.

Ramsay, A. J., and Ramshaw, I. A. Cytokine enhancement of immune responses important for immunocontraception. *Reprod. Fertil. Dev.* (1997), **9**, 91–97.

Raposo, G., Nijman, H. W., Stoorvogel, W., Leijendekker, R., Harding, C. V., Melif, C. C., and Geuze, H. J. B lymphocytes secrete antigen-presenting vesicles. *J. Exp. Med.* (1996), **183**, 1161–1172.

Ray, N. B., Ewalt, L. C., and Lodmell, D. L. Nanogram quantities of plasmid DNA encoding the rabies virus glycoprotein protect mice against lethal rabies virus infection. *Vaccine* (1997), **15**, 892–895.

Raz, E., Carson, D. A., Parker, S. E., Parr, T. B., Abai, A. M., Aichinger, G. Gromkowski, S. H., Singh, M., Lew, D., Yankauckas, M. A., Baird, S. M., and Rhodes, G. H. Intradermal gene immunization: The possible role of DNA uptake in the induction of cellular immunity to viruses. *Proc. Natl. Acad. Sci. USA* (1994), **91**, 9519–9523.

Raz, E., Dudler, J., Lotz, M., Baird, S. M., Berry, C. C., Eisenberg, R. A., and Carson, D. A. Modulation of disease activity in murine systemic lupus erythematosus by cytokine gene delivery. *Lupus* (1995), **4**, 286–292.

Raz, E., and Spiegelberg, H. L. Deviation of the allergic IgE to an IgG response by gene immunotherapy. *Int. Rev. Immunol.* (1999), **18**, 271–289.

Raz, E., Tighe, H., Sato, Y., Corr, M., Dudler, J. A., Roman, M., Swain, S. L., Spiegelberg, H. L., and Carson, D. A. Preferential induction of a Th1 immune response and inhibition of specific IgE antibody formation by plasmid DNA immunization. *Proc. Natl. Acad. Sci. USA* (1996), **93**, 5141–5145.

Raz, E., Watanabe, A., Baird, S. M., Eisenberg, R. A., Parr, T. B., Lotz, M., Kipps, T. J., and Carson, D. A. Systemic immunological effects of cytokine genes injected into skeletal muscle. *Proc. Natl. Acad. Sci. USA* (1993), **90**, 4523–4527.

Refaeli, Y., van Parjis, L., London, C. A., Tschopp, J., and Abbas, A. K. Biochemical mechanisms of IL-2-regulated Fas-mediated T cell apoptosis. *Immunity* (1998), **8**, 615–623.

Restifo, N. P., and Wang, M. Antigen processing and presentation. In *Tumor Immunology* (A. G. Dalgeish and M. Browning, eds.). Cambridge University Press, Cambridge, UK, (1996), p. 39.

Reuman, P. D., Paganini, C. M. A., Ayoub, E. M., and Small, P. A. Maternal–infant transfer of influenza-specific immunity in mouse. *J. Immunol.* (1983), **130**, 932–936.

Revillard, J.-P. (Ed.). Cytokines. *Int. Rev. Immunol.* (1998), **16**, 205–456.

Rice, J., King, C. A., Spellerberg, M. B., Fairweather, N., and Stevenson, F. K. Manipulation of pathogen-derived genes to influence antigen presentation via DNA vaccines. *Vaccine* (1999), **17**, 3030–3038.

Richmond, J. F., Mustafa, F., Lu, S., Santoro, J. C., Weng, J., O'Connell, M., Fenyo, E. M., Hurwitz, J. L., Montefiori, D. C., and Robinson, H. L. Screening of HIV-1 env glycoproteins for the ability to raise neutralizing antibody using DNA immunization and recombinant vaccinia virus boosting. *Virology* (1997), **230**, 265–274.

Ridge, J. P., Fuchs, E. J., and Matzinger, P. Neonatal tolerance revisited: Turning of T cells with dendritic cells. *Science* (1996), **271**, 1723–1726.

Rigby, M. A., Hosie, M. J., Willett, B. J., Mackay, N., McDonald, M., Cannon, C., Dunsford, T., Jarrett, O., and Neil, J. C. Comparative efficiency of feline immunodeficiency virus infection by DNA inoculation. *AIDS Res. Hum. Retrovir.* (1997), **13**, 405–412.

Robinson, H. L., Boyle, C. A., Feltquate, D. M., Morin, M. J., Santoro, J. C., and Webster, R. G. DNA immunization for influenza virus: Studies using hemagglutinin- and nucleoprotein-expressing DNAs. *J. Infect. Dis.* (1997), **176**(Suppl. 1), S50–S55.

Robinson, H. L., Hunt, L. A., and Webster, R. G. Protection against a lethal influenza virus challenge by immunization with a hemagglutinin-expressing plasmid DNA. *Vaccine* (1993), **11**, 957–960.

Robinson, H. L., Montefiori, D. C., Johnson, R. P., Manson, K. H., Kalish, M. L., Rizvi, T. A., Lu, S., Hu, S. L., Mazzara, G. P., Panicali, D. L., Herndon, J. G., Glickman, R., Candido, M. A., Lydy, S. L., Wyand, M. S., and McClure, H. M. Neutralizing antibody-independent containment of immunodeficiency virus challenges by DNA priming and recombinant pox virus booster immunizations. *Nat. Med.* (1999), **5**, 526–534.

Rocken, M., and Shevach, E. M., Immune deviation—the third dimension of non-deletional T cell tolerance. *Immunol. Rev.* (1996), **149**, 175–194.

Rodriguez, F., Zhang, J., and Whitton, J. L. DNA immunization: Ubiquitination of a viral protein enhances cytotoxic T-lymphocyte induction and antiviral protection but abrogates antibody induction. *J. Virol.* (1997), **71**, 8497–8503.

Roman, L. M., Simons, L. F., Hammer, R. E., Sambrook, J. F., and Gething, M. J. The expression of influenza virus hemagglutinin in the pancreatic beta cells of transgenic mice results in autoimmune diseases. *Cell* (1990), **61**, 383–396.

Roman, M., Martin-Orozco, E., Goodman, J. S., Nguyen, M.-D., Sato, Y., Korhblut, R. S., Richman, D. D., Carson, D. A., and Raz, E. Immunostimulatory DNA sequences function as T helper-1 promoting adjuvants. *Nat. Med.* (1997), **3**, 849–854.

Rosato, A., Zambon, A., Milan, G., Ciminale, V., D'Agostino, D. M., Macino, B., Zanovello, P., and Collavo, D. CTL response and protection against P815 tumor challenge in mice immunized with DNA expressing the tumor-specific antigen P815A. *Hum. Gene Ther.* (1997), **8**, 1451–1458.

Rossi, P., Moschese, V., Broliden, P. A., Fundaro, C., Quinti, I., Plebani, A., Giaquinto, C., Tovo, P. A., Ljunggren, K., Rosen, J., Wigzel, H., Jondal, M., and Wahren, B. Presence of maternal antibodies to HIV-1 envelope glycoprotein gp120 epitopes correlates with the uninfected status of children born to seropositive mothers. *Proc. Natl. Acad. Sci. USA* (1989), **86**, 8055–8058.

Rothel, J. S., Waterkeyn, J. G., Strugnell, R. A., Wood, P. R., Seow, H. F., Vadolas, J., and Lightowlers, M. W. Nucleic acid vaccination of sheep: Use in combination with a conventional adjuvanted vaccine against *Taenia ovis. Immuno. Cell. Biol.* (1997), **75**, 41–46.

Rothenberg, E., and Triglia, D. Clonal proliferation unlinked to TdT synthesis in thymocytes of young animals. *J. Immunol.* (1983), **130**, 1627–1634.

Rothstein, A., and Vastola, P. Homologous monoclonal antibodies induce idiotype suppression in neonates through maternal influence and in adults exposed during fetal and neonatal life. *J. Immunol.* (1984), **133**, 1151–1154.

Rouse, R. J., Nair, S. K., Lydy, S. L., Bowen, J. C., and Rouse, B. T. Induction *in vitro* of primary cytotoxic T-lymphocyte responses with DNA encoding herpes simplex virus proteins. *J. Virol.* (1994), **68**, 5685–5689.

Roy, K., Mao, H. Q., Huang, S. K., and Leong, K. W. Oral gene delivery with chitosan-DNA nanoparticles generate immunologic protection in a murine model of peanut allergy. *Nat. Med.* (1999), **5**, 387–391.

Rubinstein, L. J., Victor-Kobrin, C. B., and Bona, C. The function of idiotypes and anti-idiotypes on the development of the immune repertoire. *Dev. Comp. Immunol.* (1984), **3**, 109–116.

Rubinstein, L. J., Yeh, M., and Bona, C. Idiotype-antiidiotype network: II. Activation of salient clones by treatment at birth with idiotypes is associated with the expansion of idiotype-specific T cells. *J. Exp. Med.* (1982), **156**, 506–521.

Ruiz, P. J., Garren, H., Ruiz, I. U., Hirschberg, D. L., Nguyen, L. V., Karpuj, M. V., Cooper, M. T., Mitchell, D. J., Fathman, C. G., and Steinman, L. Suppressive immunization with DNA encoding a self-peptide prevents autoimmune disease: Modulation of T cell costimulation. *J. Immunol.* (1999), **162**, 3336–3341.

Sadlack, B., Lohler, J., Schorle, H., Klebb, G., Haber, H., Sickel, E., Noelle, R. J., and Horak, I. Generalized autoimmune disease in interleukin-2-deficient mice is triggered by an uncontrolled activation and proliferation of CD4+ T cells. *Eur. J. Immunol.* (1995), **25**, 3053–3059.

Sagodıra, S., Iochmann, S., Mevelec, M. N., Dimier-Poisson, I., and Bout, D. Nasal immunization of mice with *Cryptosporidium parvum* D induces systemic and intestinal immune responses. *Parasite Immunol.* (1999), **21**, 507–516.

Saito, T., Sherman, G. J., Kurocohchi, K., Guo, Z. P., Donets, M., Yu,, M. Y., Berzofsky, J. A., Akatsuka, T., and Feinstone, S. M. Plasmid-DNA based immunization for hepatitis C virus structural proteins: Immune responses in mice. *Gastroenterology* (1997), **112**, 1321–1330.

Sakaguchi, M., Nakamura, H., Sonoda, K., Hamada, F., and Hirai, K. Protection of chickens from Newcastle disease by vaccination with a linear plasmid DNA expressing the F protein of newcastle disease virus. *Vaccine* (1996), **14**, 747–752.

San, H., Yang, Z. Y., Pompili, V. J., Jaffe, M. L., Plautz, G. E., Xu, L., Felgner, J. H., Wheeler, C. J., Felgner, P. L., Gao, X., et al. Safety and short term toxicity of a novel cationic lipid formulation for human gene therapy. *Hum. Gene Ther.* (1993), **4**, 781–788.

Sarvas, H., Kurikka, S., Seppala, I. J., Makela, P. H., and Makela, O. Maternal antibodies partially inhibit an active antibody response to routine tetanus toxoid immunization. *J. Infect. Dis.* (1992), **165**, 977–979.

Sarzotti, M., Dean, T. A., Remington, M. P., Ly, C. D., Furth, P. A., and Robbins, D. S. Induction of cytotoxic T cell responses in newborn mice by DNA immunizatiọn. *Vaccine* (1997), **15**, 795–797.

Sarzotti, M., Robbins, D. S., and Hoffman, P. M. Induction of protective CTL response in newborn mice by a murine retrovirus. *Science* (1996), **271**, 1726–1728.

Sasaki, S., Fukushima, J., Hamajima, K., Ishii, N., Tsuji, T., Xin, K. Q., Mohri, H., and Okuda, K. Adjuvant effect of Ubenimex on a DNA vaccine for HIV-1. *Clin. Exp. Immunol.* (1998a), **111**, 30–35.

Sasaki, S., Hamajima, K., Fukushima, J., Ihata, A., Ishii, N., Gorai, I., Hirahara, F., Mohri, H., and Okuda, K. Comparison of intranasal and intramuscular immunization against human immunodeficiency virus Type I with a DNA-monophosphoryl lipid A adjuvant vaccine. *Infect. Immunol.* (1998b), **66**, 823–826.

Sasaki, S., Tsuji, T., Hamajima, K., Fukushima, J., Ishii, N., Kaneko, T., Xin, K. Q., Mohri, H., Aoki, I., Okubo, T., Nishioka, K., and Okuda, K. Monophosphoryl lipid A enhances both humoral and cell-mediated immune responses to DNA vaccination against human immunodeficiency virus type I. *Infect. Immunol.* (1997), **65**, 3520–3528.

Sato, Y., Roman, M., Tighe, H., Lee, D., Corr, M., Nguien, M.-D., Silverman, G., Lotz, M., Carson, D., and Raz, E. Immunostimulatory DNA sequences are necessary for effective intradermal gene immunization. *Science* (1996), **273**, 352–354.

Sawa, T., Miyazaki, H., Pittet, J. F., Widdicombe, J. H., Gropper, M. A., Hashimoto, S., Conrad, D. J., Folkesson, H. G., Debs, R., Forsayeth, J. R., Fox, B., and Wiener-Kronish, J. P. Intraluminal water increases expression of plasmid DNA in rat lung. *Hum. Gene Ther.* (1996), **7**, 933–941.

Schimizu, T., Koyama, S., and Iwafuchi, N. Nuclear uptake of DNA by Ehrlich ascites-tumor cells. *Biochim. Biophys. Acta* (1962), **55**, 795–798.

Schirmbeck, R., Bohm, W., Ando, K., Chisari, F. V., and Reimann, J. Nucleic acid vaccination primes hepatitis B virus surface antigen-specific cytotoxic T lymphocytes in nonresponder mice. *J. Virol.* (1995), **69**, 5929–5934.

Schirmbeck, R., Bohm, W., and Reimann, J. DNA vaccination primes MHC Class-I restricted, simian virus 40 large tumor antigen-specific CTL in H-2d mice that reject syngeneic tumors. *J. Immunol.* (1996), **157**, 3550–3558.

Schmaljohn, C., Vanderzanden, L., Bray, M., Custer, D., Meyer, B., Li, D., Rossi, C., Fuller, D., Haynes, J., and Huggins, J. Naked DNA vaccines expressing the prM and E genes of Russian spring–summer encephalitis virus and Central European encephalitis virus protect mice from homologous and heterologous challenge. *J. Virol.* (1997), **71**, 9563–9569.

Schneider, J., Gilbert, S. C., Blanchard, T. J., Hanke, T., Robson, K. J., Hannan, C. M., Becker, M., Sinden, R., Smith, G. L., and Hill, A. V. Enhanced immunogenicity for CD8$^+$ T cell induction and complete protective efficacy of malaria DNA vaccination by boosting with modified vaccinia virus Ankara. *Nat. Med.* (1998), **4**, 397–402.

Schrijver, R. S., Langedijk, J. P., Keil, G. M., Middel, W. G., Maris-Veldhuis, M., Van Oirschot, J. T., and Rijsewijk, F. A. Immunization of cattle with a BHV1 vector vaccine or a DNA vaccine both coding for the G protein of BRSV. *Vaccine* (1997), **15**, 1908–1916.

Sedegah, M., Hedstrom, R., Hobart, P., and Hoffman, S. L. Protection against malaria by immunization with plasmid DNA encoding circumsporozoite protein. *Proc. Natl. Acad. Sci. USA* (1994), **91**, 9866–9870.

Sedegah, H., Jones, T. R., Kaur, M., Hedstrom, R., Hobart, P., Tine, J. A., and Hoffman, S. L. Boosting with recombinant vaccinia increases immunogenicity and protective efficacy of malaria DNA vaccine. *Proc. Natl. Acad. Sci. USA* (1998), **95**, 7648–7653.

Seeger, C., Ganem, D., and Varmus, H. E. The cloned genome of ground squirrel hepatitis virus is infectious in the animal. *Proc. Natl. Acad. Sci. USA* (1984), **81**, 5849–5852.

Segal, B. M., and Sehvach, E. M. IL-12 unmasks latent autoimmune diseases in resistant mice. *J. Exp. Med.* (1996), **184**, 771–775.

Selby, M. J., Doe, B., and Walker, C. M. Virus-specific cytotoxic T-lymphocyte activity elicited by coimmunization with human immunodeficiency virus Type 1 genes regulated by the bacteriophage T7 promoter and T7 RNA polymerase protein. *J. Virol.* (1997), **71**, 7827–7831.

Seo, S. H., Wang, L., Smith, R., and Collisson, E. W. The carboxyl-terminal 120-residue polypeptide of infectious bronchitis virus nucleocapsid induces cytotoxic T lymphocytes and protects chickens from acute infection. *J. Virol.* (1997), **71**, 7889–7894.

Shain, R. D., and Cebra, J. J. Rise in inulin-sensitive B cells during ontogeny can be prematurely stimulated by thymus-dependent and thymus-independent antigens. *Infect. Immunol.* (1981), **32**, 211–215.

Sharma, S., Miller, P. W., Stolina, M., Zhu, L., Huang, M., Paul, R. W., and Dubinett, S. M. Multicomponent gene therapy vaccines for lung cancer: Effective eradication of established murine tumors *in vivo* with interleukin-7/herpes simplex thymidine kinase-transduced autologous tumor and *ex vivo* activated dendritic cells. *Gene Ther.* (1997), **4**, 1361–1370.

Sheridan, J. F., Smith, C. C., Manak, M. M., and Aurelian, L. J. Prevention of rotavirus-induced diarrhea in neonatal mice born to dams immunized with empty capsids of simian rotavirus SA-11. *J. Infect. Dis.* (1984), **149**, 434–443.

Shimizu, T., Koyama, S., and Iwafuchi, M. Nuclear uptake of deoxyribonucleic acid by Ehrlich ascites tumor cells. *Biochim. Biophys. Acta.* (1962), **55**, 795–798.

Shiver, J. W., Davies, M. E., Perry, H. C., Freed, D. C., and Liu, M. A. Humoral and cellular immunity elicited by HIV-1 vaccination. *J. Pharm. Sci.* (1996), **85**, 1317–1324.

Shiver, J. W., Davies, M. E., Yasutomi, Y., Perry, H. C., Freed, D. C., Letvin, N. L., and Liu, M. A. Anti-HIV env immunity elicited by nucleic acid vaccines. *Vaccine* (1997), **15**, 884–887.

Siegrist, C. A., Barrios, C., Martinez, X., Brandt, C., Berney, M., Cordoba, M., Kovarik, J., and Lambert, P.-H. Influence of maternal antibodies on vaccine responses: Inhibition of antibody but not T cell responses allows successful early prime-boost strategies in mice. *Eur. J. Immunol.* (1998), **28**, 4138–4148.

Sigal, N. H., Pickard, A. R., Metcalf, E. S., Gearhart, P. J., and Klinman, N. R. Expression of phosphrylcholine-specific B cells during murine development. *J. Exp. Med.* (1977), **146**, 933–948.

Silva, C. L. New vaccines against tuberculosis. *Braz. J. Med. Biol. Res.* (1995), **28**, 843–851.

Simon, M. M., Gern, L., Hauser, P., Zhong, W., Nielsen, P. J., Kramer, M. D., Brenner, C., and Wallich, R. Protective immunization with plasmid DNA containing the outer surface lipoprotein A gene of *Borrelia burgdorferi* is independent of an eukaryotic promoter. *Eur. J. Immunol.* (1996), **26**, 2831–2840.

Sin, J. I., Sung, J. H., Suh, Y. S., Lee, A. H., Chung, J. H., and Sung, Y. C. Protective immunity against heterologous challenge with encephalomyocarditis virus by VP1 DNA vaccination: Effect of coinjection with a granulocyte-macrophage colony stimulator factor gene. *Vaccine* (1997), **15**, 1827–1833.

Singh, R. R., Hahn, B. H., and Sercarz, E. Neonatal peptide exposure can prime T cells and subsequently induced their immune deviation. *J. Exp. Med.* (1996), **183**, 1613–1621.

Sirard, J.-C., Fayolle, C., Chastellier, C., Mock, M., Leclerc, C., and Berche, P. Intracytoplasmic delivery of Listeriolysine O by a vaccinal strain of *Bacillus anthracis* induces CD8-mediated protection against *Listeria monocytogenes. J. Immunol.* (1997), **159**, 4453–4443.

Sizemore, D. R., Branstrom, A. A., and Sadoff, J. C. Attenuated *Shigella* as a DNA delivery vehicle for DNA-mediated immunization. *Science* (1995), **270**, 299–302.

Sizemore, D. R., Branstrom, A. A., and Sadoff, J. C. Attenuated bacteria as a DNA delivery vehicle for DNA-mediated immunization. *Vaccine* (1997), **15**, 804–807.

Sjolander, A., Baldwin, T. M., Curtis, J. M., and Handman, E. Induction of a Th1 immune response and simultaneous lack of activation of a Th2 response are required for generation of immunity to leishmaniasis. *J. Immunol.* (1998), **160**, 3949–3957.

Slater, J. E., and Colberg-Poley, A. A DNA vaccine for allergen immunotherapy using the latex allergen Hev b 5. *Arh. Paul Erlich Inst. Bundesamt Sera Impfstoffe Frankf. A.M.* (1997), **91**, 230–235.

Smith, L. E., Rodrigues, M., and Russell, D. G. The interaction between CD8 T Cells and Leishmania-infected macrophages. *J. Exp. Med.* (1991), **174**, 499–505.

Smith, S. C., and Allen, P. M. Expression of myosine-Class II MHC complexes in normal myocardium occurs before induction of autoimmune myocarditis. *Proc. Natl. Acad. Sci. USA* (1992), **89**, 9131–9135.

Sornasse, T., Larenas, P. V., Davies, K. A., deVries, J. E., and Yssel, H. Differentiation and stability of Th1 and 2 cells derived from naive human neonatal CD4 T cells analyzed at the single cell level. *J. Exp. Med.* (1996), **184**, 473–481.

Sparwasser, T., Koch, E. S., Vabulas, R. M., Heeg, K., Lipford, G. B., Ellwart, J. W., and Wagner, H. Bacterial DNA and immunostimulatory CpG oligonucleotides trigger maturation and activation of murine dendritic cells. *Eur. J. Immunol.* (1998), **28**, 2045–2054.

Sparwasser, T., Miethke, T., Lipford, G., Borschert, K., Hacker, H., Heeg, K., and Wagner, H. Bacterial DNA causes septic shock. *Nature* (1997a), **386**, 336–337.

Sparwasser, T., Miethke, T., Lipford, G., Erdmann, A., Hacker, H., Heeg, K., and Wagner, H. Macrophages sense pathogens via DNA motifs: Induction of tumor necrosis factor-alpha-mediated shock. *Eur. J. Immunol.* (1997b), **27**, 1671–1679.

Spellerberg, M. B., Zhu, D., Thompsett, A., King, C. A., Hamblin, T. J., and Stevenson, F. K. DNA vaccines against lymphoma: Promotion of anti-idiotypic antibody response induced by single chain Fv genes by fusion to tetanus toxin fragment C. *J. Immunol.* (1997), **159**, 1885–1892.

Stacey, K. J., Jester, D. P., Sweet, M. J., and Hume, D. A. Macrophage activation by immunostimulatory DNA. *Curr. Top. Microbiol. Immunol.* (2000), **247**, 41–58.

Stan, A. C., Casares, S., Brumeanu, T.-D., Klinman, D. M., and Bona, C. A. CpG motifs of DNA vaccines induce the expression of chemokines and MHC class II molecules on myocytes. *Eur. J. Immunol.* (2000), submitted.

Starnbach, M. N., and Bevan, M. J. Cells infected with Yersinia present an epitope to class I MHC-restricted CTL. *J. Immunol.* (1994), **153**, 1603–1612.

Stasney, J., Cantarow, A., and Paschkis, K. E. Production of neoplasms by fractions of mammalian neoplasms. *Cancer Res.* (1950), **10**, 775–782.

Steinman, R. M., The dendritic cell system and its role in immunogenicity. *Annu. Rev. Immunol.* (1991), **9**, 271–296.

Stevenson, F. K., Zhu, D., King, K. A., Ashworth, L. J., Kumar, S., and Hawkinds, R. E. Idiotypic DNA vaccines against B-cell lymphoma. *Immunol. Rev.* (1995), **145**, 211–228.

Stewart, M. J., Plautz, G. E., Del Buono, L., Yang, Z. Y., Xu, L., Gao, X., Huang, L., Nabel, E. G., and Nabel, G. J. Gene transfer *in vivo* with DNA-liposome complexes: Safety and acute toxicity in mice. *Hum. Gene Ther.* (1992), **3**, 267–275.

Stocker, B. A., and Newton, S. M. C. Immune response to epitopes inserted in Salmonella flagellin. *Int. Rev. Immunol.* (1994), **11**, 167–178.

Stopeck, A. T., Hersh, E. M., Brailey, J. L., Clark, P. R., Norman, J., and Parker, S. E. Transfection of primary tumor cells and tumor cell lines with plasmid DNA/lipid complexes. *Cancer Gene Ther.* (1998), **5**, 119–126.

Stover, C. K., de la Cruz, V. F., Fuerst, T. R., Burlein, J. E., Benson, L. A., Bennett, L. T., Bansal, L. T., Young, J. F., Lee, M. H., and Hattful, G. F. New use of BCG for recombinant vaccines. *Nature* (1991), **351**, 456–460.

Strugnell, R. A., Drew, D., Mercieca, J., DiNatale, S., Firez, N., Dunstan, S. J., Simmons, C. P., and Vadolas, J. DNA vaccines for bacterial infections. *Immunol. Cell. Biol.* (1997), **75**, 364–369.

Subauste, C. S., Koniaris, A. H., and Remington, J. S. Murine CD8 cytotoxic T lymphocytes lyse *Toxoplasama gondii* infected cells. *J. Immunol.* (1991), **147**, 3955–3959.

Sun, Q. D., Gots, M., Mayermann, G., and Wekerle, H. Resistance to experimental autoimmune encephalomyelitis induced by tolerization to myelin basic protein. *Eur. J. Immunol.* (1989), **19**, 373–380.

Sun, S., Beard, C., Yi, A. K., Jones, P., and Sprent, J. Mitogenicity of DNA from different organisms for murine B cells. *J. Immunol.* (1997), **159**, 3119–3125.

Sun, W. H., Burkholder, J. K., Sun, J., Culp, J., Turner, J., Lu, X. G., Pugh, T. D., Ershler, W. B., and Yang, N. S. *In vivo* cytokine gene transfer by gene gun reduces tumor growth in mice. *Proc. Natl. Acad. Sci. USA* (1995), **92**, 2889–2893.

Sundaram, P., Tigelaar, R. E., and Brandsma, J. L. Intracutaneous vaccination of rabbits with the cottontail rabbit papillomavirus (CRPV) L1 gene protects against virus challenge. *Vaccine* (1997), **15**, 664–671.

Sundaram, P., Tigelaar, R. E., Xiao, W., and Brandsma, J. L. Intracutaneous vaccination of rabbits with the E6 gene of cottontail rabbit papillomavirus provides partial protection against virus challenge. *Vaccine* (1998), **16**, 613–623.

Suter, M., Lew, A. M., Grob, P., Adema, G. J., Ackermann, M., Shortman, K., and Fraefel, C. BAC-VAC, a novel generation of (DNA) vaccines: A bacterial artificial chromosome (BAC) containing a replication-competent packaging-defective virus genome induces protective immunity against herpes simplex virus 1. *Proc. Natl. Acad. Sci. USA* (1999), **96**, 12697–12702.

Sutterwala, F. S., Noel, G. J., Salgame, P., and Mosser, D. M. Reversal of proinflammatory responses by ligating the macrophage Fcγ receptor type I. *J. Exp. Med.* (1998), **188**, 217–222.

Svanholm, C., Bandholz, L., Lobell, A., and Wigzell, H. Enhancement of autobody responses by DNA immunization using expression vectors mediating efficient antigen secretion. *J. Immunol. Meth.* (1999), **228**, 121–130.

Svanholm, C., Lowenadler, B., and Wigzell, H. Amplification of T-cell and antibody responses in DNA-based immunization with HIV-1 Nef by co-injection with a GM-CSF expression vector. *Scand. J. Immunol.* (1997), **46**, 298–303.

Sweet, C., Bird, A., Jakeman, K., Coates, D. M., and Smith., H. Production of passive immunity in neonatal ferrets following maternal vaccination with killed influenza virus. *Immunology* (1987a), **60**, 83–89.

Sweet, C., Jakeman, K. J., and Smith, H. Role of milk-derived IgG in passive maternal protection of neonatal ferrets against influenza. *J. Gen. Virol.* (1987b), **68**, 2681–2686.

Syrengelas, A. D., Chen, T. T., and Levy, R. DNA immunization induces protective immunity against B-cell lymphoma. *Nat. Med.* (1996), **2**, 1038–1041.

Syrengelas, A. D., and Levy, R. DNA vaccination against the idiotype of a murine B cell lymphoma and the mechanism of tumor protection. *J. Immunol.* (1999), **162**, 4790–4795.

Szalay, G., Hess, J., and Kaufmann, S. H. Presentation of listeria monocytogenes antigens by major histocompatibility complex class II to CD8 cytotoxic T lymphocytes of lysteriolysin secretion and virulence. *Eur. J. Immunol.* (1994), **24**, 1471–1477.

Tacket, C. O., Roy, M. J., Widera, G., Swain, W. F., Broome, S., and Edelman, R. Phase 1 safety and immune response studies of a DNA vaccine encoding hepatitis B surface antigen delivered by a gene delivery device. *Vaccine* (1999), **17**, 2826–2829.

Tan, J., Newton, C. A., Djeu, J. Y., Gutsch, D. E., Chang, A. E., Yang, N. S., Klein, T. W., and Hua, Y. Injection of complementary DNA encoding interleukin-12 inhibits tumor establishment at a distant site in a murine renal carcinoma model. *Cancer Res.* (1996), **56**, 3399–3403.

Tang, D. C., Devit, C., and Johnston, S. A. Genetic immunization is a simple method for eliciting an immune response. *Nature* (1992), **356**, 152–154.

Taylor, P. M., and Askonas, B. A. Influenza nucleoprotein-specific clones are protective *in vivo*. *Immunology* (1986), **58**, 417–420.

Taylor, P. M., Davey, J., Howland, K., Rothbard, J. B., and Askonas, B. A. Class I MHC molecules rather than other mouse genes dictate influenza epitope recognition by cytotoxic T cells. *Immunogenetics* (1987), **26**, 267–274.

Tedeschi, V., Akatsuka, T., Shih, J. W., Battegay, M., and Feinstone, S. M. A specific antibody response to HCV E2 elicited in mice by intramuscular inoculation of plasmid DNA containing coding sequences for E2. *Hepatology* (1997), **25**, 459–462.

Thierry, A. R., Rabinovich, P., Peng, B., Mahan, L. C., Bryant, J. L., and Gallo, R. C. Characterization of liposome-mediated gene delivery: Expression, stability and pharmacokinetics of plasmid DNA. *Gene Ther.* (1997), **4**, 226–237.

Tighe, H., Corr, M., Roman, M., and Raz, E. Gene vaccination: Plasmid DNA is more than just a blueprint. *Immunology Today* (1998), **19**, 89–97.

Tivol, E. A., Borriello, F., Schweitzer, A. N., Lynch, W. P., Bluestone, J. A., and Sharpe, A. H. Loss of CTLA-4 leads to massive lymphoproliferation and fatal multiorgan tissue destruction, revealing a critical negative regulatory role of CTLA-4. *Immunity* (1995), **3**, 541–547.

Tobery, T. W., and Siliciano, R. F. Targeting of HIV-1 antigens for rapid intracellular degradation enhances cytotoxic T lymphocyte recognition and the induction of *de novo* CTL responses *in vivo* after immunization. *J. Exp. Med.* (1997), **185**, 909–920.

Toda, S., Ishii, N., Okada, E., Kusakabe, K. I., Arai, H., Hamajima, K., Gorai, I., Nishioka, K., and Okuda, K. HIV-1-specific cell mediated immune responses induced by DNA vaccination were enhanced by mannan-coated liposomes and inhibited by anti-interferon gamma antibody. *Immunology* (1997), **92**, 111–117.

Tokunaga, T., Yamamoto, H., Shimada, S., Abe, H., Fukada, T., Fujisawa, Y., Furutani, Y., Yano, O., Kataoka, T., Sudo, T., Makiguchi, N., and Suganuma, T. Antitumor activity of DNA fraction from *Mycobacterium bovis* BCG: I. Isolation, physicochemical characterization, and antitumor activity. *J. Natl. Cancer Inst.* (1984), **72**, 955–1002.

Tokushige, K., Wakita, T., Pachuk, C., Moradpour, M., Weiner, D. B., Zurawski, V. R., Jr., and Wands, J. R. Expression and immune response to hepatitis C virus core DNA-based vaccine constructs. *Hepatology* (1996), **24**, 14–20.

Tolley, N. D., Tsunoda, I., and Fujinami, R. S. DNA vaccination against Theiler's murine encephalomyelitis virus leads to alterations in demyelinating disease. *J. Virol.* (1999), **73**, 993–1000.

Tomkinson, J. L., and Stein, C. A. Patterns of intracellular compartmentalization, trafficking and acidification of 5'-fluoresce in labeled phosphodiester and phosphothioate oligodeoxynucleotides in HL60 cells. *Nucleic Acids Res.* (1994), **22**, 4268–4275.

Torres, C. A., Iwasaki, A., Barber, B. H., and Robison, H. L. Differential dependence on target site tissue for gene gun and intramuscular DNA immunizations. *J. Immunol.* (1997), **158**, 4529–4532.

Townsend, A. R. M., Rothbard, J., Gotch, F. M., Bahadur, G., Wraith, D., and McMichael, A. J. The epitopes of influenza nucleoprotein recognized by cytotoxic T lymphocytes can be defined with short synthetic peptides. *Cell* (1986), **44**, 956–958.

Trinchieri, G. Proinflammatory and immunoregulatory functions of Interleukin-12. *Int. Rev. Immunol.* (1998), **16**, 365–397.

Triyatni, M., Jilbert, A. R., Qiao, M., Miller, D. S., and Burrell, C. J. Protective efficacy of DNA vaccines against duck hepatitis B virus infection. *J. Virol.* (1998), **72**, 84–94.

Tsuji, T., Fukushima, J., Hamajima, K., Ishii, N., Aoki, I., Bukawa, H., Ishigatsubo, Y., Tani, K., Okubo, T., Dorf, M. E., and Okuda, K. HIV-1-specific cell mediated immunity is enhanced by co-inoculation of TCA3 expression plasmid with DNA vaccine. *Immunology* (1997a), **90**, 1–6.

Tsuji, T., Hamajima, K., Fukushima, J., Xin, K. Q., Ishii, N., Aoki, I., Ishigatsubo, Y., Tani, K., Kawamoto, S., Nitta, Y., Miyazaki, J., Koff, W. C., Okubo, T., and Okuda, K. Enhancement of cell-mediated immunity against HIV-1 induced by coinooculation of plasmid-encoded HIV-1 antigen with plasmid expressing IL-12. *J. Immunol.* (1997b), **158**, 4008–4013.

Tsuji, T., Hamajima, K., Ishii, N., Aoki, I., Fukushima, J., Xin, K. Q., Kawamoto, S., Sasaki, S., Matsunaga, K., Ishigatsubo, Y., Tani, K., Okubo, T., and Okuda, K. Immunomodulatory effects of a plasmid expressing B7-2 on human immunodeficiency virus-1-specific cell-mediated immunity induced by a plasmid encoding the viral antigen. *Eur. J. Immunol.* (1997c), **27**, 782–787.

Tsunoda, I., Tolley, N. D., Theil, D. J., Whitton, J. L., Kobayashi, H., and Fujinami, K. Exacerbation of viral and autoimmune animal models for multiple sclerosis by bacterial DNA. *Brain Pathol.* (1999), **9**, 481–493.

Tumpey, T. M., Elner, V. M., Chen, S. H., Oakes, J. E., and Lausch, R. N. Interleukin-10 treatment can suppress stromal keratitis induced by herpes simplex virus type 1. *J. Immunol.* (1994), **153**, 2258–2265.

Tuting, T., Wilson, C. C., Martin, D. M., Kasamon, Y. L., Rowles, J., Ma, D. I., Slingluff, C. L., Jr., Wagner, S. N., van der Bruggen, P., Baar, J., Lotze, M. T., and Storkus, W. J. Autologous human monocyte-derived dendritic cells genetically modified to express melanoma antigens elicit primary cytotoxic T cell responses *in vitro*: Enhancement by cotransfection of genes encoding the Th1-biasing cytokines IL-12 and IFN-alpha. *J. Immunol.* (1998), **160**, 1139–1147.

Ugen, K. E., Boyer, J. D., Wang, B., Bagarazzi, M., Javadian, A., Frost, P., Merva, M. M., Agadjanyan, M. G., Nyland, S., Williams, W. V., Coney, L., Ciccarelli, R., and Weiner, D. B. Nucleic acid immunization of chimpanzees as a prophylactic/immunotherapeutic vaccination model for HIV-1: Prelude to a clinical trial. *Vaccine* (1997a), **15**, 927–930.

Ugen, K. E., Srikantan, V., Goedert, J. J., Nelson, R. P., Williams, W. W., and Weiner, D. B. Vertical transmission of human immunodeficiency virus type I: Seroreactivity by maternal antibodies to the carboxyl region of gp41 envelope glycoprotein. *J. Infect. Dis.* (1997b), **175**, 63–69.

Uhr, J. W., and Moller, G. Regulatory effect of antibody on the immune response. *Adv. Immunol.* (1968), **8**, 81–127.

Ulmer, J. B., Deck, R. R., DeWitt, C. M., Donnelly, J. J., and Liu, M. A. Generation of MHC class-I restricted cytotoxic T lymphocytes by expression of a viral protein in muscle cells: Antigen presentation by non-muscle cells. *Immunology* (1996), **89**, 59–67.

Ulmer, J. B., Donnelly, J. J., Parker, S. E., Rhodes, G. H., Felgner, P. L., Dwarki, V. J., Gromkowski, S. H., Deck, R. R., DeWitt, C. M., Friedman, A., Hawe, L. A., Leander, K. R., Martinez, D., Perry, H. C., Shriver, J. W., Montgomery, D. L., and Liu, M. A. Heterologous protection against influenza by injection of DNA encoding a viral protein. *Science* (1993), **259**, 1745–1749.

Ulmer, J. B., Liu, M. A., Montgomery, D. L., Yawman, A. M., Deck, R. R., DeWitt, C. M., Content, J., and Huygen, K. Expression and immunogenicity of *Mycobacterium tuberculosis* antigen 85 by DNA vaccination. *Vaccine* (1997), **15**, 792–794.

Vahlsing, H. L., Yankauckas, M. A., Sawdey, M., Gromkowski, S. H., and Manthorpe, M. Immunization with plasmid DNA using a pneumatic gun. *J. Immunol. Meth.* (1994), **175**, 11–22.

Van Parijs, L., Ibraghimov, A., and Abbas, A. K. The roles of costimulation and Fas in T cell apoptosis and peripheral tolerance. *Immunity* (1996), **4**, 321–328.

Waine, G. J., Yang, W., Scott, J. C., McManus, D. P., and Kalinna, B. H. DNA-based vaccination using *Schistosoma japonicum* (Asian blood-fluke) genes. *Vaccine* (1997), **15**, 846–848.

Waisman, A., Ruiz, P. J., Hirschberg, D. L., Gelman, A., Oksenberg, J. R., Brocke, S., Mor, F., Cohen, I. R., and Steinman, L. Suppressive vaccination with DNA encoding a variable region gene of the T-cell receptor prevents autoimmune encephalomyelitis and activates Th2 immunity. *Nat. Med.* (1996), **2**, 899–905.

Wang, B., Boyer, J., Srikantan, V., Coney, L., Carrano, R., Phan, C., Merva, M., Dang, K., Agadjanyan, M., and Gilbert, L. DNA inoculation induces neutralizing immune responses against human immunodeficiency Type 1 in mice and nonhuman primates. *DNA Cell. Biol.* (1993a), **12**, 799–805.

Wang, B., Boyer, J., Srikantan, V., Ugen, K., Gilbert, L., Phan, C., Dang, K., Merva, M., Agadjanyan, M. G., Newman, M., Carrano, R., McCallus, D., Coney, L., Williams, W., and Weiner, D. B. Induction of humoral and cellular immune responses to the human immunodeficiency Type 1 virus in nonhuman primates by *in vivo* DNA inoculation. *Virology* (1995), **211**, 102–112.

Wang, B., Dang, K., Agadjanyan, M. G., Srikantan, V., Li, F., Ugen, K. E., Boyer, J., Merva, M., Williams, W. V., and Weiner, D. B. Mucosal immunization with a DNA vaccine induces immune responses against HIV-1 at a mucosal site. *Vaccine* (1997a), **15**, 821–825.

Wang, B., Ugen, K. E., Srikantan, V., Agadjanyan, M. G., Dang, K., Refaeli, Y., Sato, A. I., Boyer, J., Williams, W. V., and Weiner, D. B. Gene inoculation generates immune responses against human immunodeficiency virus Type 1. *Proc. Natl. Acad. Sci. USA* (1993b), **90**, 4156–4160.

Wang, H., and Shlomchik, M. J. Maternal Ig mediates neonatal tolerance in rheumatoid factor transgenic mice but tolerance breaks down in adult mice. *J. Immunol.* (1998), **160**, 2263–2271.

Wang, R., Doolan, D. L., Le, T. P., Hedstrom, R. C., Coonan, K. M., Charoenvit, Y., Jones, T. R., Hobart, P., Margalith, M., Ng, J., Weiss, W. R., Sedegah, M., de Taisne, C., Norman, J. A., and Hoffman, S. L. Induction of antigen-specific cytotoxic T lymphocytes in human by a malaria DNA vaccine. *Science* (1998a), **282**, 476–480.

Wang, Y., Xiang, Z., Pasquini, S., and Ertl, H. Immune response to neonatal immunization. *Virology* (1997b), **228**, 278–284.

Wang, Y., Xiang, Z., Pasquini, S., and Ertl, H. C. J. Effect of passive immunization or maternally transferred immunity on the antibody response to a genetic vaccine to rabies virus. *J. Virol.* (1998b), **72**, 1790–1796.

Ward, G., Rieder, E., and Mason, P. W. Plasmid DNA encoding replicating foot-and-mouth disease virus genomes induces antiviral immune responses in swine. *J. Virol.* (1997), **71**, 7442–7447.

Warner, J. F., Jolly, D., Mento, S., Galpin, J., Haubrich, R., and Merritt, J. Retroviral vectors for HIV immunotherapy. *Ann. N.Y. Acad. Sci.* (1995), **772**, 105–116.

Warrens, A. N., Zhang, J. Y., Sidhu, S., Watt, D. J., Lombardi, G., Sewry, C. A., and Lechler, R. I. Myoblasts fail to stimulate T cells but induce tolerance. *Int. Immunol.* (1994), **6**, 847–853.

Watanabe, A., Raz, E., Kôhsaka, H., Tighe, H., Baird, S. M., Kipps, T. J., and Carson, D. A. Induction of antibodies to a Vk region by gene immunization. *J. Immunol.* (1993), **151**, 2871–2877.

Watanabe, M., Naito, M., Sasaki, E., Sakurai, M., Kuwana, T., and Oishi, T. Liposome-mediated DNA transfer into chicken primordial germ cells *in vivo*. *Mol. Reprod. Dev.* (1994), **38**, 268–274.

Wechsler, R. J., and Monroe, J. G. Immature B lymphocytes are deficient in the src-family kinases p59 fyn and p55 fgr. *J. Immunol.* (1995), **154**, 1919–1929.

Weiller, I. J., Weiller, E., Springer, R., and Cosenza, H. Idiotype suppression by maternal influence. *Eur. J. Immunol.* (1977), **7**, 591–597.

Weiner, G. J., Liu, H. M., Wooldridge, J. E., Dahle, C. E., and Krieg, A. M. Immunostimulatory oligodeoxynucleotides containing the CpG motif are effective as immune adjuvants in tumor antigen immunization. *Proc. Natl. Acad. Sci. USA* (1997), **94**, 10833–10837.

Weiss, R., Durnberger, J., Mostbock, S., Scheiblhofer, S., Hartl, A., Breitenbach, M., Strasser, P., Dorner, F., Livey, I., Crowe, B., and Thalhamer, J. Improvement of the immune response against plasmid DNA encoding OspC of *Borrelia* by an ER-targeting leader sequence. *Vaccine* (1999), **18**, 815–824.

Weissert, R., Lobell, A., de Graaf, K. L., Eltayeb, S. Y., Andersson, R., Olsson, M., and Wigzell, H. Protective DNA vaccination against organ-specific autoimmunity is highly specific and discriminates between single amino acid substitutions in the peptide autoantigen. *Proc. Natl. Acad. Sci. USA* (2000), **97**, 1689–1694.

Wells, D. J. Improved gene transfer by direct plasmid injection associated with regeneration in mouse skeletal muscle. *FEBS Lett.* (1993), **332**, 179–182.

Wells, D. J., and Goldspink, G. Age and sex influence expression of plasmid DNA directly injected into mouse skeletal muscle. *FEBS Lett.* (1992), **306**, 203–205.

Wheeler, C. J., Felgner, P. L., Tasi, Y. J., Marshal, J., Sukhu, L., Doh, S. G., Hartikka, J., Nietupski, J., Manthorpe, M., Nichols, M., Plewe, M., Liang, X., Norman, J., Smith, A., and Cheng, S. H. A novel cationic lipid greatly enhances plasmid DNA delivery and expression in mouse lung. *Proc. Natl. Acad. Sci. USA* (1996), **93**, 11454–11459.

Wildbaum, G., and Karin, N. Augmentation of natural immunity to a pro-inflammatory cytokine (TNF-alpha) by targeted DNA vaccine confers long-lasting resistance to experimental autoimmune encephalomyelitis. *Gene Ther.* (1999), **6**, 1128–1138.

Wiley, D. C., Skehel, J. J., and Waterfield, M. Evidence from studies with a cross-linking reagent that the hemagglutinin is a trimer. *Virology* (1979), **79**, 446–448.

Will, H., Cattaneo, R., Koch, H. G., Darai, G., Schaller, H., Schellekens, H., van Eerd, P. M., and Deinhard, F. Cloned HBV DNA causes hepatitis in chimpanzees. *Nature* (1982), **299**, 740–742.

Williams, R. S., Johnston, S. A., Riedy, M., DeVit, M. J., McElligott, S. G., and Sanford, J. C. Introduction of foreign genes into tissues of living mice by DNA-coated microprojectiles. *Proc. Natl. Acad. Sci. USA* (1991), **88**, 2726–2730.

Williams, W. V., Fang, Q., Von Feldt, J. M., Boyer, J. D., Luchi, M., Wang, B., and Weiner, D. B. Immunotherapeutic strategies targeting rheumatoid synovial T-cell receptors by DNA inoculation. *Immunol. Res.* (1994), **13**, 145–153.

Winkler, M., Demeur, C., Dewasme, G.,. and Urbain, J. Immunoregulatory role of maternal idiotypes. *J. Exp. Med.* (1980), **152**, 1024–1035.

Wolff, J. A., Dowty, M. E., Jiao, S., Repetto, G., Berg, R. K., Ludtke, J. J., Williams, P., and Slautterback, D. B. Expression of naked plasmids by cultured myotubes and entry of plasmids into T tubules and caveolae of mammalian skeletal muscle. *J. Cell. Sci.* (1992a), **103**, 1249–1259.

Wolff, J. A., Ludtke, J. J., Acsadi, G., Williams, P., and Jani, A. Long-term persistence of plasmid DNA and foreign gene expression in mouse muscle. *Hum. Mol. Genet.* (1992b), **1**, 363–369.

Wolff, J. A., Malone, R. W., Williams, P., Chong, W., Acsadi, G., Jani, A., and Felgner, P. L. Direct gene transfer into mouse muscle *in vivo*. *Science* (1990), **247**, 1465–1468.

Wolff, J. A., Williams, P., Acsadi, G., Jiao, S., Jani, A., and Chong, W. Conditions affecting direct gene transfer into rodent muscle *in vivo*. *Biotechniques* (1991), **11**, 478–485.

Wooldridge, J. E., Ballas, Z., Krieg, A. M., and Weiner, G. J. Immunostimulatory oligodeoxynucleotides containing CpG motifs enhance the efficacy of monoclonal antibody therapy of lymphoma. *Blood* (1997), **89**, 2994–2998.

Wu, Z. Q., Drayton, D., and Pisetsky, D. S. Specificity and immunochemical properties of antibodies to bacterial DNA in sera of normal human subjects and patients with systemic lupus erythematosus. *Clin. Exp. Immunopathol.* (1997), **109**, 27–31.

Xiang, Z. Q., and Ertl, H. C. Manipulation of the immune response to a plasmid-encoded viral antigen by coinoculation with plasmids expressing cytokines. *Immunity* (1995a), **2**, 129–135.

Xiang, Z. Q., and Ertl, H. C. Transfer of maternal antibodies results in inhibition of specific immune responses in the offspring. *Virus Res.* (1992), **24**, 297–314.

Xiang, Z. Q., He, Z., Wang, Y., and Ertl, H. C. The effect of interferon-gamma on genetic immunization. *Vaccine* (1997), **15**, 896–898.

Xiang, Z. Q., Spitalnik, S. L., Cheng, J., Erikson, J., Woyczyk, B., and Ertl, H. C. Immune responses to nucleic acid vaccines to rabies virus. *Virology* (1995b), **209**, 569–579.

Xiang, Z. Q., Spitalnik, S., Tran, M., Wunner, W. H., Cheng, J., and Ertl, H. C. Vaccination with a plasmid vector carrying the rabies virus glycoprotein gene induces protective immunity against rabies virus. *Virology* (1994), **199**, 132–140

Xiong, S., Gerloni, M., and Zanetti, M. Engineering vaccines with heterologous B and T cell epitopes using immunoglobulin genes. *Nature Biotech.* (1997a), **15**, 882–885.

Xiong, S., Gerloni, M., and Zanetti, M. *In vivo* role of B lymphocytes in somatic transgenic immunization. *Proc. Natl. Acad. Sci. USA* (1997b), **94**, 6352–6357.

Xu, D., and Liew, F. Y. Genetic vaccination against leishmaniasis. *Vaccine* (1994), **12**, 1534–1536.

Xu, D., and Liew, F. Y. Protection against leishmaniasis by injection of DNA encoding a major surface glycoprotein, gp63, of *L. major. Immunology* (1995), **84**, 173–176.

Xu, L., Sanchez, A., Yang, Z., Nabel, E. G., Nichol, S. T., and Nabel, G. J. Immunization for Ebola virus infection. *Nat. Med.* (1998), **4**, 37–42.

Yakubov, L. A., Deeva, E. A., Zarytkova, V. F., Ivanova, E., Ryte, A. S., Yurchenko, L. V., and Vlasov, V. V. Mechanism of oligonucleotide uptake by cells: Involvement of specific receptors? *Proc. Natl. Acad. Sci. USA* (1989), **86**, 6454–6458.

Yamamoto, S., Yamamoto, T., Kataoka, T., Kuramoto, E., Yano, O., and Tokunaga, T. Unique palindromic sequences in synthetic oligonucleotides are required to induce IFN and augment IFN-mediated NK activity. *J. Immunol.* (1992), **148**, 4072–4076.

Yang, K., Mustafa, F., Valsamakis, A., Santoro, J. C., Griffin, D. E., and Robinson, H. L. Early studies on DNA-based immunizations for measles virus. *Vaccine* (1997), **15**, 888–891.

Yang, N. S., Burkholder, J., Roberts, B., Martinell, B., and McCabe, D. *In vivo* and *in vitro* gene transfer to mammalian somatic cells by particle bombardment. *Proc. Natl. Acad. Sci. USA* (1990), **87**, 9568–9572.

Yang, W., Waine, G. J., and McManus, D. P. Antibodies to *Schistosoma japonicum* (Asian bloodfluke) paramyosin induced by nucleic acid vaccination. *Biochem. Biophys. Res. Commun.* (1997), **212**, 1029–1039.

Yankauckas, M. A., Morrow, J. E., Parker, S. E., Abai, A., Rhodese, G. H., Dwarki, V. J., and Gromkowski, S. H. Long term anti-nucleoprotein cellular and humoral immunity is induced by intramuscular injection of plasmid DNA containing NP gene. *DNA Cell. Biol.* (1993), **12**, 771–776.

Yasutomi, Y., Robinson, H. L., Lu, S., Mustafa, F., Lekutis, C., Arthos, J., Mullins, J. L., Voss, G., Manson, K., Wyand, M., and Letvin, N. L. Simian immunodeficiency virus-specific cytotoxic T-lymphocyte induction through DNA vaccination of rhesus monkeys. *J. Virol.* (1996), **70**, 678–681.

Yellen, A. J., Glenn, W., Sukhatame, V. P., Cao, X., and Monroe, J. G. Signaling through surface IgM in tolerance-susceptible immature murine B lymphocytes. *J. Immunol.* (1991), **146**, 1446–1454.

Yi, A.-K., Chace, J. H., Cowdery, J. S., and Krieg, A. M. IFNγ promotes IL-6 and IgM secretion in response to CpG motifs in bacterial DNA and oligodeoxynucleotides. *J. Immunol.* (1996a), **156**, 5558–5564.

Yi, A.-K., Klinman, D. M., Martin, T. L., Matson, S., and Krieg, A. M. Rapid immune activation by CpG motifs in bacterial DNA. *J. Immunol.* (1996b), **157**, 5349–5402.

Yi, A.-K., Hornbeck, P., Lafrenz, D. E., and Krieg, A. M. CpG DNA rescue of murine B lymphoma cells from anti-IgM-induced growth arrest and programmed cell death is associated with increased expression of c-myc and bcl-xL. *J. Immunol.* (1996c), **157**, 4918–4925.

Yi, A.-K., and Krieg, A. M. CpG DNA rescue from anti-IgM-induced WEH1 B lymphoma apoptosis. *J. Immunol.* (1998), **160**, 1240–1248.

Yokoyama, M., Hassett, D. E., Zhang, J., and Whitton, J. L. DNA immunization can stimulate florid local inflammation, and the antiviral immunity induced varies depending on injection site. *Vaccine* (1997), **15**, 553–560.

Yokoyama, M., Zhang, J., and Whitton, J. L. DNA immunization confers protection against lethal lymphocytic choriomeningitis virus infection. *J. Virol.* (1995), **69**, 2684–2688.

Yokoyama, W. M. Natural killer cell receptors. *Curr. Opin. Immunol.* (1998), **10**, 298–305.

York, Y. A.., Rog, C., Andrews, D. W., Riddel, S. R., Graham, F. L., and Johnson, D. C. A cytosolic herpes simplex virus protein inhibits antigen presentation to CD8 T lymphocytes. *Cell* (1994), **77**, 525–535.

Youssef, S., Wildbaum, G., and Karin, N. Prevention of experimental autoimmune encephalomyelitis by MIP-1alpha and MCP-1 naked DNA vaccines. *J. Autoimmun.* (1999), **13**, 21–29.

Zaghouani, H., Kristal, M., Kuzu, H., Moran, T., Shah, H., Kuzu, Y., Schulman, J., and Bona, C. Cells expressing a heavy chain gene carrying a viral T cell epitope are lysed by specific cytolytic T cells. *J. Immunol.* (1992), **148**, 3604–3609.

Zaghouani, H., Kuzu, Y., Kuzu, H., Daian, C., and Bona, C. Engineered immunoglobulin molecules as vehicle for viral epitopes. *Int. Rev. Immunol.* (1993a), **10**, 265–278.

Zaghouani, H., Steinman, R., Nonacs, R., Shah, H., Gerhard, W.. and Bona, C. Presentation of a viral T cell epitope expressed in the CDR3 region of a self immunoglobulin molecule. *Science* (1993b), **259**, 224–227.

Zarozinski, C. C., Fynan, E. F., Selin, L. K., Robinson, H. L., and Welsh, R. M. Protective CTL-dependent immunity and enhanced immunopathology in mice immunized by particle bombardment with DNA encoding an internal virion protein. *J. Immunol.* (1995), **154**, 4010–4017.

Zhang, D., Yang, X., Berry, J., Shen, C., McClarty, G., and Brunham, R. C. DNA vaccination with the major outer-membrane protein gene induces acquired immunity to *Chlamydia trachomatis* (mouse pneumonitis) infection. *J. Infect. Dis.* (1997), **176**, 1035–1040.

Zhao, T. M., Robinson, M. A., Bowers, F. S., and Kindt, T. J. Infectivity of chimeric human T-cell leukemia virus type I molecular clones assessed by naked DNA inoculation. *Proc. Natl. Acad. Sci. USA* (1996), **93**, 6653–6658.

Zhong, W., Wiesmuller, K. H., Kramer, M. D., Wallich, R., and Simon, M. M. Plasmid DNA and protein vaccination of mice to the outer surface protein A of *Borrelia burgdorferi* leads to induction of T helper cells with specificity for a major epitope and augmentation of protective IgG antibodies *in vivo*. *Eur. J. Immunol.* (1996), **26**, 2749–2757.

Zhou, X., Berglund, P., Rhodes, G., Parker, S. E., Jondal, M., and Liljestrom, P. Self-replicating Semliki Forest virus RNA as recombinant vaccine. *Vaccine* (1994), **12**, 1510–1514.

Zhu, N., Liggitt, D., Liu, Y., and Debs, R. Systemic gene expression after intravenous DNA delivery into adult mice. *Science* (1993), **261**, 209–211.

Zhu, X., Stauss, H. J., Ivanyi, J., and Vordermeier, H. M. Specificity of CD8[+] T cells from subunit-vaccinated and infected H-2b mice recognizing the 38 kDa antigen of *Mycobacterium tuberculosis*. *Int. Immunol.* (1997a), **9**, 1669–1676.

Zhu, X., Venkataprasad, N., Thangaraj, H. S., Hill, M., Singh, M., Ivanyi, J., and Vordermeier, H. M. Functions and specificity of T cells following nucleic acid vaccination of mice against *Mycobacterium tuberculosis*. *J. Immunol.* (1997b), **158**, 5921–5926.

Zimmermann, S., Egeter, O., Hausmann, S., Lipford, G. B., Rocken, M., Wagner, H., and Heeg, K. CpG oligo-deoxynucleotides trigger protective and curative Th1 responses in lethal murine leishmaniasis. *J. Immunol.* (1998), **160**, 3627–3630.

Index

A48 IdX, 137; *see also* Anti-A48 idiotypic
    antibodies
Adjuvants, 17, 25
Allergic conditions, DNA vaccines in, 99–101
ampR gene, 26
Anergy, 109
Anti-A48 idiotypic antibodies, 125, 126
Anti-DNA antibodies, 9
Anti-DNA antibody titers, 106
Anti-influenza virus response; *see also* Influenza
    effect of maternal antibodies on, 139–140
Antigen 85 complex (Ag85), 87, 88
Antigen delivery, 102–103
Antigen presenting cells (APCs), 7, 20, 35–36, 43,
        45, 49, 52
    professional, 2, 22, 35–36, 44, 51–53, 110, 119
    residential and remote, 35, 43, 44, 46
    from skin, 40
    transfecting, 110
    transfer between various types of, 46
Antigen transfer, 46, 47
Antigen transfer hypothesis, 45
Antihemagglutinin (anti-HA) antibodies, 128, 136
Aphtovirus, 66
Apoptosis, 28
Arenaviridae, 63
Attenuation, 53
Autoimmune diseases
    DNA vaccination against, 101–104, 107–108
    Th1-mediated, organ-specific, 106
Autoimmunity, risk of, 52, 99, 108
Avihepadnavirus, 75

B7-2, 22
B-cell epitopes, 7
B-cell receptors (BCR), 112, 113
B-cell vaccines eliciting neutralizing antibodies, 6
B-cells, 1–2, 28, 30–31, 44

B-cells (*cont.*)
    neonatal vs. adult, 123–124
Bacillus Calmette–Guérin (BCG), 86, 87
Bacterial antigens, DNA-based immunization with,
        85–90
Bacterial artificial chromosomes (BAC), 13
Bacterial cells, penetration of foreign DNA into, 36
Bacterial DNA, 27, 108
    as antigen and immune modulator, 99
Bacterial-mediated delivery of plasmids, 13
Biolistic DNA administration, 15–17
Black fever, 91
Borrelia burgdorferi, 88–89
Bovine respiratory syncytial virus (BRSV), 61, 66
"Broad vaccines," 54
Brucella abortus, 89

Cancer: *see* Tumors
Carcinoembryonic antigen (CEA), 113–114
Cardiovirus, 66
Cationic lipids, formulation of DNA with, 15
Cationic liposomes, 18
Chimeric viruses, 7
Chlamydia trachomatis, 89
Circumsporozoite protein (CSP), 91–93
Cloned DNA (cDNA), 88
Clostridium tetani, 89, 90
Coronaviridae, 67
Coronaviruses, 67
Co-stimulatory factors, molecules, 21, 23
Cowdria ruminantium, 89
CpG, 26, 46
CpG motifs, 26, 27, 54, 101, 107, 108
CpG nucleotides, 46
CpG ODN, 27, 28, 46, 101, 107
    effect on production of cytokines by antigen-
        presenting cells, 31
    inducing secretion of IL-6 by *B*-cells, 30–31

175

DATE DUE